## DATE DUE

# Dermatologic Therapy in Current Practice

# Dermatologic Therapy in Current Practice

Edited by

## Ronald Marks
FRCP, FRCPath
*Emeritus Professor of Dermatology,*
*University of Wales College of*
*Medicine, Cardiff, UK*

and

## James J Leyden
MD
*Professor of Dermatology, University of*
*Pennsylvania Hospital, Philadelphia,*
*USA*

## Martin Dunitz

© 2002, Martin Dunitz Ltd, a member of the Taylor & Francis group

First published in the United Kingdom in 2002 by
Martin Dunitz Ltd
The Livery House
7–9 Pratt Street
London NW1 0AE

| | |
|---|---|
| Tel: | +44-(0)20-7482-2202 |
| Fax: | +44-(0)20-7267-0159 |
| E-mail: | info.dunitz@tandf.co.uk |
| Website: | http://www.dunitz.co.uk |

Although every effort has been made to ensure that drug doses and other information are presented accurately in this publication, the ultimate responsibility rests with the prescribing physician. Neither the publishers nor the authors can be held responsible for errors or for any consequences arising from the use of information contained herein. For detailed prescribing information or instructions on the use of any product or procedure discussed herein, please consult the prescribing information or instructions on the use of any product or procedure discussed herein, please consult the prescribing information or instructional material issued by the manufacturer.

A CIP catalogue record for this book is available from the British Library

ISBN 1-85317-344-4

Distributed in the USA by
Fulfilment Center
Taylor & Francis
7625 Empire Drive
Florence, KY 41042, USA
Toll Free Tel: 1-800-634-7064
Email: cserve@routledge nv.com

Distributed in Canada by
Taylor & Francis
74 Rolark Drive
Scarborough
Ontario M1R 4G2, Canada
Toll Free Tel: 1-877-226-2237
Email: tal fran@istar.ca

Distributed in the rest of the world by
ITPS Limited
Cheriton House
North Way, Andover
Hampshire SP10 5BE, UK
Tel: +44 (0)1264 332424
Email: reception@itps.co.uk

Composition by Scribe Design, Gillingham, Kent, UK
Printed and bound in Spain by E. G. ZURE SA

# Contents

# Preface

Dermatologists are better known for their clinical diagnostic skills rather than for their effective therapies – but hopefully we are on the threshold of a new era. There has been an explosion in our understanding of the nature of skin disease. Admittedly, we have some way to go – atopic dermatitis and psoriasis still keep their cards pretty close to their chest – but as a specialty we can be pleased with recent progress. Pharmacology too has moved ahead, and this twin pronged advance – pharmacological science and the pathogenesis of disease – has resulted in novel therapies and new hope for dermatology patients.

This book contains commentaries and reviews on some of the more important advances in the treatment of skin disorders which we hope is of practical interest to our readers. Authors were invited to focus particularly on issues of practical clinical importance, and to present their data in prose that was both concise and enjoyable to read. We trust that the readership will agree.

*Ronald Marks*
*James J Leyden*

# List of contributors

Robert Baran, MD
Le Grand Palais
42 rue des Serbes
06400 Cannes
France

Leslie S Baumann, MD
Cedars Medical Center
1295 NW 14th Street, Suite K
Miami FL 33125
USA

René Chatelain, MD
Klinik und Poliklinik für Dermatologie
und Allergologie
Ludwig-Maximilians-Universität
München
Fraunlobstr. 32
80337 München
Germany

Irina Daza, MD
Policlinica Barquisimeto
Av. Los Leones Consultorio 17
Barquisimeto 3002 Lara
Venezuela

James Ferguson, MD, FRCP
Photobiology Unit
Department of Dermatology
Ninewells Hospital and Medical School
Dundee DD1 9SY
UK

Christoph C Geilen, MD, PhD
Freie Universität Berlin
Universitätsklinikum Benjamin Franklin
Klinik und Poliklinik für Dermatologie
Fabeckstr. 60-62
14195 Berlin
Germany

Clive EH Grattan, MA, MD, FRCP
Dermatology Department
Norfolk and Norwich NHS Health
Care Trust
West Norwich Hospital
Bowthorpe Road
Norwich NR2 3TU
UK

Carla Hary, MD
Klinik und Poliklinik für Dermatologie
und Allergologie
Ludwig-Maximilians-Universität
München
Fraunlobstr. 32
80337 München
Germany

Kristen M Kelly, MD
Department of Dermatology
Medical Science I, Room C340
University of California
Irvine CA 92697-2400
USA

Francisco A Kerdel, MD, MBBS
Department of Dermatology
and Cutaneous Surgery
University of Miami
Miami FL 33125
USA

Anne Kobza Black, MD, FRCP
St John's Institute of Dermatology
King's College London
St Thomas' Campus
St Thomas' Hospital
London SE1 7EH
UK

Birger Konz, MD
Klinik und Poliklinik für Dermatologie
und Allergologie
Ludwig-Maximilians-Universität
München
Fraunlobstr. 32
80337 München
Germany

Konstantin Krasagakis, MD
Freie Universität Berlin
Universitätsklinikum Benjamin Franklin
Klinik und Poliklinik für Dermatologie
Fabeckstr. 60-62
14195 Berlin
Germany

Gary Lask, MD
Division of Dermatology
UCLA School of Medicine
Los Angeles CA 90024
USA

Melissa Lazarus, MD
Cedars Medical Center
1295 NW 14th Street, Suite K
Miami FL 33125
USA

Donna Lee, MD
Division of Dermatology
UCLA School of Medicine
Los Angeles CA 90024
USA

James J Leyden, MD
Department of Dermatology
University of Pennsylvania Hospital
2 Maloney Building
3600 Spruce Street
Philadelphia PA 19104
USA

Annia C Lourenço, MD
Av Silva Jardim, 1364/1204
80250-200 Curitiba-PR
Brazil

Nicholas J Lowe, MD, FRCP, FACP
Cranley Clinic
3 Harcourt House
Cavendish Square
London W1M 9AD
UK

Christiane Machado, MD
Cedars Medical Center
1295 NW 14th Street, Suite K
Miami FL 33125
USA

Ronald Marks, FRCP, FRCPath
Skin Care Cardiff Limited
23 Blenheim Road
Penylan
Cardiff CF2 5DS
UK

Constantinos E Orfanos, MD
Freie Universität Berlin
Universitätsklinikum Benjamin Franklin
Klinik und Poliklinik für Dermatologie
Fabeckstr. 60-62
14195 Berlin
Germany

Bianca Maria Piraccini, MD
Istituto di Clinica Dermatologica
Università degli studi di Bologna
Policlinico S Orsola
Via G Massarenti, 1
Bologna 40138
Italy

Gerd Plewig, MD
Klinik und Poliklinik für Dermatologie
und Allergologie
Ludwig-Maximilians-Universität
München
Fraunlobstr. 32
80337 München
Germany

Barry I Resnik, MD
Department of Dermatology and
Cutaneous Surgery
University of Miami
Miami FL 33101
USA

Sorrel S Resnik, MD
Department of Dermatology and
Cutaneous Surgery
University of Miami
Miami FL 33101
USA

David T Roberts, MB, ChB,
FRCP(Glasg)
Department of Dermatology
South Glasgow University Hospitals
Southern General Hospital
Govan Road
Glasgow G51 4TF
UK

Peter M Steijlen, MD
Department of Dermatology
University of Nijmegen
6500 HB Nijmegen
The Netherlands

Antonella Tosti, MD
Istituto di Clinica Dermatologica
Università degli studi di Bologna
Policlinico S Orsola
Via G Massarenti, 1
Bologna 40138
Italy

Peter van de Kerkhof, MD
Department of Dermatology
University of Nijmegen
6500 HB Nijmegen
The Netherlands

Julian Verbov, MD, FRCP, FRCPCH
Department of Dermatology
Royal Liverpool Children's Hospital
Alder Hey
Eaton Road
Liverpool L12 2AP
UK

Gerald D Weinstein, MD
Department of Dermatology
Medical Science I, Rm C340
University of California, Irvine
Irvine CA 92697
USA

# 1

# Advances in the drug treatment of skin disease

*Ronald Marks and James J Leyden*

## Introduction

The last 30–40 years has seen major improvement in the way that patients with skin disease are treated. For the most part the treatment is not only different – it is also very much better. In this chapter we have arbitrarily chosen topics where the new agents in question have made major impacts on the prognosis and quality of the life of patients with common skin disorders.

The last two decades of the 20th Century have seen great changes in the way that the major pharmaceutical companies have tackled the issues of drug discovery. There can be few human enterprises in which so much resource has been invested with so little tangible return. This is not a criticism – the fact is that the task is difficult and we are now in an era of diminishing returns. In addition to which the regulatory requirements and restrictions imposed by both national and international bodies make the introduction of new drugs a tortuous and ponderous task.

## Vitamin D analogues

Vitamin $D_3$ (calciferol) was noted to have a marked effect on epidermal differentiation long before its use was contemplated for psoriasis. The oral form was reported to a marked therapeutic effect in psoriasis by Hollick from Boston who did much to promote research in this area.[1] However, not all reported studies of the oral compound have found a significant degree of benefit.[2] Topical vitamin $D_3$ was investigated intensively and found to have an inarguable and striking therapeutic activity with relatively little in the way of significant adverse effects.[3] Not unexpectedly the major concern was whether sufficient vitamin D penetrated into the circulation to cause hypercalcaemia. For all practical purposes it can be said that serum calcium of the trial patients remained unchanged and that all the parameters of bone metabolism investigated were unaltered. A less, but nonetheless significant problem – skin irritation with burning discomfort, erythema and scaling – occurred in 10–15% of patients and is the main drawback to its use topically. This irritation was of the same order as that seen with the topical retinoids, but probably rather less than that experienced with dithranol preparations. Despite results of clinical trials, topical vitamin $D_3$ itself has not been (and almost certainly never will be) introduced into the market and one can only presume that it was felt that the development of vitamin $D_3$ analogues would provide too much competition for healthy commercial independence.

Calcipotriol is the vitamin $D_3$ analogue that has proved most successful thus far. In a concentration of 50 µg/g it is available as an ointment, a cream and a scalp lotion. In clinical trials it regularly significantly improves approximately 65% of patients[4] and has proven more successful than 0.1% betamethasone-17-valerate[5] ointment and to be equal to or more successful than dithranol treatment.[6] In addition, calcipotriol has proved safe and successful when used over periods for as long as a year.[7] It has also been found safe and effective for use in children under the age of 12.

Its greatest use has been in the treatment of typical plaque type psoriasis of extensor surfaces, but because of its potential for irritation, until recently it has not generally been employed for more sensitive areas of the skin such as the face, the genitalia and the flexural areas. With greater experience there has been a much greater readiness to use calcipotriol cautiously on some of the more easily irritated sites and recently it has been successfully used with topical steroids in sensitive areas.[8] Use of the specially formulated scalp lotion has also proved quite successful with concurrent use of medium potency topical corticosteroids (it can also be given to patients for flexural lesions). Calcipotriol has also been used successfully together with PUVA treatment.[9]

Currently only one other vitamin $D_3$ analogue, tacalcitol, is licensed for the treatment of psoriasis and available on prescription in Europe. This agent is certainly effective[10] but does not appear to be as potent as calcipotriol. It certainly does not cause as much skin irritation as calcipotriol and is particularly useful for those fair-skinned subjects (often of Celtic ancestry) whose skin is very easily irritated and for the treatment of flexural sites.

Yet other vitamin $D_3$ analogues have been submitted to clinical trial and are likely to be licensed in the near future.

The way in which these vitamins $D_3$ analogues work is not known for certain. They appear to bind with the nuclear vitamin $D_3$ receptor which is structurally close by the nuclear receptor complex and the corticosteroid receptor and appear to promote normal epidermal differentiation and reduce the heightened epidermal cell production seen in psoriasis.[11,12] Whether any or all of these actions of the drugs are primary effects or merely epiphenomena is not yet clear. It is of considerable interest that the actions of the vitamin $D_3$ analogues are quite similar to those of the retinoids and it may be that similar therapeutic pathways are travelled by both groups of drugs.

As calcipotriol is a new potent agent for the treatment of psoriasis it is perhaps not altogether surprising that clinicians have used it to treat patients with other epidermal disorders in which epidermal differentiation is deficient and scaling is prominent. It has proved quite effective in improving the skin of patients with different types of severe ichthyosis.[13] It was particularly helpful for patients with non-bullous ichthyosiform erythroderma and those with sex-linked ichthyosis.

The topical vitamin $D_3$ analogues are an interesting and important new group of agents and it seems likely that further developments in this area will yield even more active drugs for psoriasis.

## Cyclosporin

Cyclosporin represents one of the major therapeutic advances in medicine in the past 25 years. This cyclic polypeptide selectively inhibits lymphokine secretion by activated T cells and prevents secretion of interleukin-2 necessary to activate B cells, thereby preventing maturation into antibody- or autoantibody-producing cells.[14,15] Major advances in organ transplantation occurred with the discovery of this molecule and over the past 20 years this drug has been shown to have major utility in severe psoriasis, atopic dermatitis and other destructive inflammatory disorders such as pyoderma gangrenosum. Unfortunately, neither cyclosporin nor its metabolites have been found effective in topical formulations. The

future, however, is bright for topical immunosuppressive therapy with preparations of topical macrolides.

Cyclosporin is a highly non-polar lipophilic molecule and the initial dosage form was an oil-based formulation that required emulsification by bile salts and digestion by pancreatic enzymes prior to absorption. Consequently, bioavailability was quite variable. A more recent formulation which forms a homogeneous microemulsion immediately on contact with gastrointestinal fluids provides increased bioavailability and in contrast to original formulations provides a linear response over a wide range of doses.[16-18]

While cyclosporin can be used safely in several dermatological disorders, both acute and chronic side-effects can develop. Acute side-effects of gastrointestinal upset, fatigue, headache and musculoskeletal discomfort are influenced by concentration and tend to resolve after several weeks without treatment. More persistent and clinically significant chronic side-effects include hirsutism, gingival hyperplasia, hypertension, renal toxicity and drug–drug interaction because of its effect on the cytochrome P-450 system. Patients need to be monitored for changes in blood pressure and kidney function. With any long-term use of an immunosuppressive agent the risk of developing a cancer is at least theoretically possible. In dermatological uses of cyclosporin the relatively low dose (compared to transplant doses) and brief or intermittent use minimizes their risk.

Tacrolimus, a topical macrolide immunosuppressive agent has recently been approved by the FDA. This molecule is more potent than cyclosporin in inhibiting T-cell activation. Studies have shown marked benefit in atopic dermatitis particularly in more severe cases which are resistant to corticosteroid treatment.[19–23] Another similar agent on the horizon is ascomycin which also has shown promise in patients with severe eczema.[24–26] Both of these agents do not produce skin atrophy, a clear advantage over topical corticosteroids.

## Psoriasis

Psoriasis is the disease in which cyclosporin has been most extensively used and studied. Numerous double-blind, placebo-controlled studies have demonstrated benefit in both plaque-stage and pustular psoriasis. Doses of 3 to 5 mg/kg induce remission in large numbers of patients with high rates of relapse on discontinuation.[18,28–30] For this reason, many have advocated long-term, lower dose suppression therapy. Such regimens have been shown to be effective and safe although monitoring for hypertension and renal toxicity must be done. More recently, use of cyclosporin as a 'crisis buster' has been proposed.[18] Doses of 5.0 mg/kg per day are predictably effective in controlling severe flares of psoriasis including erythrodermic flares. Unlike methotrexate which can be associated with rare acute catastrophic side-effects

such as a rapid drop in blood count or fulminant hepatitis, cyclosporin is free of acute severe side-effects. Once an acute flare is reversed, cyclosporin is continued while other modalities such as acitretin, phototherapy, methorexate and topical agents are introduced. The aim is to gradually taper the cyclosporin. Another major use of cyclosporin is for patients who have been unresponsive to other therapies with the same goal of withdrawing cyclosporin once the psoriasis is under control and restarting other agents or maintenance therapy. In some patients, long-term cyclosporin is the only way of controlling their disease.

## Atopic dermatitis

Atopic dermatitis can be a severe generalized debilitating process which is unresponsive to therapies except prolonged use of systemic corticosteroids. Numerous studies have demonstrated that relatively brief courses of cyclosporin can induce long-term remissions or reduce the inflammatory state to a point where previously ineffective agents are now sufficient to control the process.[17,30–44] The future of immunotherapy in atopic dermatitis is clearly in topical therapy with tacrolimus and other macrolides.

# Antifungal agents

The discovery and development of griseofulvin in the late 1950s ended the wide epidemics of fungal infection of the scalp as well as providing a therapy for infections of other body areas. The next 20 years brought the development of a large number of topical agents starting with tolnaftate and haloprogin, leading on to the explosion of the imidazoles and finally the allylamines.

The development of systemic agents was much slower. In the early 1980s, ketoconazole, an imidazole, was introduced and represented a major advance, particularly in view of its broad spectrum of activity and usefulness in a variety of systemic infections. Ketoconazole, however, did not improve our ability to treat tinea capitis or onychomycosis, the Achilles' heel of griseofulvin. There was, however, some increased benefit to the treatment of recalcitrant skin infections particularly those of the hands and feet. A major step forward occurred with the development of the triazoles and terbinafine.[47-49]

## Fluconazole

Fluconazole is a triazole and the first of its class to be licensed for clinical use. Because of its water solubility it can be used intravenously and gastrointestinal absorption does not require gastric acidity. The water solubility also results in high penetration into cerebrospinal fluid. This drug is widely distributed in body tissues, including the nail bed and the nail plate and appears to be eliminated more slowly from skin and nails than from plasma.

The antifungal activity of fluconazole results from its ability to inhibit fungal cytochrome P-450-dependent 14-α-demethylase, a key enzyme in ergosterol cell wall synthesis. The spectrum of activity encourages a variety of yeasts as well as dermatophytes. The pharmacokinetics of fluconazole result in high and sustained concentrations in skin and nails which exceed those achieved in plasma. Its low molecular weight and high water solubility result in high bioavailability. This agent has been extensively studied in onychomycosis and shown to be effective when pulsing regimens of 150 to 300 mg once weekly are employed till clearing.[47-49] This agent has not yet been approved by the US FDA for use in nail or skin infections, but is available for systemic infection.

## Itraconazole

Itraconazole is another triazole which is more active in vitro than ketoconazole. It is very effective in animal models and highly effective in a variety of systemic fungal infections such as candidiasis, histoplasmosis, blastomycosis and sporotrichosis. This drug is poorly water soluble and its bioavailability improves when taken with a fatty meal. Due to its lipophilicity, itraconazole concentrates in fat and is also seen in high levels in skin and nails. This agent has been shown to be highly effective in treating cutaneous yeast and dermatophyte infections and particularly effective when used in pulse dosing for the treatment of onychomycosis.[50–54]

Itraconazole inhibits ergosterol synthesis at the demethylation step converting lanosterol to 14-demethyl lanosterol. This activity results in gradual leakage of cell contents through a damaged cell wall and a so-called 'fungistatic' effect occurs. Because the enzyme inhibited is cytochrome P-450 dependent, the possibility of drug interaction with drugs which are metabolized by this system is an important consideration in its use.

## Terbinafine

Terbinafine is an allylamine which acts on squalene epoxidase, a much earlier step in cell wall synthesis, and is therefore highly toxic at very low concentrations and exerts a so-called 'fungicidal' effect. This drug is also widely distributed and concentrates in skin and nails. This agent has been extensively studied in skin and nail infections.[55,56] In head to head studies, terbinafine has proven to be more effective than itraconazole in onychomycosis possibly because of its fungicidal effects at very low concentrations.[57] Squalene epoxidase is not an enzyme belonging to the cytochrome P-450 system so that, in contrast to azoles, allylamines have no intrinsic tendency to inhibit these enzymes. Drug-drug interactions are not a problem with this agent.

All three drugs represent major advances in antifungal therapy. To date, the vast majority of studies have revolved around the treatment of onychomycosis. A much more important area from the points of view of morbidity and public health is that of tinea capitis. The massive epidemics of the pre-1950s have disappeared, yet tinea capitis remains an extremely common infectious disease. These new agents are under study in this highly important disease process and it is likely that one or more will prove to be highly effective and safe for this indication.[58]

# New topical retinoids

Retinoid therapy began in the 1970s with the demonstration that retinoic acid, now called tretinoin, was useful in the treatment of acne and the so-called disorders of keratinization. In the 1960s, the systemic retinoids isotretinoin and etretinate were approved for the treatment of acne and psoriasis.

Retinoids appear to exert their biological effects through multiple gene regulatory mechanisms.[59–65] Gene transplantation can be activated by the binding of retinoids with the promoter regions of specific genes, and retinoids can also indirectly repress the activity of other nuclear transcription factors such as AP1. The discovery and characterization of retinoid receptors has led to both a better understanding of their actions as well as providing a methodology for screening potential new therapeutic agents. There are six known retinoid receptors belonging to two families, the retinoic acid receptor (RAR) and the retinoid X receptor (RXR) families. Each family has three subtypes α, β and γ. For activation of gene transcription, RARs must form heterodimers with RXR, while RXRs can function as homodimers. RXRs can also form functional heterodimers with vitamin $D_3$ and thyroid hormone receptors.

The multiplicity of retinoid receptors coupled with the variety of possibilities for receptor heterodimerizations and homodimerizations probably account for the ability of retinoids to influence a wide range of biological responses. Currently, a goal of several pharmaceutical companies is to target disease therapy with receptor- and function-selective retinoids in order to try to minimize adverse effects. In skin, the predominant RAR subtype is RARγ. The hope is that a retinoid that binds selectively to a particular subtype will have biological effects only in the tissues in which that subtype is expressed and the target gene of the receptor subtype.

## Adapalene

Adapalene is an aromatic acid derivative which has an affinity profile for RARβ and γ with low affinity for RARα and does not bind to cytosolic retinoic acid binding proteins. In in vitro and animal model systems, adapalene has been shown to have a variety of effects on cell differentiation and

proliferation, as well as anti-inflammatory and comedolytic effects. Moreover, adapalene is lipophilic and concentrates in sebaceous follicles. Furthermore, in human patch testing studies, adapalene has been shown to have a much lower irritant potential than topical tretinoin at therapeutic concentrations. All of these characteristics make this molecule a strong candidate for acne therapy.[66-68] Subsequently, multicentred, controlled clinical trials have shown that adapalene gel 0.1% is superior to 0.03% and therapeutically equivalent to 0.025% tretinoin gel.[68-70] Both agents produce a 40–50% reduction in non-inflammatory comedones and inflammatory papules and pustules after 12 weeks of therapy. Adapalene is better tolerated than tretinoin gel. Studies comparing adapalene gel with different concentrations and cream formulations of tretinoin have not been done.

Adapalene is clearly an effective topical retinoid for the treatment of acne and represents an example of how a basic science understanding of pharmacological effects can be utilized to develop new therapeutic agents.

## Tazarotene

Tazarotene is a member of a novel, conformationally rigid class of retinoids, the acetylenic retinoids. Tazarotene itself does not bind to RARs but its free acid metabolite, tazarotenic acid, has a high affinity with the rank order of affinity being RARβ>RARγ>RARα>.

Neither tazarotene nor tazarotenic acid bind with RXRs. This agent has been approved for treating both psoriasis and acne.[71-72] Most studies to date have been in the former.

Psoriasis involves a complex multi-faceted pathophysiology with immunologically mediated inflammation, abnormal differentiation and proliferation of keratinocytes the most prominent abnormalities. Tazarotene appears to influence all of these pathogenic factors. In human studies, tazarotene has been shown to reverse the overexpression of differentiation markers such as involucrin, keratinocyte transglutaminase, migration inhibitory protein and skin-derived antileukoproteinase as well as a replacement of keratins K6 and K16 seen in hyperproliferative disorders with K1 and K10. Furthermore, the increased expression of interleukin-6, a potent autocrine growth factor for keratinocytes and interleukin-8 a chemotactic factor for neutrophils and lymphocytes is suppressed. The levels of transforming growth factor-α and epidermal growth factor receptor which are increased in psoriasis are also suppressed.

Tazarotene appears to modulate psoriasis by inducing or down-regulating the markers of abnormal differentiation and proliferation as well as through anti-inflammatory effects. Controlled clinical trials have demonstrated that once-daily tazarotene 0.05% and 0.1% gel formulations are effective. Significant clinical improvement is seen in approximately 60% of patients after 12 weeks of therapy with 50–60% of those improved maintaining that improvement 12 weeks after discontinuation of tazarotene. Local irritation occurs in some, but can be suppressed by topical corticosteroids. The latter are commonly employed and large clinical trials have shown that the addition of medium or high potency topical corticosteroid once daily alternating with tazarotene also used once daily produces a more rapid and greater benefit with superior tolerability. Likewise, the combination of tazarotene with ultraviolet (UV) B phototherapy has proved to be more effective than either alone[73] and reduces the total UV dose required for clearance.

## Topical retinoids and photodamage

One of the major advances in the decade of the 1990s has been the use of topical tretinoin in photodamaged skin. Following the initial uncontrolled clinical studies, numerous controlled studies have verified the benefit of tretinoin in reducing fine wrinkling, mottled hyperpigmentation and surface roughness.[74-77] The most profound effects are seen in the dyspigmentation in dysplasia of photodamage.[78] Long-term studies have shown epidermal thickening, hypergranulosis, reduction in dermal hyaluronic acid and synthesis of new collagen subepidermally which correlates with long-term clinical improvement. A proposed mechanism for the action of tretinoin in photodamaged skin involves the observation that

UVB-induced AP-1 binding is reduced by 70% and that coincident with this there is a reduction of UVB-induced collagenase activity.[79-82] These activities may not only help reverse damage, but also may prevent further tissue damage. It is clear that the multiplicity of gene effects produced by tretinoin can help reverse some of the damage due to chronic UV injury, which probably includes damage to multiple genes which control skin function.

# Interferons in the treatment of skin diseases

The interferons are a group of small molecular weight proteins (15–20 kDa approximately) that are produced by several cell types after specific types of stimulation. They were first described by Isaacs and Lindermann in 1957 as proteins in vital cell culture fluids that blocked further production of virus particles. Apart from their important effects on viral replication, the interferons have a vital role in immunoregulation and have a marked effect on the growth of tumours. Three types of interferon are recognized, each one produced by different cell types and each with its individual structure, receptors and biological effects, although these may be quite closely related. The three types, interferon-α (IFN-α) produced by macrophages which has many isoforms IFN-β produced by fibroblasts, and IFN-γ produced by T lymphocytes. The interferon molecules are too large for gastrointestinal absorption or absorption percutaneously and need to be injected systemically or intralesionally to obtain a biological effect. They are now produced by recombinant technology and are significantly expensive. They all produce unpleasant adverse side-effects.

## Non-melanoma skin cancer

There have been several studies of the effects of IFNs on basal cell cancers (BCC), squamous cell carcinomas, Bowen's disease and solar keratoses. The overall impression from reading reports of these studies and having conducted one ourselves[83] is that intralesional IFN (recombinant IFN alpha-2b) is often effective and may be regarded as an alternative to more conventional therapies. This modality has particular use for some patients. Elderly frail subjects, those with large, difficult to remove, lesions and those who do not want surgical treatment should be considered for intralesional IFN. In a controlled study of intralesional IFN alpha-2b $1/5 \times 10^6$ i.u. three times per week for 3 weeks compared to placebo in patients with biopsy-proven BCC, 81% of those treated with IFN remained tumour free at 1 year as opposed to 20% in the placebo group.[84] In the Cardiff study,[85] 20 patients with biopsy-proven solar keratoses or Bowen's disease were treated with either IFN alpha-2b intralesionally $1 \times 10^6$ i.u. twice weekly for 4 weeks or 5% 5-fluorouracil twice daily for 2 weeks. Complete resolution had taken place in nine of ten patients by 8 weeks in the IFN-treated group and in all ten by 16 weeks. All lesions treated with 5-fluorouracil had resolved by 8 weeks. Histologically both groups showed considerable inflammation, but there was more basal cell liquefaction degeneration and lichenoid change in the IFN-treated patients. Large keratoacanthomas and verrucous carcinoma have also been treated successfully with IFN. Some 16 studies have been published of the effects of IFN in epithelial tumours and precancers with an overall success rate of 80–85%. Clearly this is a useful, if somewhat expensive, method of treatment for some groups of difficult patients and difficult lesions.[85]

## Viral warts

Viral warts are only trivial ailments for those who don't have them. Although most disappear within one year, there are some that continue to give rise to pain, discomfort, limitation of movement and embarrassment for much longer periods. Multiple tender plantar warts and the presence of myriads of plane warts over the face and neck are two such situations that are beyond the surgical assistance of cryotherapy and may benefit from interferon treatment. Multiple, large, recalcitrant genital warts are another example. recombinant IFN-α has been used both intralesionally and systemically. IFN-α administered in doses of $10^6$ i.u./day subcutaneously or intralesionally three times weekly for 3 weeks produced remission in 30–80%

compared to 15–50% in the placebo-treated group.[86,87] However, a multicentre, double-blind placebo-controlled study of $1.5 \times 10^6$ i.u. of IFN-α three times weekly for 4 weeks failed to show superiority of the IFN compared to placebo in patients with recurrent genital warts.[88] There are several reports of the successful use of topical IFN for different types of wart and others describing the particular usefulness of IFN combined with other sorts of treatment.

It is clear that the last words on the treatment of warts with IFNs have not yet been written. While it seems to be the case that some type of IFN treatment may be effective in some patients, we need to have better evidence of which regimen is effective in which clinical situation as we are dealing with an expensive treatment with a potential for unpleasant adverse side-effects.

## Atopic dermatitis

There is a desperate need for new treatments for patients with severe atopic dermatitis and although IFN-γ itself may not be suitable for all as an alternative treatment, some similar agent or analogue may well prove useful.[89] The basis of the use of IFN-γ stems from the finding that the balance of T-helper lymphocyte subpopulations is disturbed in atopic dermatitis. There appears to be an emphasis on the TH2 subpopulation rather than the TH1 subset. TH2 cells secrete interleukin-4 (IL-4) and IL-5 as their predominant lymphokines while TH1 cells secrete IFN-γ as their major 'chemical messenger'. There is, therefore, an apparent deficiency of IFN-γ at least at the theoretical level. The strong influence of IL-4 and IL-5 may well account for the high IgE levels in atopic dermatitis.

Studies using subcutaneous IFN-γ in patients with severe atopic dermatitis have resulted in significant improvement in many patients and a decrease in IgE levels in some others.[90,91] One stringently performed study by Hanifin and colleagues[92] was especially convincing. They employed a dose of 50 μg/m² body surface subcutaneously daily over a 12-week period in a randomized double-blind placebo-controlled trial. The clinical state of these patients was evaluated using short ordinal scales for the symptoms and each of the physical signs. The results were unequivocal – there was a substantial clinical improvement with a reduction of about 50% in the scores overall in some 45% of IFN-treated patients compared with 22% controls. For the most part the side-effects of the IFN therapy have been tolerable and subcutaneous IFN-γ on a daily basis must be regarded as an alternative treatment for severely affected patients whose disease is refractory to other types of treatment.

with an increased recurrence-free interval compared to placebo and that it is the only adjuvant treatment to show a significant therapeutic benefit in randomized controlled clinical trials.[10] Two studies in particular suggest that disease-free interval rather than overall survival is significantly increased by administration of 'low-dose' IFN alpha-2a. The first is that of Pehamberger et al[93] in which 311 patients with stage II disease were treated for 1 year and the second that of Grob et al[94] who treated 489 patients with stage II malignant melanoma for 18 months. High-dose regimens using IFN alpha-2b have also resulted in significantly increased disease-free intervals and strong suggestions of improvement in overall survival for patients with stage III disease and nodal metastases (in one study the overall survival time was increased from 2.8 to 3.8 years).[95,96] However, it is clear that more carefully controlled studies will have to be performed as the latest studies are much less certain concerning benefit.[93] It is certain that IFN-γ does not provide any benefit and that the adverse side-effects of IFN-α in the doses employed are quite unpleasant and potentially dangerous.

## Melanoma

IFN-α has been used in a variety of ways for melanoma at all stages and for melanoma in situ. The only clear messages that emerge from the many studies are that its use is associated

## Miscellaneous disorders

One or several of the IFNs have been used for numerous skin disorders and it is not possible to comment on them all. Perhaps it is worthwhile mentioning that IFN alpha-2b has been successfully used to treat keloids and seems to give better results than intralesional triamcinolone.[97] Behçet's disease has been reported to respond to both IFN alpha-2b and IFN-γ.[98,99]

For further details of the uses of interferons, a comprehensive review of the clinical uses of the interferons by Rubzczak and Schwartz[100] can be recommended to readers.

# References

1.  Holick MF, Formmer JE, McNeil SC et al, Photometabolism of 7-dihydrocholesterol to previtamin $D_3$ in skin of rats exposed to ultraviolet irradiation. *Biochemistry* 1977: 18; 107–114.

2.  Siddiqui MA, Al-Khawajah MM, Vitamin $D_3$ and psoriasis: a randomised, double-blind placebo-controlled study. *J Dermatol Treat* 1990: 1; 243–5.

3.  van de Kerkhof PCM, van Harten J, Verjans H, A long term assessment of the safety and tolerability of calcitriol ointment in the treatment of chronic plaque psoriasis. *J Dermatol Treat* 1996: 7(Suppl 1); S11–S14.

4.  Ashcroft DM, Wanlo AL, Williams HC, Griffiths CEM, Systematic review of comparative efficacy and tolerability of calcipotriol in treating chronic plaque psoriasis. *Br Med J* 2000: 320; 963–7.

5.  Cunliffe WJ, Berth Jones J, Claudy A et al, Comparative study of calcipotriol (MC 903) ointment and betamethasone-17-valerate ointment in patients with psoriasis vulgaris. *J Am Acad Dermatol* 1993: 26; 736–43.

6.  Berth-Jones J, Chu AC, Dodd WH et al, A multicentre, parallel group comparison of calcipotriol ointment and short contact dithranol therapy in chronic plaque psoriasis. *Br J Dermatol* 1992: 127; 266–71.

7.  Poyner T, Hughes W, Dass BK et al, Long term treatment of chronic plaque psoriasis with calcipotriol. *J Dermatol Treat* 1993: 4; 173–77.

8.  Lebwohl M, Topical application of calcipotriene and corticosteroids: Combination regimens. *J Am Acad Dermatol* 1997: 37; S55–S58.

9.  Koo J, Calcipotriol/calcipotriene (Dovonex/Daivonex) in combination with phototherapy: A review. *J Am Acad Dermatol* 1997: 37; S59–S61.

10.  Veien NK, Bjerke JR, Rossmann-Ringdahl I, Jakobsen HB, Once daily treatment of psoriasis with tacalcitol compared with twice daily treatment with calcipotriol: a double-blind trial. *Br J Dermatol* 1997: 137; 581–86.

11.  Bikle DD, Vitamin D: A calciotropic hormone regulating calcium-induced keratinocyte differentiation. *J Am Acad Dermatol* 1997: 37; S42–S52.

12.  Kragballe K, Treatment of psoriasis by the topical application of the novel cholecalciferol analogue calcipotriol (MS 903). *Arch Dermatol* 1989: 125; 1647–52.

13.  Thiers BH, The use of topical calcipotriene/calcipotriol in conditions other than plaque type psoriasis. *J Am Acad Dermatol* 1997: 37; S69–S71.

14.  Anonymous, Sandimmun for severe atopic dermatitis. *Chem Drug* 1993: 240; 948.

15.  Camp RD, Reitamo S, Friedmann PS et al, Cyclosporine A in severe therapy

resistant atopic dermatitis: report of an international workshop, April 1993. *Br J Dermatol* 1993: 129; 217–20.

16. Chawla M, Ali M, Marks R et al, Comparison of the steady state pharmacokinetics of the two formulations of cyclosporin in patients with atopic dermatitis. *Br J Dermatol* 1996: 15(Suppl 48); 9–14.

17. Granlund H, Erkko P, Sinisalo M, Reitamo S, Cyclosporin in atopic dermatitis: time to relapse and effect of intermittent therapy. *Br J Dermatol* 1995: 132(1); 106–12.

18. Koo JY, Neoral in psoriasis therapy: toward a new perspective. *Int J Dermatol* 1997: 36(Suppl 1); 25–9.

19. Rothe MJ, Grant-Kels JM, Atopic dermatitis: an update. *J Am Acad Dermatol* 1996: 35; 1–13.

20. Ruzicka T, Bieber T, Schöpf E et al, A short-term trial of tacrolimus ointment for atopic dermatitis. The European Tacrolimus Multicenter Atopic Dermatitis Study Group. *N Engl J Med* 1997: 337; 816–21.

21. Alaiti S, Kang S, Fiedler VC et al, Tacrolimus (FK506) ointment for atopic dermatitis. A phase 1 study in adults and children. *J Am Acad Dermatol* 1998: 38; 69–76.

22. Ruzicka T, Assmann T, Homey B, Tacrolimus. The drug for the turn of the Millennium? *Arch Dermatol* 1999: 135; 574–80.

23. Zabawski EJ, Costner M, Cohen JB, Cockerell CJ, Tacrolimus: pharmacology and therapeutic uses in dermatology. *Int J Dermatol* 2000: 39; 721–7.

24. Harper J, Green A, Scott G et al, First experience of topical SDZ ASM 981 in children with atopic dermatitis. *Br J Dermatol* 2001: 144; 781–7.

25. Queille-Roussel C, Paul C, Duteil L et al, The new topical ascomycin derivative SDZ ASM 981 does not induce skin atrophy when applied to normal skin for 4 weeks: A randomised double-blind controlled study. *Br J Dermatol* 2001: 144, 507–13.

26. Griffiths CEM, Ascomycin: an advance in the management of atopic dermatitis. *Br J Dermatol* 2001: 144; 679–81.

27. Ellis CN, Fradin MS, Messana JM et al, Cyclosporine for plaque-type psoriasis. Results of multidose, double-blind trial. *N Engl J Med* 1991: 324(5); 277–84.

28. Koo JY, A randomised, double-blind study comparing the efficacy, safety and optimal dose of the two formulations of cyclosporin, Neoral and Sandimmun in patients with severe psoriasis. OLP302 Study Group. *Br J Dermatol* 1998: 139; 88–95.

29. Mizoguchi M, Kawaguchi K, Ohsuga Y et al, Cyclosporin ointment for psoriasis and atopic dermatitis. *Lancet* 1992: 339(8801); 1120.

30. Berth-Jones J, Finlay AY, Zaki I et al, Cyclosporine in severe childhood atopic dermatitis: a multicenter study. *J Am Acad Dermatol* 1996: 34(6); 1016–21.

31. Berth-Jones J, Graham-Brown RA, Marks R et al, Long term efficacy and safety of cyclosporine in severe adult atopic dermatitis. *Br J Dermatol* 1997: 136; 76–81.

32. de Prost Y, Bodemer C, Teillac D et al, Double-blind randomised placebo controlled trial of local cyclosporine in atopic dermatitis. *Arch Dermatol* 1989: 125(4); 570.

33.   de Prost Y, Bodemer C, Teillac D et al, Randomised double-blind placebo controlled trial of local cyclosporin in atopic dermatitis. *Acta Derm Venereol Suppl (Stockh)* 1989: 144; 136–8.

34.   Gaig P, Alijotas J, Lopez A et al, Cyclosporine A in atopic dermatitis. *Allergol Immunopathol (Madr)* 1993: 21(5); 169–72.

35.   Gold MH, Picascia DD, Roenigk HH Jr et al, Treatment resistant atopic dermatitis controlled with cyclosporine A. *Int J Dermatol* 1989: 28(7); 481–2.

36.   Ishii E, Yamamoto S, Sakai R et al, Production of interleukin-5 and the suppressive effect of cyclosporin A in childhood severe atopic dermatitis. *J Pedatr* 1996: 128(1); 152–5.

37.   Korstanje MJ, van de Staak WJ, Cyclosporin maintenance therapy of severe atopic dermatitis. *Acta Derm Venereol* 1991: 71(4); 356–7.

38.   Mandara G, Ranno C, Gugliemo F et al, A case of paediatric severe atopic dermatitis (AD) treated successfully with low cyclosporin A (Cya) dosage. *Ann Allergy Asthma Immunol* 1997: 78(1); 153.

39.   Munro CS, Levell NJ, Shuster S, Friedmann PS, Maintenance treatment with cyclosporin in atopic eczema. *Br J Dermatol* 1994: 130; 376–80.

40.   Taylor RS, Cooper KD, Headington JT et al, Cyclosporine therapy for severe atopic dermatitis. *J Am Acad Dermatol* 1989: 21(3 part 1); 580–3.

41.   van Joost T, Heule F, Korstanje M et al, Cyclosporin in atopic dermatitis: a multicentre placebo-controlled study. *Br J Dermatol* 1994: 130(5); 634–40.

42.   van Joost T, Kozel MM, Tank B et al, Cyclosporin in atopic dermatitis. Modulation in the expression of immunologic markers in lesional skin. *J Am Acad Dermatol* 1992: 27(6 part 1); 922–8.

43.   Zaki I, Emerson R, Allen BR, Treatment of severe atopic dermatitis in childhood with cyclosporin. *Fr J Dermatol* 1996: 136(Suppl 48); 21–4.

44.   Zonneveld IM, De Rie MA, Beljaards RC et al, The long term safety and efficacy of cyclosporin in severe refractory atopic dermatitis: a comparison of two dosage regimens. *Br J Dermatol* 1996: 135(Suppl 48); 15–20.

45.   Saay MS, Dismuker WE, Azole antifungal agents: emphasis on new triazoles. *Antimicrob Agents Chemother* 1985: 31; 1756–60.

46.   Bimbaum JE, Pharmacology of the allylamines. *J Am Acad Dermatol* 1990: 23; 782–5.

47.   Scher RK, Breneman D, Savin R et al, Once weekly fluconazole (150, 300 or 450 mg) in the treatment of distal subungual onychomycosis of the toenail. *J Am Acad Dermatol* 1998: 38(6 part 2); S77–86.

48.   Drake L, Babel D, Stewart M et al, Once weekly fluconazole (150, 300 or 450 mg) in the treatment of distal subungual onychomycosis of the fingernail. *J Am Acad Dermatol* 1998: 38(6 part 2); S87–94.

49.   Rich P, Scher RK, Breneman D et al, Phamacokinetics of three doses of once weekly fluconazole (150, 300, 450 mg) in distal subungual onychomycosis. *J Am Acad Dermatol* 1988: 38; S103–9.

50.   Alcantra R, Garibay JM, Intraconazole therapy in dermatomycosis and vagina candidiasis: efficacy and adverse effects

profile in a large multicenter study. *Adv Ther* 1998: 5(6); 326–33.

51.  Bourlond A, Lachapelle JM, Aussems J et al, Double-blind comparison of itraconazole with griseofulvin in the treatment of tinea corporis and tinea cruris. *Int J Dermatol* 1989: 28(6); 410–12.

52.  Degreef H, Marien K, De Veylder H et al, Itraconazole in the treatment of dermatophytoses: a comparison of two daily dosages. *Rev Infect Dis* 1987: 9(Suppl 1); S104–6.

53.  Hay RJ, Clayton YM, Moore MK, Midgely G, Itraconazole in the management of chronic dermatophytosis. *J Am Acad Dermatol* 1990: 23(3 part 2); 551–64.

54.  Andre J, De Doncker P, Ginter G et al, Intermittent pulse therapy with itraconazole in onychomycosis: an update (abstract). 54th Annual Meeting, American Academy of Dermatology, Washington DC, 10–15 February 1996.

55.  de Backer M, de Keyser P, de Vroey C, Lesaffre E, A 12 week treatment for dermatophyte toe onychomycosis: terbinadine 250 mg/day vs intraconazole 2000 mg/day – a double blind comparative trial. *Br J Dermatol* 1996: 134 (Suppl 136); 16–17.

56.  Brautigam M, Nolting S, Schopf RE, Weidinger G for the Seventh Lamisil German Onychomycosis Study Group, Randomised double-blind comparison of terbinafine and itraconazole for treatment of toenail tinea infection. *BMJ* 1995: 311; 919–21.

57.  Evans GE, Sigurgeirsson B, Double-blind randomised study of continuous terbinafine compared with intermittent itraconazole in the treatment of onychomycosis. *Br Med J* 1999: 318; 1031–5.

58.  Leyden JJ, Update on tinea capitis and new anti-fungal therapies. *Pediatr Infect Dis* 1999: 18(2); 215–16.

59.  Chambon P, The retinoid signalling pathway: molecular and genetic analyses. *Cell Biol* 1994: 5; 115–25.

60.  Charpentier B, Bernardon JM, Eustache J et al, Synthesis, structure affinity relationships and biological activities of ligands binding to retinoic acid receptor subtypes. *J Med Chem* 1995: 38; 4993–5006.

61.  Bernard BA, Bernardon JM, Delescluse C et al, Identification of synthetic retinoids with selectivity for human retinoic acid receptor γ. *Biochem Biophys Res Commun* 1992: 186; 977–83.

62.  Darmon M, Rocher M, Cavey MT et al, Biological activity of retinoids correlates with affinity for nuclear receptors but not for cytosolic binding protein. *Skin Pharmacol* 1988: 1; 161–75.

63.  Bouclier M, Luginbuhl B, Shroot B et al, Arachidonic acid induced ear oedema in four strains of rats and mice: a comparative study of anti-inflammatory drugs. *Agents Actions* 1990: 29; 62–4.

64.  Bouclier M, Shroot B, Dionisius V et al, A rapid and simple test system for the evaluation of the inhibitory activity of topical retinoids on cellotape stripping induced ODC activity in the hairless rat. *Dermatologica* 1984: 169; 242–3.

65.  Elder JT, Astrom, Pettersson U et al, Differential regulation of retinoic acid receptors and binding proteins in human skin. *J Invest Dermatol* 1992: 98; 673–9.

66.  Griffiths CEM, Elder JT, Bernard BA et al, Comparison of CD 271 (adapalene) and all trans retinoic acid in human skin: dissociation of epidermal effects and

CRABP-II mRNA expression. *J Invest Dermatol* 1992: 101; 325–8.

67.    Shroot B, Michel S, Pharmacology and chemistry of adapalene. *J Am Acad Dermatol* 1997: 36; S96–103.

68.    Jamoulie JC, Grandjean L, Lamaud E et al, Follicular penetration and distribution of topically applied CD 271, a new naphthoic acid derivative intended for topical acne treatment. *J Invest Dermatol* 1990: 94; 731.

69.    Verschoore M, Poncet M, Czernielewski J, Adapalene 0.1% gel has low skin irritation potential. *J Am Acad Dermatol* 1997: 36; S104–9.

70.    Cunliffe WJ, Caputo R, Dreno B et al, Clinical efficacy and safety comparison of adapalene gel and tretinoin gel in the treatment of acne vulgaris: Europe and US multicenter trials. *J Am Acad Dermatol* 1997: 36; S126–34.

71.    Chandraratna R, Tazarotene: the first receptor-selective topical retinoid for the treatment of psoriasis. *J Am Acad Dermatol* 1997: 37; S12–17.

72.    Duric M, Nagpal S, Asano AT et al, Molecular mechanisms of tazarotene action in psoriasis. *J Am Acad Dermatol* 1997: 37; S18–24.

73.    Koo J, Tazarotene in combination with phototherapy. *J Am Acad Dermatol* 1998: 39; S144–8.

74.    Kligman AM, Grove GL, Hirose R et al, Topical tretinoin for photoaged skin. *J Am Acad Dermatol* 1985: 15; 836–59.

75.    Weiss JS, Ellis CN, Headington JT et al, Topical tretinoin improves photoaged skin: a double-blind vehicle controlled study. *JAMA* 1988: 259; 527–32.

76.    Lever L, Kumar P, Marks R, Topical retinoic acid for treatment of solar damage. *Br J Dermatol* 1990: 122; 91–8.

77.    Leyden JJ, Grove GL, Grove MJ et al, Treatment of photodamaged facial skin with topical tretinoin. *J Am Acad Dermatol* 1989: 21; 638–44.

78.    Rafal ES, Griffiths CEM, Ditre CM et al, Topical tretinoin (retinoic acid) treatment for liver spots associated with photodamage. *N Engl J Med* 1992: 326; 368–74.

79.    Kang S, Fisher GJ, Voorhees JJ, Photoaging and topical tretinoin. *Arch Dermatol* 1997: 133; 1280–1.

80.    Gilchrist BA, turning back the clock: retinoic acid modifies intrinsic aging charges. *J Clin Invest* 1994: 94; 1711–12.

81.    Griffiths CEM, Russman AN, Majmuder G et al, Restoration of collagen formation in photodamaged human skin by tretinoin (retinoic acid). *N Engl J Med* 1993: 329; 530–55.

82.    Bhawan J, Gonzalez-Serva A, Nehal K et al, Effects of tretinoin on photodamaged skin: a histologic study. *Arch Dermatol* 1991: 127; 666–72.

83.    Shuttleworth D, Marks R, A comparison of the effects of intralesional interferon α-2b and topical 5% 5-fluorouracil cream in the treatment of solar keratoses and Bowen's disease. *J Dermatol Treat* 1989: 1; 65–8.

84.    Cornell RC, Greenway HT, Tucker SB et al, Intralesional interferon therapy for basal cell carcinoma. *J Am Acad Dermatol* 1990: 23; 694–700.

85.    Stadler R, Interferons in dermatology. Present day standard. *Dermatol Clin* 1998: 16; 377–98.

86.  Reichmann RC, Oakes D, Bonnez W et al, Treatment of condyloma acuminatum with three different interferons administered intralesionally. *Ann Intern Med* 1988: 108; 675–9.

87.  Vance JC, Bart BJ, Hansen RC et al, Intralesional recombinant alpha-2-interferon for the treatment of patients with condylomata acuminata or verruca plantaris. *Arch Dermatol* 1986: 122; 272–4.

88.  Eron LJ, Alder MB, O'Rourke JM et al, Recurrence of condylomata acuminata following cryotherapy is not prevented by systemically administered interferon. *Genitourin Med* 1993: 69; 91–3.

89.  Reinhold U, Wehrmann W, Kukel S et al, The influence of interferon gamma and interleukin-4 on IgE production in B-lymphocytes of patients with atopic dermatitis: a possible criterion for selections of patients for interferon therapy. *Acta Derm Venereol (Stockh)* 1990: 71; 484–7.

90.  Reinhold U, Wehrmann W, Kukel S et al, Recombinant interferon gamma therapy for atopic dermatitis. *Lancet* 1990: 1; 1282 (letter).

91.  Hanifin JM, Schneider LC, Donald YM et al, Recombinant interferon gamma therapy for atopic dermatitis. *J Am Acad Dermatol* 1993: 28; 189–97.

92.  Russell-Jones R, Interferon-α therapy for melanoma. *Clin Exp Dermatol* 2000: 25; 1–6.

93.  Pehamberger H, Soyer H, Steiner A et al, Adjuvant interferon alpha-2a treatment in resected primary stage II cutaneous melanoma. *J Clin Oncol* 1998: 16; 1425–9.

94.  Grob J, Dreno B, Salmoniere P et al, Randomised trial of interferon-alpha 2a as adjuvant therapy in resected primary melanoma thicker than 1.5 mm without clinically detectable node metastases. *Lancet* 1998: 351; 1905–10.

95.  Kirkwood J, Strawderman M, Ernstoff M et al, Interferon alpha-2b adjuvant therapy of high resected cutaneous melanoma: the Eastern Cooperative Oncology Group Trial EST 1684. *J Clin Oncol* 1996: 14; 7–17.

96.  Cole B, Gelber R, Kirkwood J et al, Quality of life adjusted survival analysis of interferon alpha-2b adjuvant treatment of high risk resected cutaneous melanoma in an Eastern Cooperative Oncology Group Study. *J Clin Oncol* 1996: 14; 2666–73.

97.  Berman B, Flores F, Recurrence rates of excised keloids treated with postoperative triamcinolone acetonide injections or interferon alpha-2b injections. *J Am Acad Dermatol* 1997: 37; 755–7.

98.  Azizlerli G, Sarica R, Köse A et al, Interferon alpha-2a in the treatment of Behçet's disease. *Dermatol* 1996: 19; 239–41.

99.  Mahrle G, Schultze HJ, Recombinant inteferon gamma (rIFN-gamma) in dermatology. *J Invest Dermatol* 1990: 95; 132S–7S.

100.  Ruszczak Z, Schwartz RA, Interferons in dermatology: biology, pharmacology and clinical applications. In: *Advances in Dermatology* 1998: Vol 13, Mosby-Year Book Inc.

# 2

## Management approaches to atopic dermatitis

*Julian Verbov*

## Introduction

Atopic dermatitis (AD) is a common inherited likely polygenic chronic inflammatory skin disease. A recent study identified two chromosomal regions showing evidence for both association and linkage with AD.[1] Prevalence has been increasing over the past 30 years or more in the industrialized world and figures from different countries show prevalences of 12–26% in children up to 12 years[2] and 2–10% in adults. I believe even these figures may be underestimates because many mildly affected individuals do not seek medical help and thus are not included in the figures. There is commonly a family history of one or more of asthma, AD and allergic rhinitis in affected individuals. Parental history appears to be the most valuable predictive parameter of AD.[3] However,

exposures associated with social class seem to be as important as genetic factors in determining childhood eczema.[4,5] In atopics, responses to common allergens result in generation of helper T lymphocytes of the so-called Th2 type in preference to those of Th1 type. However, there is more to AD than allergy[6] and its role must not be overemphasized. We do not have a cure but we can make the skin and life itself more pleasant for the affected individual and his/her family.

Atopic dermatitis usually appears in the first year of life but uncommonly before the age of 3 months. It is typically irritant and erythematous with papules and vesicles often initially appearing over the face (Figs 2.1 to 2.6) and scalp. The barrier function of atopic skin is impaired leading to generally dry skin. However, dominant ichthyosis vulgaris is also often associated with AD. Atopic skin has an increased susceptibility to colonization with *Staphylococcus aureus*. Staphylococcal superantigens can lead to release of mediators and cytokines causing inflammation. Such antigens can reduce the effectiveness of applied corticosteroids.[7] The role of staphylococcal superantigens in AD has been reviewed recently.[8]

In the management of AD, a thorough personal and family history is essential. Examination of the patient will confirm the diagnosis and adequate time must be spent explaining the condition to parents and to patients (if of a suitable age). AD causes 'the itching you have, and the scratching

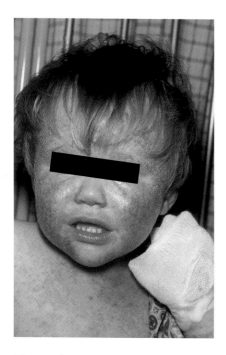

## Figure 2.1

Male 18-month-old with scratched secondarily infected eczema.

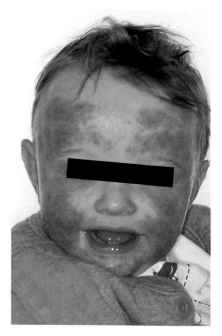

## Figure 2.2

Male 1-year-old with marked facial involvement.

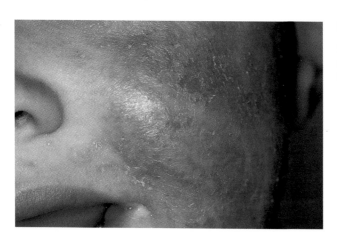

## Figure 2.3

Close-up of left cheek of infant shown in Fig. 2.2.

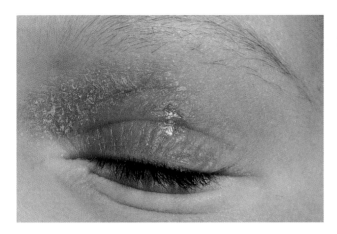

### Figure 2.4
Eyelid involvement.

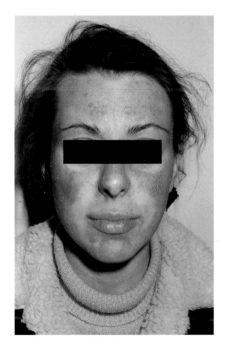

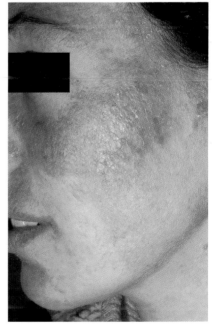

### Figure 2.5
Adult female with facial involvement.

### Figure 2.6
Same patient as in Fig. 2.5 showing close-up of left side of face.

you do'. Patients should be encouraged to rub the affected skin or adjacent to such skin rather than to scratch the actual eczema. Affected individuals should avoid wool next to the skin and cotton is recommended. Nails should be kept short. The itch of AD and treatment options have been discussed in a recent article.[9]

Topical applications are of prime importance in management. These include liberal use of emollients, and application of tar preparations, corticosteroids, antiseptics, antibiotics and other antibacterial agents, and more recently immunosuppressive agents such as tacrolimus. Systemic drugs include antibiotics, antihistamines, and in carefully selected patients, cyclosporin, azathioprine, methotrexate and corticosteroids. Enquiry about possible use of evening primrose oil and Chinese herbs by patients or their parents is common, particularly when they feel that the usually prescribed medications have not helped; these and other alternative treatments are mentioned later.

Dietary advice includes encouragement of breastfeeding. Breastfeeding for 6 months or more may delay the onset of AD but is unlikely to affect the natural history of the disease. There is insufficient evidence that dietary manipulation in adults or in the majority of children reduces symptom severity in AD. For severe unresponsive eczema in infants and young children regimens avoiding suspected foods can be tried but if no clear benefit is obtained they should not be continued for more than 3–4 weeks. Careful monitoring with the aid of a dietician is essential with such diets.

Peanut allergy, which can be severe and potentially fatal,[10] rarely resolves in older children and adults, but may resolve in some young children who become sensitized early in life.[11] Prick testing and the RAST (radioallergosorbent) test for detecting and measuring circulating antibodies are generally not very helpful in young children, being difficult to interpret because of the common false-positive reactions.

Occupations such as hairdressing, engineering, nursing and gardening should generally be avoided in AD, even if the eczema is dormant at the time of application to work, because of the danger of reactivation of eczema, particularly over the hands.

In managing patients with AD explanation about the nature of the disease and general measures such as avoidance of provoking factors are important. Reinforcement through parent/patient meetings with nursing staff and contact with the National Eczema Society provide additional support. The management of an individual patient must take the patient's relevant background into account, which includes consideration of personal and family circumstances as well as atopy. Management of AD has been extensively discussed.[12,13]

In assessing new therapies for AD, double-blind randomized controlled trials are important, if possible, because of the fluctuating nature of the disease and significant placebo effects.

Accurate assessment of disease activity and severity is difficult because of the lack of objective measures. Objective recording of patient symptoms, or disability scores, may be difficult to interpret.

# Topical applications

## Emollients

The mainstay of management remains adequate use of emollients. This means repeated liberal application of a particular preparation to soften and moisturize the skin. It should be appreciated that an individual patient will often have a preference for a particular emollient. Emollients do have an intrinsic mild antipruritic action. Ointments are in general more effective than creams. However, creams are more popular in adults because they are not greasy. Emollient bath products and emollients used as soap substitutes are important. Even after bathing or showering with a suitable emollient product, the skin should have emollient immediately applied to prevent drying. Emollients for the bath or shower may have one or more antibacterial agents added; such agents are particularly useful when secondary skin infection is a problem.

## Corticosteroids

The appearance of hydrocortisone in the early 1950s revolutionized the treatment of eczema and topical corticosteroids remain of great importance in the management of AD. They are classified in the UK as mildly potent (e.g. hydrocortisone 1%), moderately potent (e.g. clobetasone butyrate 0.05%), potent (e.g. betamethasone valerate 0.1%), and very potent (e.g. clobetasol propionate 0.05%). This classification indicating potency is useful and should always be considered in the individual patient. The aim in AD should be to reduce the itching and minimize the eruption. The aim is to use a steroid that will control the eczema but will be safe to use. Applying the preparation thinly and in calculated amounts is important. A fingertip unit system is one way to do this.[14] Too-frequent application of a too-potent a steroid over wide areas of skin are likely to damage the skin, and absorption can produce osteopenia, cataracts, hypothalamic-pituitary-adrenal suppression and Cushing's syndrome.

Steroid applications are generally prescribed for use once or twice daily. Often treatment should be commenced with a more potent steroid and as the condition improves a steroid of weaker potency is prescribed. In a child, moderately and mildly potent preparations should generally be the ones prescribed with the more potent preparations being reserved for adults. The face and flexures of a child should generally be treated with a mildly potent steroid only. Topical steroid applications may be combined with an antibiotic or other antibacterial agent if, as is often the case, secondary skin infection is present. Skin infection is a trigger for further spread of eczema.

## Tar preparations

Tar-containing creams, ointments, and shampoos still have a place in the management of some eczema patients.

## Bandaging

Bandaging of limbs with moist zinc oxide or coal tar paste-impregnated occlusive cotton bandages is very useful, particularly in children. Such bandages, often changed twice weekly, allow the inflamed skin to heal and prevent the individual directly attacking the skin. Wet wraps are also useful in young children with severe uncontrolled eczema. In one system a potent steroid (one part) diluted with an emollient (nine parts) is applied to the limbs and/or the trunk which are then covered with damp elasticated tubular bandage shaped into sleeves, vest etc., and another layer of dry, shaped lightweight bandage is then applied. Damp wraps can be applied twice daily or remoistened as they become dry. Application of wraps is time consuming, but such therapy for a flare of AD is often helpful in youngsters. Use of steroids under such occlusive wet dressings should normally be short-term, and both efficacy and safety have to be assessed.[15]

# Systemic drugs

## Antihistamines

Although antihistamines may not influence the itch significantly[16] these drugs do have a definite role in AD. They should be readily prescribed in a dosage adequate to reduce the itching. The older more sedative antihistamines are most effective but their use is often restricted in the older individual because of the necessity to be fully awake at school, at work, or when driving. A non-sedating antihistamine such as cetirizine can be prescribed to provide some relief, albeit minor, for the unfortunate older patient. I tend to prescribe hydroxyzine or chlorpheniramine in infants and hydroxyzine, chlorpheniramine or trimeprazine in children over 2 years old. Clemastine is also useful and has the advantage of a sucrose-free elixir formulation. There is also a sugar-free solution of cetirizine.

## Antibiotics

There should be no hesitation in prescribing short courses of a suitable oral antibiotic when bacterial skin infection is marked.

Most herpes simplex infections in AD patients are neither widespread nor severe but widespread infection, eczema herpeticum (Figs 2.7 and 2.8), is most important to diagnose. It requires oral or intravenous aciclovir. Such infection is usually a primary herpes infection. Individuals with AD

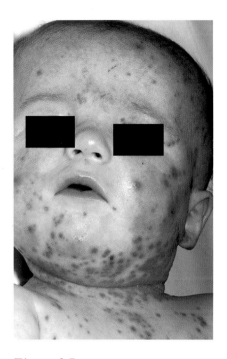

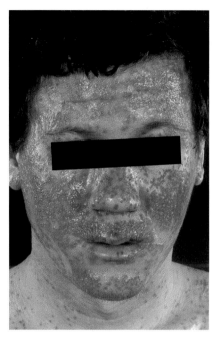

**Figure 2.7**

Eczema herpeticum in a 6-month-old male.

**Figure 2.8**

Eczema herpeticum in a young adult male.

should avoid close contact with people with active cold sores because of the danger of acquiring widespread herpetic infection. For instance, a child with AD should not bathe with a sibling who has a cold sore.

## Attacking the environment

Such measures include not smoking, controlling pets and airborne pet allergens, using covers for mattresses, pillows and duvets, removing carpets, keeping pets out of bedrooms, reducing indoor humidity and bathing or showering in the morning. All of the above will contribute to improving an affected individual. The role of the house-dust mite in precipitating AD is unclear. However, daily vacuuming of bedroom carpets with an effective cleaner and the use of certain bed covers have been shown to reduce house-dust mite allergen and result in clinical improvement in many patients with severe AD.[17] Changing the environment by admission to hospital is often helpful when outpatient treatment of AD fails. Over the years, indoor ventilation has decreased and the rate at which indoor air is exchanged for fresh air in a modern house is ten times lower than it was 30 years ago, with a considerable increase in humidity and in the concentrations of indoor pollutants and airborne allergens.[18]

# Inoculations

Although hygienic measures in modern societies may be partly responsible for the increased occurrence of atopic diseases in these populations,[19] inoculations should still be encouraged in children with AD. Children allergic to eggs do not appear to be at greater risk for anaphylaxis in response to MMR vaccine than other children.

# Prognosis

There is a tendency for AD to improve with increasing age, and figures indicate 65% clearance at the age of 11 years, and 74% clearance at the age of 16 years.[20] However, as these authors found, there may be recurrences in adolescence and early adulthood. Many young adults with hand eczema give a history of AD in childhood.

# Unconventional approaches

The efficacy of evening primrose oil in treating AD remains doubtful. A recent double-blind placebo-controlled study in Sweden found no significant benefit in 60 atopic children.[21] Topical sodium cromoglycate has been reported to be of some benefit in AD[22] but properly controlled studies are required. I have not found high dose oral vitamin C to be of benefit. Chinese herbal treatment has been promoted as a treatment for AD and much has been written in the lay press on its benefits. Such herbs, used orally, have been subject to two useful double-blind placebo-controlled studies,[23,24] in which more benefit was seen with the active treatment. However, the active pharmacological agents have not been identified and the mechanism of action of such herbs is unclear. Reports of serious side-effects including kidney and liver toxicity with such preparations have appeared.[25] The evidence base for efficacy is not sufficient and there is doubt about the safety of this treatment.[26]

In a recent paper,[27] in which γ-linoleic acid, Chinese herbal tea, diets eliminating antigens, pseudoallergens, metal salts and sodium, and bioresonance were considered, the authors concluded that none of the treatments provided unequivocally convincing evidence of efficacy even when double-blind placebo-controlled studies were available. A significant corticosteroid content in some Chinese medications, both oral and topical, has also regularly been found.

Doxepin, a tricyclic antidepressant, is available as a topical preparation containing doxepin 5% for the relief of pruritus in eczema. However, it is absorbed percutaneously which limits its value.[9]

# Severe resistant AD

## *Immunomodulators*

### Cyclosporin

Cyclosporin (*ciclosporin*) is a macrolide immunosuppressive agent which acts by altering the cytokine gene transcription, thus inhibiting T-cell activation and modulating the cell-mediated immune response.[28] Cyclosporin may work in AD by altering interleukin (IL-4) transcription and monocyte IL-10 production, possibly promoting Th1 cytokine profiles.[29] Sowden et al[30] showed that in adults with AD, oral cyclosporin given for 8 weeks significantly reduced skin activity and extent compared to placebo, and there have been other controlled trials. There have also been open studies in children[31] and in adults.[32] Short-term cyclosporin therapy (maximum 8 weeks) is currently regularly prescribed in intractable disease and, in general, should be given for no more than 3–6 months. Relapse following withdrawal of cyclosporin is usual so that ultraviolet (UV) radiation, for instance, should be introduced as cyclosporin is tapered.

Use of cyclosporin should be limited to patients with severe refractory disease because of nephotoxicity, hypertension and the potential risk of malignancies occurring with such therapy. Topical cyclosporin is ineffective in treating AD.

### Tacrolimus

Trials of the topical macrolide immunosuppressive agent tacrolimus (FK506) an inhibitor of calcineurin, have been encouraging.[33] Tacrolimus is 10–100 times more potent than cyclosporin in inhibiting T-cell activity. It also has greater skin penetration than cyclosporin.[34] Studies have shown it to be safe and effective both in adults and in children in a topical formulation.[35-37] A burning sensation at the site of application is the most common side-effect. Perhaps it will become an alternative to topical corticosteroids. There are recent reviews of the pharmacology and therapeutic uses of tacrolimus in dermatology.[38,39]

### SDZ ASM 981

Like cyclosporin and tacrolimus, this drug is an immunosuppressive. It is derived from the macrolactam ascomycin. It has an anti-inflammatory action and acts as a cytokine inhibitor, suppressing T-cell proliferation and antigen-specific activation. Recent trials of topical SDZ ASM 981 in adults[40] and children[41] are encouraging. In addition, it does not appear to produce skin atrophy.[42] A useful editorial on ascomycin has appeared[43] and a review of topical immunomodulators in childhood AD.[44]

## Methotrexate

This drug, which inhibits the enzyme dihydrofolate reductase, essential for the synthesis of purines and pyrimidines, has had some success in AD when used in relatively low dosage, e.g. 2.5 mg daily for four consecutive days a week. The regimen is altered according to patient response. The drug has to be carefully monitored during treatment, and investigations before starting treatment include full blood count, and both renal and liver function tests.

## Azathioprine

This is a synthetic purine analogue and can be effective in AD.[45] A disadvantage is that it takes 6–8 weeks to exert its action and monitoring for toxicity is essential. Pretreatment determination of thiopurine methyltransferase (TPMT) activity levels may predict patients with deficiency of the enzyme and thus at risk for bone marrow toxicity.[46]

## Interferon gamma (IFN-γ)

This is a cytokine produced primarily by T cells with a Th0/Th1 profile which plays an important regulatory role in immune function. IFN-γ promotes proliferation of Th1 cells and decreases IgE levels and eosinophil counts. Subcutaneous IFN-γ does reduce the severity

of AD. Side-effects of this very expensive drug include 'flu-like symptoms and alteration in liver function tests. Hanifin et al[47] showed greater improvement in erythema and excoriation scores than in placebo-treated patients; interestingly no reduction in serum IgE was found. Improvement in clinical severity parameters has also been seen in other studies.[48,49]

## Intravenous immunoglobulin (IVIg)

This has been used in management of AD but it is very expensive and its efficacy is, as yet, unproven.

## Mycophenolate mofetil

This has not been thoroughly tested in AD. Mycophenolic acid inhibits de novo purine biosynthesis, resulting in blockage of proliferative responses of T and B lymphocytes.[50] It may have inhibitory effects on cytokine production and thus reduce the inflammatory response.[51] No significant benefit was seen in a recent small open trial of mycophenolate mofetil[52] and clearly randomized controlled studies are necessary.

## Anti-inflammatory agents

These include antihistamines (mentioned earlier), UV radiation which also has a recognized place in non-refractory AD, phosphodiesterase inhibitors, leukotriene receptor antagonists, thalidomide and thymopentin.

## Ultraviolet radiation

UV phototherapy can be beneficial in AD. Both UVA and UVB or a combination of the two have been used, and narrow-band UVB (TL01) may also be effective.[53] Psoralen UVA (PUVA) has a small place in severe AD but possible long-term adverse effects must be carefully considered. Extracorporeal photochemotherapy (photophoresis) using UVA irradiation of enriched leucocytes in the presence of methoxsalen has been shown to be effective in some patients with severe AD in a recent open trial.[54] A review of phototherapy for AD has recently appeared.[55]

## Phosphodiesterase inhibitors (PDEIs)

Atopic leucocytes have increased intracellular PDE activity which causes deficient cyclic AMP levels: This deficit results indirectly in increased cytokine and mediator release.[56] Topical and systemic PDEIs are expected to be developed over the next few years. Safety combined with effectiveness is the aim.

## Leukotriene receptor antagonists

Such drugs interfere with leukotriene-induced chemotaxis, vascular permeability and airway constriction and are used in asthma. Four patients have been reported whose AD improved when treated with oral zafirlukast.[57] A pilot study of zileuton, another leukotriene antagonist, in six adult patients, showed encouraging results.[58] However, the anti-inflammatory effects are not proven in AD as yet, and controlled studies are necessary. Side-effects and drug interactions are possible. Regarding the latter, zafirlukast can inhibit the hepatic microsomal cytochrome P450 isoenzymes CYP2C9 and CYP3A at therapeutic concentrations.[59]

## Thalidomide

Work needs to be done to discover whether this drug with its inherent dangers has any place in the management of severe AD.

## Thymopentin

This is a synthetic pentapeptide derived from the thymic hormone, thymopoietin. It enhances production of Th1 cytokines and suppresses Th2 cytokines. A double-blind trial showed a reduction in clinical severity of AD.[60]

## Conclusion

In practical terms, with regard to the management of AD, mild eczema may just require regular application of emollients. Most patients with AD will be controlled by liberal use of emollients, cautious use of topical corticosteroids, relevant use of topical antibiotics or other antibacterials, short courses of oral antibiotics and regular use of oral antihistamines. However, severe eczema may require severe treatment, and other modalities, as mentioned above, are then required.

# The importance of research

Sad miserable infant
obliged to accept
an unfortunate existence.
Lack of itch eludes him
Itch, scratch, rub –
his daily bread.
"Deliver me from this evil"
he would cry
if insight permitted.

Sad miserable family
sharing the quantity of suffering
yet unwilling to accept
the unfortunate fate of the individual.
"Speedily deliver us all from this evil"
they cry.

Caring doctor
appreciates life's quality.
Provides emollience first
yet accepts drug therapy.
Concedes prognosis to a Higher
Authority
supporting an obligatory push from
earth.

*(This poem regarding AD first appeared in the* British Journal of Dermatology *(Verbov J, BJD 1996: 135; 668) and is published with permission of the Editors of the* British Journal of Dermatology*)*

# References

1.   Beyer K, Nickel R, Freidhoff L et al, Association and linkage of atopic dermatitis with chromosome 13q 12-14 and 5q 31-33 markers. *J Invest Dermatol* 2000: 115; 906–8.

2.   Friedmann PS, Allergy and the skin II Contact and atopic eczema. *BMJ* 1998: 316; 1226–9.

3.   Beyer K, Wahn U, Is atopic dermatitis predictable? *Pediatr Allergy Immunol* 1999: 10 (Suppl 12); 7–10.

4.   Williams HC, Strachan DP, Hay RJ, Childhood eczema: disease of the advantaged? *BMJ* 1994: 308; 1132–5.

5.   Harris JM, Cullinan P, Williams HC et al, Environmental associations with eczema in early life. *Brit J Dermatol* 2001; 144: 795–802.

6.   Schäfer T, Krämer U, Vieluf D et al, The excess of atopic eczema in East Germany is related to the intrinsic type. *Br J Dermatol* 2000: 143; 992–8.

7.   McFadden J, What is the role of *Staphylococcus aureus* in atopic eczema? *CME Bull Dermatol* 1999: 2; 4–6.

8.   Skov L, Baadsgaard O, Bacterial superantigens and inflammatory skin diseases. *Clin Exp Dermatol* 2000: 25; 57–61.

9.   Greaves M, Mast cell mediators other than histamine induced pruritus in atopic dermatitis patients – a dermal microdialysis study. *Br J Dermatol* 2000: 142; 1079–83.

10.   Sicherer SH, Sampson HA, Peanut and tree nut allergy. *Curr Opin Pediatr* 2000: 12; 567–73.

11.   Hourihane JO'B, Roberts SA, Warner JO, Resolution of peanut allergy: case-controlled study. *BMJ* 1998: 316; 1271–5.

12.   McHenry PM, Williams HC, Bingham EA, Management of atopic eczema: Joint Workshop of the British Association of Dermatologists and the Research Unit of the Royal College of Physicians of London. *BMJ* 1998: 310; 843–7.

13. Sidbury R, Hanifin JM, Old, new, and emerging therapies for atopic dermatitis. *Dermatol Clin* 2000: 18; 1–11.

14. Long CC, Finlay AY, The fingertip unit – a new practical measure. *Clin Exp Dermatol* 1991: 316; 444–7.

15. Wolkerstorfer A, Visser RL, de Waard-van der spek FB et al, Efficacy and safety of wet-wrap dressings in children with severe atopic dermatitis: influence of corticosteroid dilution. *Br J Dermatol* 2000: 143; 999–1004.

16. Hägermark Ö, Wahlgren C-F, Itch in atopic dermatitis: the role of histamine and other mediators and the failure of antihistamine therapy. *Dermatol Ther* 1996: 1; 75–82.

17. Friedmann PS, Dust mite avoidance in atopic dermatitis. *Clin Exp Dermatol* 1999: 24; 433–7.

18. Woodcock A, Custovic A, Avoiding exposure to indoor allergens. *BMJ* 1999: 316; 1075–8.

19. Gereda JE, Leung DYM, Thatayatikom A et al, Relation between house-dust endotoxin exposure, type 1 T-cell development and allergen sensitisation in infants at high risk of asthma. *Lancet* 2000: 355; 1680–3.

20. Williams HC, Strachan DP, The natural history of childhood eczema: observations from the British 1958 birth cohort study. *Br J Dermatol* 1998: 139; 834–9.

21. Hederos C-A, Berg A, Epogam evening primrose oil treatment in atopic dermatitis and asthma. *Arch Dis Child* 1996: 75; 494–7.

22. Moore C, Ehlayel MS, Junprasert J, Sorensen RU, Topical sodium cromoglycate in the treatment of moderate to severe atopic dermatitis. *Ann Allergy Asthma Immunol* 1998: 81; 452–8.

23. Sheehan MP, Atherton DJ, A controlled trial of traditional Chinese medicinal plants in widespread non-exudative atopic eczema. *Br J Dermatol* 1992: 126; 179–84.

24. Sheehan MP, Rustin MH, Atherton DJ et al, Efficacy of traditional Chinese herbal therapy in adult atopic dermatitis. *Lancet* 1992: 340; 13–17.

25. Harper J, Traditional Chinese medicine for eczema. *BMJ* 1994: 308; 489–90.

26. Armstrong NC, Ernst E, The treatment of eczema with Chinese herbs: a systematic review of randomized clinical trials. *Br J Clin Pharmacol* 1999: 48; 262–4.

27. Worm M, Henz BM, Novel unconventional therapeutic approaches to atopic eczema. *Dermatology* 2000: 201; 191–5.

28. Liu J, FK506 and cyclosporin, molecular probes for studying intracellular signal transduction. *Immunol Today* 1993: 14; 290–5.

29. Campbell DE, Kemp AS, Cyclosporine restores cytokine imbalance in childhood atopic dermatitis. *J Allergy Clin Immunol* 1997: 99; 857–9.

30. Sowden JM, Berth-Jones J, Ross JS et al, Double-blind controlled, crossover study of cyclosporin in adults with severe refractory atopic dermatitis. *Lancet* 1991: 338; 137–40.

31. Berth-Jones J, Finlay AY, Zaki I et al, Cyclosporine in severe childhood atopic dermatitis: a multicenter trial. *J Am Acad Dermatol* 1996: 34; 1016–21.

32. Berth-Jones J, Graham-Brown RAC, Marks R et al, Long-term efficacy and safety of cyclosporin in severe adult atopic dermatitis. *Br J Dermatol* 1997: 136; 76–81.

33. Rothe MJ, Grant-Kels JM, Atopic dermatitis: an update. *J Am Acad Dermatol* 1996: 35; 1–13.

34. Goto T, Kino S, Hatanaka H et al, FK506: historical perspectives. *Transplant Proc* 1991: 23; 2713–17.

35. Ruzicka T, Bieber T, Schöpf E et al, A short-term trial of tacrolimus ointment for atopic dermatitis. The European Tacrolimus Multicenter Atopic Dermatitis Study Group. *N Engl J Med* 1997: 337; 816–21.

36. Boguniewicz M, Fiedler VC, Raimer S et al, A randomised vehicle-controlled trial of tacrolimus ointment for treatment of atopic dermatitis in children. *J Allergy Clin Immunol* 1998: 102; 637–44.

37. Alaiti S, Kang S, Fiedler VC et al, Tacrolimus (FK506) ointment for atopic dermatitis. A phase 1 study in adults and children. *J Am Acad Dermatol* 1998: 38; 69–76.

38. Ruzicka T, Assmann T, Homey B, Tacrolimus. The drug for the turn of the Millennium? *Arch Dermatol* 1999: 135; 574–80.

39. Zabawski EJ, Costner M, Cohen JB, Cockerell CJ, Tacrolimus: pharmacology and therapeutic uses in dermatology. *Int J Dermatol* 2000: 39; 721–7.

40. Luger T, Van Leent EJM, Graeber M et al, SDZ ASM 981: an emerging safe and effective treatment for atopic dermatitis. *Br J Dermatol* 2001: 144; 788–94.

41. Harper J, Green A, Scott G et al, First experience of topical SDZ ASM 981 in children with atopic dermatitis. *Br J Dermatol* 2001: 144; 781–7.

42. Queille-Roussel C, Paul C, Duteil L et al, The new topical ascomycin derivative SDZ ASM 981 does not induce skin atrophy when applied to normal skin for 4 weeks: A randomised double-blind controlled study. *Br J Dermatol* 2001: 144; 507–13.

43. Griffiths CEM, Ascomycin: an advance in the management of atopic dermatitis. *Br J Dermatol* 2001: 144; 679–81.

44. Paller AS, Use of nonsteroidal topical immunomodulators for the treatment of atopic dermatitis in the pediatric population. *J Pediatr* 2001: 138; 163–8.

45. Chu T, The role of systemic therapy in severe atopic eczema. *CME Bull Dermatol* 1999: 2; 23–8.

46. Snow JL, Gibson LE, A pharmacogenic basis for the safe and effective use of azathioprine and other thiopurine drugs in dermatologic patients. *J Am Acad Dermatol* 1995: 32; 114–16.

47. Hanifin JM, Schneider LC, Leung DY et al, Recombinant interferon-gamma therapy for atopic dermatitis. *J Am Acad Dermatol* 1993: 28; 189–97.

48. Schneider LC, Baz Z, Zarcone C, Zurakowski D, Long-term therapy with recombinant interferon-gamma (rIFN-gamma) for atopic dermatitis. *Ann Allergy Asthma Immunol* 1998: 80; 263–8.

49. Stevens SR, Hanifin JM, Hamilton T et al, Long-term effectiveness and safety of recombinant human interferon gamma therapy for atopic dermatitis despite unchanged serum IgE levels. *Arch Dermatol* 1998: 134; 799–804.

50. Engui EM, Mirkovitch A, Allison AC, Lymphocyte-selective anti-proliferative and immunosuppressive effects of mycophenolic acid in mice. *Scand J Immunol* 1991: 33; 175–83.

51.   Kitchen JE, Pomeranz MK, Pak G et al, Rediscovering mycophenolic acid: a review of its mechanism, side-effects and potential uses. *J Am Acad Dermatol* 1997: 37; 445–9.

52.   Hansen ER, Buus S, Deleuran M, Andersen KE, Treatment of atopic dermatitis with mycophenolate mofetil. *Br J Dermatol* 2000: 143; 1324–6.

53.   Hudson-Peacock MJ, Diffey BL, Farr PM, Narrow-band UVB phototherapy for severe atopic dermatitis. *Br J Dermatol* 1996: 135; 332.

54.   Prinz B, Michelsen S, Pfeiffer C, Plewig G, Long-term application of extra-corporeal photochemotherapy in severe atopic dermatitis. *J Am Acad Dermatol* 1999: 40; 577–82.

55.   Krutmann J, Phototherapy for atopic dermatitis. *Clin Exp Dermatol* 2000: 25; 552–8.

56.   Hanifin JM, Chan SC, Cheng JB et al, Type 4 phosphodiesterase inhibitors have clinical and in vitro anti-inflammatory effects in atopic dermatitis. *J Invest Dermatol* 1996: 107; 51–6.

57.   Carucci JA, Washenik K, Weinstein A et al, The leukotriene antagonist zafirlukast as a therapeutic agent for atopic dermatitis. *Arch Dermatol* 1998: 134; 785–6.

58.   Woodmansee DP, Simon RA, A pilot study examining the role of zileuton in atopic dermatitis. *Ann Allergy Asthma Immunol* 1999: 83; 548–52.

59.   Dempsey OJ, Leukotriene receptor antagonist therapy. *Postgrad Med J* 2000: 76; 767–73.

60.   Leung DYM, Hirsch RL, Schneider L et al, Thymopentin therapy reduces the clinical severity of atopic dermatitis. *J Allergy Clin Immunol* 1990: 85; 927–33.

# 3

# Advances in acne therapy

*James J Leyden*

## Introduction

Acne vulgaris is the most common skin disease and as such it is fitting that major advances have occurred in the treatment of this disorder in the past 25 years. A great deal has been learned about the pathophysiology of the disease that has led to use of three major classes of therapeutic agents, i.e. retinoids, antibiotics and hormonal drugs. Before the treatment advances of the past 25 years, many variants of acne were not treated successfully. Now rational and effective treatments exist for all forms of the disease.

## Acne pathophysiology

Four major areas of pathophysiology have been identified (Table 3.1):

1. Excessive sebum production
2. Abnormal desquamation of follicular epithelium

3. *Propionibacterium acnes* proliferation
4. Inflammation generated by *P. acnes* production of proinflammatory molecules

Sebum production begins in the prepubertal period when adrenal glands mature and secrete increasing amounts of adrenal androgens.[1,2] Those children with lesions of acne have elevated levels of dehydroepiandrosterone sulfate (DHEAS) and commonly go on to develop more pronounced acne. The early lesions of acne are uniformly found in the midline of the face and consist of non-inflammatory comedones. At this early stage, colonization by *P. acnes* has not yet occurred.[3-5] With gonadal development, increased sebum production occurs and *P. acnes* colonization develops.[5] Current thinking is that sebaceous glands of acne patients are over-responsive to androgens rather

---

**Table 3.1 Acne pathophysiology**

Excessive Sebum Production
linoleic acid deficiency
↓
Microcomedo
abnormal desquamation
lipid accumulation
*P. acnes* proliferation
↓        ↓
Comedones    Inflammation

than that overproduction of androgens occurs. However, patients with excessive androgen production, e.g. those with variants of the so-called polycystic ovary syndrome, frequently develop acne. The discovery that testosterone is converted to an intracellular, metabolically more active dihydrotestosterone by the enzyme 5-$\alpha$-reductase offers promise for new treatments since inhibitors of this enzyme exist. One such inhibitor, finasteride, is available for treatment of prostatic hypertrophy and shows promise for androgenetic alopecia. Sebaceous glands appear to utilize another isoenzyme, so-called type I, and topical and/or systemic inhibitors may be drugs of the future.[6,7]

For now we have several classes of drugs which inhibit sebum production and are useful for treating acne. These include estrogens, antiestrogens and isotretinoin.

## Estrogen therapy

Ethinyl estradiol given systemically at a dose of 5 $\mu$g/day will produce a 90% reduction in sebum excretion within 6 weeks.[8] This effect cannot be maintained in the face of concomitant androgen therapy, suggesting that the effect of estrogen is not at the peripheral level of the sebaceous gland.[8] Likewise systemic estrogen is associated with decreases in circulating free testosterone, suggesting that the effect of estrogen on acne may be through decreasing the amount of testosterone reaching the sebaceous gland.[9]

Many years ago Pochi and Strauss demonstrated that oral contraceptives containing 50 $\mu$g of estrogen and various progestins were beneficial in the treatment of acne and that this benefit was due to sebum suppression.[8] The sebum suppression effect is enhanced by the addition of small amounts of corticosteroids (5 to 10 mg of prednisone).[10] In recent years, oral contraceptives have evolved to pills containing lower levels of estrogen (30 to 35 $\mu$g) in combination with various progestins. The lower levels of estrogens are less predictably helpful in suppressing sebum. Moreover, the effect of the progestin may be important in view of the androgenic effects of many progestins. Oral contraceptives containing non-androgenic progestins such as norgestimate and desogestrel appear to be better choices for acne therapy.[9]

The US FDA recently approved a combination of norgestimate and ethinyl estradiol for the treatment of acne. Clinical improvements in acne are associated with a significant reduction in free testosterone and a significant increase in sex hormone-binding globulin (SHBG). In addition, norgestimate is associated with an increase in high-density lipoproteins (HDLs) while progestins with androgenic activity such as triphasic levonorgestrel reduce HDLs.[11] Interestingly, a combination of 30 to 40 $\mu$g of ethinyl estradiol with 50 to 125 $\mu$g of levonorgestrel does produce a reduction in free testosterone and an increase in SHBG levels in addition to decreasing HDLs.[11] The reduction in free testosterone and the increased SHBG were less than that seen with a triphasic combination of 35 mg of estrogen and 180 to 250 mg of norgestimate.[9] Clinical trials with estrogen plus levonorgestrel are underway and will help clarify the clinical significance of the role of the progestin in acne therapy.

## Antiandrogen therapy

In many parts of the world, the potent antiandrogen, cyproterone acetate, is available and generally used in combination with estrogen. The original combination of 50 g of estrogen in combination with 2 mg of cyproterone acetate is gradually being replaced by a 35 μg estrogen plus 2 mg cyproterone acetate. A dose response has been shown for cyproterone acetate given alone but little difference was found between 12 months of high-dose cyproterone acetate (100 mg/day) and the combination of 50 μg of estrogen and 2 mg of cyproterone acetate.[12,13]

For those patients who have a contraindication for estrogen therapy, e.g. phlebitis, breast cancer, migraine headaches, etc., spironolactone can be helpful. Doses of 100 to 200 mg/day can suppress sebum production and improve acne. Spironolactone appears to act through a peripheral antiandrogen effect.[14,15]

## Isotretinoin

Isotretinoin counteracts all areas of acne pathophysiology. Its effect on sebum production is profound and prompt.[16-18] Reductions of greater than 90% occur within a month of therapy with 1.0 mg/kg per day. As a consequence of the profound suppression of sebum, *P. acnes* levels are markedly reduced, as are gram-negative bacteria, in those who become heavily colonized by these organisms.[19] In addition, isotretinoin reverses comedogenesis and produces anti-inflammatory effects by suppressing chemotactic responses.[20] When isotretinoin therapy is discontinued, sebaceous gland function slowly returns. However, prolonged reductions in sebum production are also seen.[21] The mechanism(s) involved in the action of isotretinoin on sebaceous glands and the prolonged benefit even in those in whom sebum production returns to pretreatment levels remain unclear. Retinoids are now known to exert effects on gene transcription and affect all differentiation. This type of molecular effect has not been demonstrated in acne patients, and unlike for other retinoids, no receptor has been identified for isotretinoin.

Another possibility for the profound reduction of sebum is that isotretinoin produces a selective toxic effect on sebaceous glands. In one study, acute cell toxicity changes were seen in sebaceous glands at the electron microscopic level within one week of therapy at 1 mg/kg.[20] The prolonged clinical benefits are even less understood in terms of mechanisms. Sebum and *P. acnes* levels can return to pretreatment levels without clinical disease similar to the situation in patients who spontaneously "outgrow" acne and develop remissions. My own, totally unproved hypothesis is that in both situations, changes occur in follicular epithelial differentiation resulting in a follicular wall in which there is an orderly desquamation of corneocytes and a better barrier function resulting in a different microenvironment. This hypothesis is based on post-treatment biopsies and biopsies from patients who have entered spontaneous remission and is obviously open to criticism in terms of sampling errors and problems in quantification of such observations.

## 5α-Reductase inhibitors

In sebaceous glands and other androgen-sensitive organs, testosterone is converted into the cellularly more active dihydrotestosterone by 5-α-reductases. Two isoenzymes have been identified and differences exist from tissue to tissue in terms of which isoenzyme is active. Clearly in the prostate and terminal hair follicles, type II is active and drugs which inhibit this isoenzyme are active in prostatic hypertrophy and androgenetic alopecia. In acne, the specific isoenzyme action in abnormal sebaceous glands, i.e. those in a pilosebaceous unit engaged in acne, has not been identified. Sebaceous glands from the scalp of acne patients are controlled by type I.[6,7] The future for new drugs of this type which are useful in acne is bright.

The isoenzyme involved in abnormal sebaceous glands will be clarified and one or more of various drug candidates are likely to prove safe and effective and expand our therapeutic menu of drugs.

## Comedogenesis

The hallmark preclinical lesion of acne vulgaris is the so-called microcomedo which is the earliest stage of comedogenesis.[21] This lesion may evolve into a clinically non-inflamed lesion, i.e. an open or closed comedo or into an inflammatory lesion if *P. acnes* proliferation and the generation of inflammatory mediators occur.[21] This process is the first clinical expression of acne and typically occurs in the midline, i.e. the central forehead, nose and chin, of youngsters who subsequently go on to develop more extensive acne.

In the microcomedo there is a distension of sebaceous follicles and the accumulation of large numbers of corneocytes which appear to be shed in layers which are tightly compacted. The keratin protein pattern in acne follicles to date has not shown any differences from normal epithelium and thus this abnormality should not be referred to as abnormal keratinization but rather as an abnormality in desquamation. One intriguing finding which may be crucial in the pathophysiology of comedogenesis is the finding of decreased or absent levels of linoleic acid in the sebum and comedones of acne patients.[22] Linoleic acid is an essential fatty acid and its role in normal epithelial differentiation and desquamation is well studied for the epidermis. Linoleic acid deficiency causes hyperkeratosis of the epidermis and a faulty epidermal barrier function. Hyperkeratosis is the hallmark of comedogenesis and a faulty barrier function would facilitate delivery of proinflammatory stimuli produced by *P. acnes* into the dermis.

# Topical tretinoin and isotretinoin

Tretinoin was the first retinoid developed for topical therapy in acne. The original formulation was a hydroalcoholic solution and irritant reactions were frequent.[23] Subsequently, cream and gel formulations were developed which were better tolerated and provided a flexibility in terms of vehicle and concentration in terms of irritancy responses of individuals. Tretinoin works by normalizing the desquamation process in both the microcomedo as well as mature comedones.[23] Its effect on the microcomedo makes the environment less favorable for *P. acnes* proliferation and also enhances the delivery of other agents, e.g. topical and systemic antibiotics.[24]

Recent advances in tretinoin have centered around strategies to reduce the irritant potential without sacrificing clinical benefit. Two formulations recently approved by the FDA minimize irritant potential. Tretinoin is formulated in porous microspheres called microsponges which deliver tretinoin to the skin such that the potential for irritation is greatly reduced. Studies in sensitive-skinned individuals such as those with an atopic background and/or a rosacea tendency have shown far less in the way of either clinical signs of irritation or injury to the stratum corneum barrier function. Clinical efficacy is comparable to similar concentrations of earlier formulations. Another new formulation which minimizes irritant potential is that in which tretinoin is complexed with a complex polymer which limits delivery to the epidermis but does not interfere with delivery into sebaceous follicles.

Topical isotretinoin is available in many countries as a 0.05% gel and has been shown to be effective in reducing both non-inflammatory and inflammatory lesions. This formulation is generally viewed as less irritating than tretinoin gel but no direct comparison studies exist for therapeutic efficacy.

# Adapalene and tazarotene

With the discovery that tretinoin bonds with specific nuclear receptors, the possibility of developing an in vitro screening method for therapeutically useful molecules became a reality. These receptors, so-called $\alpha$, $\beta$, $\gamma$ and $\chi$, result in complexes which then affect gene transcription.

Adapalene is a naphthoic acid derivative which is stable in light (tretinoin is unstable), lipophilic, binds to the β and γ receptors (tretinoin binds α, β and γ) and has retinoid effects in a variety of in vitro and animal models, and these properties are similar to those of tretinoin.[24] Clinical trials have shown that adapalene is comparable to tretinoin in terms of efficacy and somewhat less prone to irritant reactions.[25] In view of this molecule's success and the discovery of tazarotene as an effective agent for treating acne through the same process, it is likely that the future will bring newer drugs with retinoid benefits. The goal is to find more effective, less-irritating drugs.

Tazarotene is a novel synthetic acetylenic retinoid. Its acid metabolite, tazarotenic acid, binds to the β and γ retinoid receptors.[26] This agent has recently been approved by the FDA for the treatment of both psoriasis and acne. Its primary point of attack appears to be similar to that of other retinoids in that it helps to normalize follicular epithelial desquamation. Clinical trials have shown a dose response improvement in acne with significant reduction in comedonal and inflammatory lesions.

# P. acnes and antibiotic therapy

The inflammation of acne is the result of overgrowth of *P. acnes* in the environment of the microcomedo and production of inflammatory mediators. In the follicular epithelium of sebaceous follicles, collections of neutrophils and lymphocytes can be found in preinflammatory and early inflammatory lesions.[21] *P. acnes* secretes a variety of chemotactic factors as well as various proinflammatory cytokines including IL-1, TNF-α and IL-8.[27–31] Disruption of the integrity of the follicular wall leads to extravasation of follicular contents into the dermis which incites acute and chronic inflammatory responses.[21] An area which needs to be studied in depth is differences in host responses to these inflammatory stimuli. Differences in the intensity of inflammation must in part be due to host response variations.

Over the past 25 years, numerous developments in the therapeutic agents aimed at reducing *P. acnes* have developed. *P. acnes* is very sensitive to a wide range of antibiotics with the exception of mupirocin and aminoglycosides. The problem of antibiotic therapy has been one of delivery of antibiotics into the lipid-rich environment of sebaceous follicles. Current data on the in vivo effect of topical and systemic agents indicate that those agents that are more lipophilic have a greater effect in reducing *P. acnes* counts, suggesting that these agents partition more effectively into sebaceous follicles. Unfortunately, no techniques have been developed which can quantify in vivo concentrations of antibiotics in sebaceous follicles.

Table 3.2 summarizes our results of measuring in vivo effects of the various topical and systemic agents currently available in the US. Of the topical agents, benzoyl peroxide, and particularly benzoyl peroxide in combination with erythromycin or glycolic acid, is the most effective topical agent with clindamycin the next most effective agent. Azelaic acid and metronidazole have no in vivo effects and their antiacne effects are due to non-antibacterial effects. For systemic agents, minocycline is clearly the most effective agent with doxycycline (a lipophilic molecule) at 200 mg equivalent to 1 g of the less-lipophilic tetracycline hydrochloride. Trimethoprim-sulfamethoxazole is also a very effective agent but is used less frequently because of the risk of severe drug reactions. Urticarial and serum sickness reactions are uncommon but appear to be more common with minocycline.

In addition to suppressing the viability of P. acnes, antibiotics also exert so-called anti-inflammatory effects. These appear to be mainly the result of interference with the metabolic activities of P. acnes whereby the ability to generate proinflammatory molecules is curtailed. For example, concentrations of antibiotics that do not influence the growth curve characteristics of P. acnes can inhibit the production of chemotactic factors, lipase production and the responsiveness of neutrophils to chemistatic stimuli can be blunted.[32,33] These effects can occur without the death of P. acnes and account for why the clinical effect of antibiotic therapy is more than just a microbiological effect.

A relatively new issue with respect to antibiotic therapy is the emergence of less-sensitive or 'resistant' strains of P. acnes.[34-36] Our group and that in Leeds in the UK described the first strains of less-sensitive P. acnes in the early and mid 1980s. At that time, recovery of less-sensitive strains was uncommon and clinical relevance was even less common. By 1997, both groups were routinely recovering these strains from acne patients. In Leeds, 70% of patients have some strains resistant to at least one antibiotic with

### Table 3.2 P. acnes reduction (logarithm base 10) after 6 weeks of therapy

| Topical | | Systemic | |
|---|---|---|---|
| Benzoyl peroxide/erythromycin | 2.5 | Tetracycline HCl (1 g) | 0.5 |
| Benzoyl peroxide/glycolic acid | 2.3 | Doxycycline (200 mg) | 1.0 |
| Benzoyl peroxide | 2.1 | Minocycline (200 mg) | 2.3 |
| Clindamycin | 1.2 | Erythromycin (1 g) | 0.5 |
| Erythromycin | 0.5–0.75 | Trimethoprim (200 mg twice daily) | 0.5 |
| Azelaic acid | No reduction | Trimethoprim/sulfamethoxazole | 1.0 |
| Metronidazole | No reduction | (twice daily) | |

more strains resistant to erythromycin than to tetracycline, and now more strains less sensitive to minocycline are being recovered. These results are similar to ours and indicate a rapidly evolving problem which is now clearly at the point of clinical relevance and may lead to less and less clinical benefit for one of the mainstays of acne therapy. The genetic basis of erythromycin resistance in *P. acnes* has been shown to be the result of three specific point mutations in 23S rRNA which forms part of the antibiotic binding site in ribosomes.[37] An important question under study is how stable these mutations are and whether or not these strains remain on skin after removal of antibiotic pressure. For individuals with strains resistant to multiple antibiotics early studies indicate that oral isotretinoin therapy is

effective in both controlling acne and eradicating the resistant strains as a result of suppression of sebum.[38] The issue of *P. acnes* resistance is likely to become an increasingly important clinical issue in the coming years and strategies for optimal antibiotic usage will have to be developed.

## Summary

Basic information on the pathophysiology of acne has led to rational therapies. We now have a menu of topical and systemic agents which can be used to counter the pathophysiological events in acne.[39] These treatments are such that all forms of acne can now be successfully treated. There is no reason for the physical and emotional scarring of acne to occur (Table 3.3).

### Table 3.3 Therapeutic advances

|  | Sebum reduction | Follicular desquamation | P. acnes reduction | Combination drugs |
|---|---|---|---|---|
| Topical | None | Tretinoin Isotretinoin Adapalene Tazarotene | Erythromycin Clindamycin Benzoyl peroxide Nadifloxacin | Benzoyl peroxide/erythromycin Benzoyl peroxide/clindamycin Erythromycin/tretinoin Clindamycin/tretinoin Benzoyl peroxide/glycolic acid |
| Systemic | Estrogen Estrogen + steroids Spironolactone Cyproterone acetate Isotretinoin | Isotretinoin | | |

# References

1. Lucky AW, Biro FM, Huster GA et al, Acne vulgaris in premenarchal girls: an early sign of puberty associated with rising levels of dehydroepiandrosterone. *Arch Dermatol* 1994: 130; 308–14.

2. Stewart ME, Downing DT, Cook JS, Hansen JR, Sebaceous gland activity and sebum dehydroepiandrosterone sulfate levels in boys and girls. *Arch Dermatol* 1992: 128; 1345–8.

3. Lavker RM, Leyden JJ, Lamellar inclusions in follicular horny cells; a new aspect of abnormal keratinization. *J Ultrastruct Res* 1979: 69: 362–70.

4. Leyden JJ, McGinley KJ, Vowels B, *Propionibacterium acnes* colonization in acne and nonacne. *Dermatology* 1998: 196: 55–8.

5. Leyden JJ, McGinley KJ, Mills OJ Jr, Kligman AM, *Propionibacterium* levels in patients with and without acne vulgaris. *J Invest Dermatol* 1974: 62; 37–41.

6. Thiboutot DM, Harris G, Cimis V et al, Activity of type I 2-alpha-reductase exhibits regional differences in isolated sebaceous glands and whole skin. *J Invest Dermatol* 1995: 105; 209–14.

7. Thiboutot DM, Knaggs H, Gilliland K, Hagari S, Activity of type 1 5-alpha-reductase is greater in the follicular infrainfundibulum compared with the epidermis. *Br J Dermatol* 1997: 136; 166–71.

8. Pochi PE, Strauss JS, Sebaceous gland suppression with ethinyl estradiol and dehydroepiandrosterone. *Arch Dermatol* 1973: 108; 210–14.

9. Redmar GP, Olson WH, Lippman JS et al, Norgestimate and ethinyl estradiol in the treatment of acne vulgaris: a randomized placebo-controlled trial. *Obstet Gynecol* 1997: 89; 615–22.

10. Pochi PE, Strauss JS, Effects of prednisone on sebaceous gland secretion. *J Invest Dermatol* 1996: 49; 456–9.

11. Janaud A, Pouffy J, Upmalis D, Daine MA, A comparison study of lipid and androgen metabolism with triphasic oral contraceptive formulations containing norgestimate or levonorgestrel. *Acta Obstet Gynecol Scand Suppl* 1992: 156; 25–30.

12. Hammerstein J, Moltz L, Schwartz U, Antiandrogens in the treatment of acne and hirsutism. *J Steroid Biochem* 1983: 19; 591–7.

13. Lehucher-Ceyrac D, Weber-Buisset M-J, Saurat J-H, Réduction de l'excrétion sébacée et amélioration de l'acné chez des patientes traitées par l'association: acétate de cyprotérone-éthinyl oestradiol. *Ann Dermatol Venereol* 1981: 108; 861–8.

14. Goodfellow A, Alaghband-Zadeh J, Carter G et al, Oral spironolactone improves acne vulgaris and reduces sebum excretion. *Br J Dermatol* 1984: 111; 209–14.

15. Burke BM, Cunliffe WJ, Oral spironolactone therapy for female patients with acne, hirsutism or androgenic alopecia. *Br J Dermatol* 1985: 112; 124–5.

16. Peck GL, Olsen TG, Yoder FW, Prolonged remissions of cystic conglobate acne with 13-cis-retinoic acid. *N Engl J Med* 1979: 300; 329–33.

17. Strauss JS, Stranieri JS, Farrell LN, The effect of marked inhibition of sebum production with 13-cis-retinoic acid on skin surface lipid composition. *J Invest Dermatol* 1980: 74; 66–7.

18. King K, Jones DH, Daltry DC, Cuncliffe WJ, A double-blind study of the

effects of 13-cis-retinoic acid on acne, sebum excretion rate and microbial population. *Br J Dermatol* 1982: 107; 583–90.

19.  Leyden JJ, McGinley KJ, Qualitative and quantitative changes in cutaneous bacteria associated with systemic isotretinoin therapy for acne conglobata. *J Invest Dermatol* 1986: 86; 390–3.

20.  Lavker RM, Leyden JJ, Kligman AM, The anti-inflammatory activity of iso-tretinoin is a major factor in the clearing of acne conglobata. In: Marks R, Plewig G (eds) *Acne and related disorders*. London: Martin Dunitz, 1989, pp. 207–217.

21.  Cunliffe WJ, Norris JFB, Isotretinoin: an explanation for its long-term benefit. *Dermatologica* 1987: 175 (Suppl 1); 133.

22.  Downing DT, Stewart ME, Wertz PW, Strauss JS, Essential fatty acids and acne. *J Am Acad Dermatol* 1986: 14; 221–5.

23.  Kligman AM, Fulton JE Jr, Plewig G, Topical vitamin A acid in acne vulgaris. *Arch Dermatol* 1969: 99; 469–76.

24.  Leyden JJ, Marples RR, Mills OH, Kligman AM, Tretinoin and antibiotic therapy in acne vulgaris. *South Med J* 1974: 67; 20–5.

25.  Shroot B, Michel S, Pharmacology and chemistry of adapalene. *J Am Acad Dermatol* 1997: 36; 5 96–103.

26.  Nagpal S, Athanikar J, Chandraranta RAS, Separation of transactivation and AP1 antagonism functions of retinoic acid receptor alpha. *J Biol Chem* 1995: 270; 923–7.

27.  Webster GF, Leyden JJ, Characterization of serum-independent poly-morphonuclear leukocyte chemotactic factors produced by *Propionibacterium acnes*. *Inflammation* 1980: 4; 261–9.

28.  Puhvel SM, Sakamoto M, The chemoattractant properties of comedonal components. *J Invest Dermatol* 1978: 71; 324–9.

29.  Webster GF, Leyden JJ, Norman ME, Nilsson UR, Complement activation in acne vulgaris: in vitro studies with *Propionibacterium acnes* and *Propionibacterium granulosum*. *Infect Immun* 1978: 22; 523–9.

30.  Puhvel SM, Hoffman IK, Sternberg TH, Presence of complement fixing antibodies to *Corynebacterium acnes* in the sera of patients with acne vulgaris. *Arch Dermatol* 1966: 93; 364–6.

31.  Vowels BR, Yang S, Leyden JJ, Induction of proinflammatory cytokines by soluble factor of *Propionibacterium acnes*: implications for chronic inflammatory acne. *Infect Immun* 1995: 63; 3158–65.

32.  Webster GF, Leyden JJ, McGinley KJ, McArthur WP, Suppression of polymorphonuclear luekocyte chemotactic factor production in *Propionibacterium acnes* by subminimal inhibitory concentrations of tetracycline, ampicillin, minocycline and erythromycin. *Antimicrob Agents Chemother* 1982: 21; 770–2.

33.  Esterly NB, Koransky JS, Furey NL, Trevisan M, Neutrophil chemotaxis in patients with acne receiving oral tetracycline therapy. *Arch Dermatol* 1984: 120; 1308–13.

34.  Leyden JJ, McGinley KJ, Cavalieri S et al, *Propionibacterium acnes* resistant to antibiotics in acne patients. *J Am Acad Dermatol* 1983: 8; 41–5.

35.  Eady EA, Cove JH, Blake J et al, Recalcitrant acne vulgaris: clinical, biochemical and microbiological investigation of patients not responding to antibiotic treatment. *Br J Dermatol* 1988: 18; 415–23.

36.   Eady EA, Jones CE, Tipper JL et al, Antibiotic resistant propionibacteria in acne: need for policies to modify antibiotic usage. *BMJ* 1993: 306; 555–6.

37.   Ross JI, Eady EA, Cove JH et al, Resistance to erythromycin and clindamycin in cutaneous propionibacteria isolated from acne patients is associated with mutations in 23S rRNA. *Antimicrob Agents Chemother* 1997: 41; 1162–5.

38.   Coates P, Adams CA, Cunliffe WJ et al, Does oral isotretinoin prevent propionibacterium acnes? *Dermatology* 1997: 195(Suppl 1); 4–9.

39.   Leyden JJ, Therapy for acne vulgaris. *N Engl J Med* 1997: 336; 1156–62.

# 4

# Update on management of acne inversa

*René Chatelain, Birger Konz, Carla Hary and Gerd Plewig*

## Historical background

In 1907 Erich Hoffmann was the first to describe perifolliculitis capitis abscedens et suffodiens (dissecting cellulitis of the scalp), but he did not connect the disease with acne.[1] In 1951 Kierland wrote an important review on 'hidrosadenitis' suppurativa, acne conglobata and dissecting cellulitis of the scalp.[2] However, he concluded that the apocrine gland was at the origin of what he called unusual pyodermas. Pillsbury et al in 1956 then connected the three diseases into a new entity termed follicular occlusion triad,[3] recognizing that the underlying pathogenetic mechanism was follicular hyperkeratinization, as in acne vulgaris, leading to distension of the infundibulum, rupture of the follicle and secondary bacterial colonization.

However, the authors still believed that the consequent destruction of the tissue was due to involvement of the apocrine glands. In 1989 the pilonidal sinus was also added to the acne triad, creating the new entity of acne tetrad, now termed acne inversa.[4,5]

The defining features of acne inversa are: (1) occurrence in adults, not juveniles as in acne vulgaris; (2) the linkage of several follicles by secondary comedones with multiple openings; (3) communicating epithelium-lined channels (dissecting cellulitis) originating from abscesses; (4) draining sinuses in intertriginous, 'inversa' areas (groin, buttocks, perianal region, breast, axillae and even extremities); and (5) hypertrophic scars followed by contraction, particularly in the axillae and groins.

## Diagnosis and differential diagnosis of acne inversa

Acne inversa is not rare, but frequently misdiagnosed especially in mono- or oligosymptomatic patients who do not present with the full tetrad picture. However, the presence of one symptom of acne tetrad should lead to a search for lesions in other areas – the neck, the entire scalp, the axillae, the groin, the mammary folds, the genitalia, the perineum, the anal region and the buttocks. Most, but not all patients have a history of acne conglobata in typical areas. Affection of the scalp can lead to scarring alopecia. Intertriginous areas may display furunculoid nodules, abscesses, draining sinuses with discharge of fetid pus, extensive tissue destruction followed by hypertrophic and sometimes monstrous scars, leading to contractions in groin and axillae. The draining sinuses may dissect deeply into subcutaneous tissue, the fascia and muscles, which then can only be revealed by radiologic techniques or during surgery. In some patients elephantiasis nostras-like swellings of the genitalia may occur.[6] Secondary gram-positive and -negative bacterial infections aggravate and sustain the disease.

Typically the patients have been affected for many years or even decades and have undergone many different therapeutic attempts to cure this devastating disease. The patients are stricken by the discharge of foul pus, the often constant appearance of painful new abscesses and contractures. Often patients are overweight with consequent intertriginous hyperhidrosis, which is an aggravating factor for the disease. In some patients abnormal sex hormone levels have been found, but the relevance of these alterations has not been clear even after multiple studies (for review see reference 7).

Due to odd variants of the disease even for dermatologists the diagnosis of acne inversa in some cases presents a challenge. Sometimes only one area is unilaterally affected. Secondary elephantiasis nostras following streptococcal infection leading to enlargement and distortion of genitalia is difficult to connect with acne inversa as the underlying cause. Axillary furuncles and

carbuncles are commonly misdiagnosed; the same occurs with perianal abscesses and rectal fistula (enteritis regionalis, ileitis terminalis Crohn), actinomycosis, tuberculosis, malignant tumors, pyoderma vegetans and in rare cases lymphogranuloma inguinale or granuloma venereum. On the scalp one has to consider gram-negative folliculitis and deep trichophytosis.

The outcome of this chronic nonselfhealing disease might lead not only to psychosocial problems and depression in patients with acne inversa but also in rare cases to squamous cell carcinoma (Marjolin ulcer), bacterial meningitis and even systemic amyloidosis (for review see references 5, 8 and 9).

## Genetics, histopathology and laboratory findings

As in acne vulgaris, in which a genetic predisposition for seborrhea is well established, in acne inversa a genetic predisposition is also of importance but less well documented, but familial occurrence has been reported.[6,10]

Acne inversa is, like acne vulgaris, a disease originating in the sebaceous follicles. In acne inversa the non-facial, intertriginous terminal follicles with pigmented, coarse hairs, often associated with apocrine sweat glands, the so-called apocrine-pilosebaceous units, are affected, leading to a secondary necrotizing process of the apocrine glands.[11] The earliest event is hyperkeratosis of the infundibulum, resulting in comedo-like horny impactions, followed by rupture of the follicle and deposition of foreign-body material (corneocytes, bacteria, hairs and sebum) in the connective tissue.[12] An inflammatory tissue reaction follows, first attracting granulocytes and mononuclear cells followed finally by granuloma formation. The reason for follicle rupture is not well understood, but friction in the intertriginous areas might be a cause. Epithelial tissue is then observed trying to encapsulate the granulomas leading eventually to epithelium-lined ducts. Secondary bacterial colonization, most often *Staphylococcus aureus*, streptococci, *Proteus mirabilis* and other gram-negative bacteria[13] intensifies the inflammatory process, leading to abscesses reaching the subcutaneous fat (septal and lobular panniculitis), destroying apocrine and eccrine sweat glands followed by pus-draining sinuses which find their way to the skin surface or through fascia into muscles (Figs 4.1 and 4.2). This chronic inflammatory

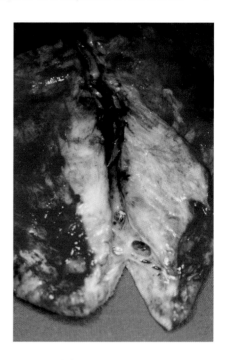

## Figure 4.1

Excised tissue with deep penetrating draining sinus.

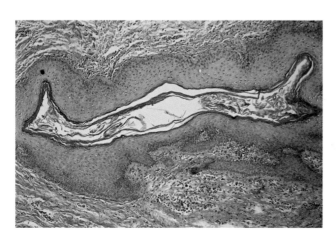

## Figure 4.2

Histologic section of acne inversa showing inflammatory infiltrate and epithelium-lined draining sinus.

tissue damage causes hypertrophic scars which might then result in contractures in axillae and groin. It is the deep penetrating, eventually epithelial-lined draining sinuses which make acne inversa such a chronic disabling disease.

Abnormal laboratory findings in patients with acne inversa all result from the chronic inflammatory process, and thus are secondary and not primary causes of the disease (elevated sedimentation rate, leukocytosis, low serum iron, abnormal serum electrophoresis). In a few patients congenital $a_1$-antitrypsin deficiency has been described, but is not found in the majority of patients.[14]

## Treatment

In contrast to acne vulgaris, which almost always heals spontaneously in early adulthood, acne inversa is a chronic, non-selfhealing disease. A wide variety of different therapeutic strategies has been tried in acne inversa, but none of them is effective, even the recently introduced isotretinoin, except extensive surgical procedures. Therefore patients, who have often had a history of many years of frustrating attempts at treatment including multiple 'abscess' incisions, have to be informed early on about surgical measures to be taken possibly at the earliest recognized stage and the uselessness of waiting. All other measures such as antibiotics or isotretinoin are just complementary.

## Diet

The rate of sebum production, keratinization in the follicles and the inflammatory processes are in general not influenced by diet. However, some patients report aggravation by various foods or alcohol, and this should be taken into consideration. Iodides and bromides are known to aggravate inflammatory processes and should therefore be avoided. Smoking is sometimes discussed as another causative factor. There is no evidence for this aside from the well-known hazards of smoking.

## Psychological advice

Acne inversa patients suffer tremendously from their chronic disease which may cause depression, social deprivation, unemployment or difficulties in sexual relationships. It may alter the personality of the patient permanently so that they suffer from psychologic disability even after successful surgical treatment. On the other hand, necessary extensive surgery especially to the genitalia and to women's mammary areas might itself lead to cosmetically unfavorable permanent results, which also require psychological help.

## Local treatment

*Cleaning and antiseborrheic measures:* although the sebum that has left the follicles and remains on the skin surface has no further effect on the course of acne, cleaning and degreasing of the skin has a complementary effect. For this purpose detergents, alcoholic solutions (ethanol 50%, isopropanol 20–40%) or grease-absorbing paper towels can be used several times daily. Alcoholic solutions might also help to keep hyperhidrous intertriginous areas dry.

*Comedolytic:* as in acne vulgaris, the earliest event in acne inversa is the retention hyperkeratosis of the infundibula of sebaceous follicles, leading to comedo formation. However, once the inflammatory processes have started leading to deep penetrating subcutaneous draining sinuses comedolytic therapy with, for example, topical tretinoin, benzoyl peroxide or UV irradiation, is of no further help.

*Antimicrobial:* topical application of antibiotics (erythromycin, clindamycin, tetracycline) is not recommended in acne inversa. Hexachlorophene or polyvinylpyrrolidone lavages or sitz baths, however, are appreciated by patients to wash off fetid pus and detritus.

*Anti-inflammatory:* as mentioned for topical antibiotics, locally applied anti-inflammatory lotions, emulsions or UV radiation have no beneficial effect in acne inversa.

*Epilation:* epilation does not prevent the inflammatory processes leading to deep penetrating sinuses and might only be of some benefit in early superficial lesions.[15]

*Radiation therapy:* nowadays anti-inflammatory radiation therapy is, due to possible severe long-term side-effects, no longer used.

## Systemic treatment

*Estrogens and antiandrogens:* for women with acne vulgaris, contraceptives containing estrogens, chlormadinone acetonate (Eunomin) or cyproterone acetate (Dianette) are recommended due to their antiseborrheic, anticomedogenic and anti-inflammatory effect on papules and pustules. Female patients with acne inversa might therefore also profit from these agents, but cure of the disease is not seen.[16,17]

*Antibiotics:* antibiotics should if possible be given according to the sensitivities, as gram-negative bacterial colonization is frequent and erythromycin or tetracycline, which are frequently used in acne vulgaris, are not effective. Third generation cephalosporins or gyrase inhibitors should be used.

*Sulfones:* we have used diaminodiphenylsulfone (dapsone) in acne inversa ourselves, but have found no long lasting effect.

*Corticosteroids:* intralesional injections of triamcinolone acetonide suspension may improve smaller inflammatory nodules as in acne conglobata. Systemic corticosteroids, usually 1 mg prednisolone/kg body weight per day for 1 or 2 weeks, is sometimes helpful when there is progressive inflammation.

*Isotretinoin:* isotretinoin has recently been introduced into acne inversa therapy. This drug has provided good anti-inflammatory effects and reduces suppuration, edema and the volume of sebaceous glands. However, by itself it is also not curative and the disease relapses after discontinuing treatment.

As mentioned previously, all the above therapeutic agents have proven unsuccessful in healing acne inversa. In milder cases, however, some of the treatments lead to significant improvement in the disease (for review see references 5, 8, 18 and 19).

## Surgery

The surgical approach is the only method for obtaining definitive cure of acne inversa. Surgery should be performed at the earliest possible stage of the disease. Deep and wide excisions far beyond clinical borders have to be performed regardless of the localization. This procedure not only requires a determined dermato-surgeon, but also a determined and well-informed patient. In some cases stepwise surgery in multiple areas is necessary resulting in long stays in hospital. For preoperative treatment antibiotics are used according to the sensitivities. Additionally, especially in extensively suppurative, inflammatory and edematous cases, we see advantages in pretreating the patients with isotretinoin for several months in order to 'dry up' the intertriginous areas and facilitate surgical excision. In highly

inflammatory lesions a pretreatment with corticosteroids (usually 1.0 mg prednisolone/kg body weight per day) for several weeks, might also be recommended. It should be mentioned that both isotretinoin and corticosteroids should be discontinued before surgery to prevent postoperative wound healing problems. In patients treated with both isotretinoin and antibiotics the possibility of pseudotumor cerebri should be taken into consideration.

Smaller superficial lesions can eventually be excised or vaporized with a $CO_2$ laser. However, this procedure is not suited for deep penetrating lesions, which sometimes are recognized only intraoperatively.[20,21] Coagulation by the laser reduces intraoperative bleeding, and the resulting wounds are generally allowed to granulate with secondary reepithelialization.

Surgical procedures depend on the extent of the lesions:

1. Simple incisions are not recommended, as these carry an almost 100% rate of recurrence.
2. Excision with primary suture, including rotation flaps or muscle flaps, is possible in smaller lesions (Figs 4.3 and 4.4). The advantage lies in the one-step surgery, and functionally and cosmetically good results. However, a higher recurrence rate is usually seen often due to insufficient area excised.[22]
3. Excision with allowance for granulation and secondary reepithelialization is suited for all types of lesions. Very often one obtains good

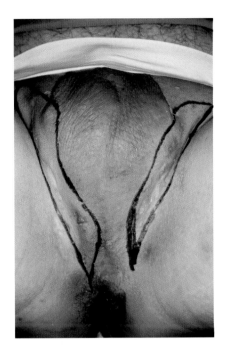

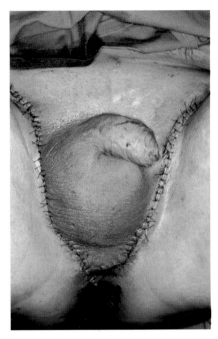

Figure 4.3

Bilateral inguinal acne inversa in a 36-year-old man. Preoperative site showing multiple furunculoid nodules and draining sinuses with purulent discharge. Marking of excision area.

Figure 4.4

Postoperative site after primary suturing.

functional and cosmetic results. Patients however are disabled by the long duration of wound healing and reepithelialization.

4. The best results are obtained by excision, temporary granulation and free grafting (split or mesh graft). This approach provides the best functional and cosmetic results in extensive lesions, but a two-step operation and long intervals between the procedures to allow for granulation of the often very deep wounds are necessary (Figs 4.5 to 4.7). For large free grafts, tissue adhesives are recommended.[23]

5. Excision and primary free grafting in a one-step procedure for extensive lesions is the most frequently used and easiest procedure. Functional and cosmetic results are good in more superficial lesions.

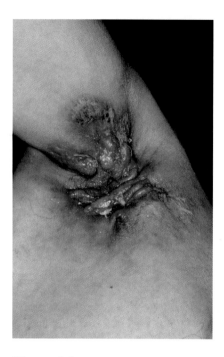

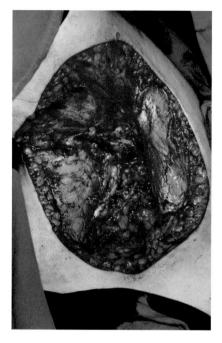

## Figure 4.5

Acne inversa of right axilla in a 40-year-old man with multiple furunculoid nodules, abscesses, draining sinuses with discharge of fetid pus, extensive tissue destruction followed by hypertrophic scarring leading to contraction.

## Figure 4.6

Deep postoperative excision site after removal of the subcutaneous fat, reaching the pectoralis major muscle. The wound was allowed a 2-week period for granulation prior to mesh grafting.

For review of surgical procedures in acne inversa see references 23–31. Even in sufficiently wide and deep excisions local recurrence rates range, depending on the anatomical site, from 5 to 50%.[24,25]

We have recently reviewed 177 patients with acne inversa, who had been treated by surgery at 322 different anatomical sites during the period of 1975–1995 in the Department of Dermatology, University of Munich.[31] Of the 177 patients 57% were men, 43% women. This frequency distribution of acne inversa between male and female patients does not reflect observations made by other authors who have reported a far higher incidence of acne inversa in women (79.2% and 91.7%).[27,28] The axillary region was

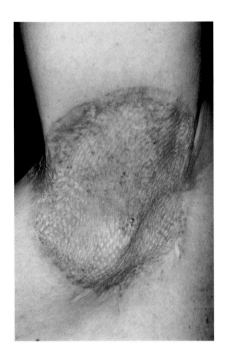

## Figure 4.7

Postoperative result 1 year after mesh grafting.

saw fewer postoperative complications (7.1% and 5.3%, respectively). As not all patients had been interviewed at the time of writing we cannot report on recurrence rates.

## Conclusion

Acne inversa is a chronic, often devastating and disabling disease, which leads to severe physical and psychological problems for the affected patients. Very often these patients undergo years or even decades of frustrating local or systemic treatments, not leading to a definitive cure, as the disease is misdiagnosed in many cases. Knowledge of the clinical picture of acne inversa especially in monosymptomatic cases leading to early diagnosis and transfer of the patient to a dermatosurgery unit at the earliest possible stage of the disease are important in obtaining a final cure of the disease.

affected in 51.2%, the genito-inguinal region was affected in 41.6%. We performed surgery with primary suture in 193 patients (60%) and free grafting, in most cases after secondary granulation, in 129 patients (40%). Postoperative complications after primary suture were similar in the axilla and the genitoinguinal region (18% and 17%, respectively), after free grafting we

## References

1. Hoffmann E, Perifolliculitis capitis abscedens et suffodiens, Sitzungsbericht. Berliner Dermatologische Gesellschaft. Sitzung am 12. November 1907. *Dermatol Z* 1908: 15; 120–35.

2. Kierland RR, Unusual pyodermas (Hidrosadenitis suppurativa, acne conglobata, dissecting cellulitis of the scalp). A review. *Minn Med* 1951: 34; 319–41.

3. Pillsbury DM, Shelley WB, Kligman AM, Bacterial infections of the skin. In: *Dermatology, 1st edn.* Philadelphia: Saunders, 1956, pp. 482–4.

4. Plewig G, Steger M, Acne inversa (alias acne triad, acne tetrad or hidradenitis suppurativa). In: Marks R, Plewig G (eds) *Acne and related disorders*. London: Martin Dunitz, 1989, pp. 345–57.

5. Jansen T, Plewig G, Acne inversa. *Int J Dermatol* 1998: 37; 96–100.

6. Fitzsimmons JS, Guilbert PR, Fitzsimmons EM, Evidence of genetic factors in hidradenitis suppurativa. *Br J Dermatol* 1985: 113; 1–8.

7. Harrison BJ, Hughes LE, Characterization of the endocrine "lesion" in hidradenitis suppurativa, In: Marks R, Plewig G (eds) *Acne and related disorders*. London: Martin Dunitz, 1989, pp. 361–3.

8. Plewig G, Kligman AM, *Acne and rosacea, 3rd edn*. Berlin: Springer, 2000, pp. 309–41.

9. Mendoca H, Rebelo C, Fernandes A et al, Squamous cell carcinoma arising in hidradenitis suppurativa. *J Dermatol Surg Oncol* 1991: 17; 830–2.

10. Fitzsimmons JS, Fitzsimmons EM, Gilbert G, Familial hidradenitis suppurativa. *J Med Gen* 1984: 21; 281–5.

11. Yu CCW, Cook MG, Hidradenitis suppurativa: a disease of follicular epithelium, rather than apocrine glands. *Br J Dermatol* 1990: 122; 763–9.

12. Plewig G, Die sogenannten rezidivierenden Schweißdrüsenabszesse und ihre chirurgische Behandlung. In: Schweiberer L (ed) Chirurgische und Plastisch-chirurgische Aspekte bei Infektionen und infizierten Defekten der Körperoberfläche, der Extremitäten und der Analregion, München: Zuckschwerdt, 1982, pp. 17–25.

13. Highet AS, Warren RE, Weekes AJ, Bacteriology and antibiotic treatment of perianal suppurative hidradenitis. *Arch Dermatol* 1988: 124; 1047–51.

14. Eberle F, Adler G, Roth SL, Pyoderma fistulans sinifica und kongenitaler Alpha-1-Antitrypsinmangel. *Hautarzt* 1980: 31; 100–4.

15. Morgan WP, Leicester G, The role of depilation and deodorants in hidradenitis suppurativa. *Arch Dermatol* 1982: 118; 101–2.

16. Mortimer PS, Dawber RPR, Gales MA, Moore MA, A double-blind controlled crossover trial of cyproterone acetate in females with hidradenitis suppurativa. *Br J Dermatol* 1986: 115; 263–8.

17. Sawers RS, Randall VA, Ebling FJG, Control of hidradenitis suppurativa in women using combined antiandrogen (cyproterone acetate) and oestrogen therapy. *Br J Dermatol* 1986: 115; 269–74.

18. Rödder-Wehrmann O, Küster W, Plewig G, Acne inversa – Diagnose und Therapie. *Hautarzt* 1991: 42; 5–8.

19. Chatelain R, Hary C, Konz B, Plewig G, Acne Inversa. In: Katsambas AD, Lotti TM (eds) *European handbook of dermatological treatments*. Berlin, Heidelberg: Springer, 1999, pp. 11–14.

20. Sherman AI, Reid R, $CO_2$ laser for suppurative hidradenitis of the vulva. *J Reprod Med* 1991: 36; 113–17.

21. Lapins J, Marcussen JA, Emtestam L, Surgical treatment of chronic hidradenitis suppurativa: $CO_2$ laser stripping – secondary intention technique. *Br J Dermatol* 1994: 131; 551–6.

22. Harrison BJ, Mudge M, Hughes LE, Recurrence after surgical treatment of hidradenitis suppurativa. *BMJ* 1987: 294; 487–9.

23. Grösser A, Surgical treatment of chronic axillary and genitocrural acne conglobata by split-thickness skin grafting. *J Dermatol Surg Oncol* 1982: 8; 391–7.

24. Harrison BJ, Mudge M, Hughes LE, Recurrence after surgical treatment of hidradenitis suppurativa. *BMJ* 1987: 294; 487–9.

25. Hughes LE, Harrison BJ, Mudge M, Surgical management of hidradenitis – principles and results. In: Marks R, Plewig G (eds) *Acne and related disorders*. London: Martin Dunitz, 1989, pp. 367–70.

26. Banerjee AK, Surgical treatment of hidradenitis suppurativa. *Br J Surg* 1992: 79; 863–6.

27. Jemec GBE, Effect of localized surgical excision in hidradenitis suppurativa. *J Am Acad Dermatol* 1988: 18; 1103–7.

28. Watson JD, Hidradenitis suppurativa – a clinical review. *Br J Plast Surg* 1985: 38; 567–9.

29. Greeley PW, Plastic surgical treatment of chronic suppurative hidradenitis. *Plast Reconstr Surg* 1951: 7143–6.

30. Bennett RG, Treatment of hidradenitis suppurativa. In: Bennet RG (ed) *Fundamentals of cutaneous surgery*. Washington: Mosby, 1987, pp. 607–14.

31. Konz B, Chatelain R, Heckmann M, Therapie der Acne inversa. In: Dummer R, Panizzon R, Burg G (eds) Fortschritte der Operativen und Onkologischen Dermatologie, Band 11, Operative und Konservative Dermatoonkologie. Berlin, Wien: Blackwell, 1996, pp. 88–97.

# 5

# Update on drugs used in the treatment of psoriasis

*Kristen M Kelly and*
*Gerald D Weinstein*

## Introduction

Psoriasis is a chronic inflammatory skin disorder with intermittent flares and clearing that affects about 2% of the population. Psoriasis is an uncomfortable and occasionally disabling disease, with a social and economic impact that is often underestimated by medical personnel.

Psoriasis has several clinical phenotypes including guttate, pustular, and arthritic variants. This review focuses mainly on the most common form, chronic plaque psoriasis.

## Clinical manifestations and history

Psoriasis can start at any time, but there are two main peaks of onset: young adults (16–22 years of age) and middle-aged adults (50–60 years of age).[1] Clinically the lesions are well demarcated with circumscribed, variably thickened, scaly plaques typically found on the elbows, knees, scalp, and sites of local trauma (Koebner's phenomenon). Relapses are common, and the frequency and severity of these episodes can be affected by exposure to exacerbating factors such as cold weather, dry humidity, infection and some drugs.

Heredity is an important factor in this disease and is probably polygenic. A study of several kindreds showed linkage to a gene localized to the distal end of chromosome 17q, but the biological effects of this gene remain to be elucidated.[2] The extent to which genetic and epigenetic factors are important is not yet understood.

## Pathophysiological features

The characteristic histological features of psoriasis are hyperproliferation of the epidermis and the presence of inflammatory cells in the epidermis and dermis. In the psoriatic epidermis, the proliferative activity of keratinocytes is increased and the migration period of keratinocytes from the basal layer to the epidermal surface as well as the duration of the cell cycle is shortened.[3]

T-cell-produced cytokines are believed to be the inducing factors for the epidermal cell abnormalities in psoriasis.[4] Evidence for this is suggested by the therapeutic effectiveness of cyclosporin and the predominance of

CD4 lymphocytes in the dermis and CD8 cells in the epidermis of affected patients. It is not yet clear whether persistent T-cell activation is stimulated by a microbial antigen or an autoimmune process.[5]

## Treatment

Psoriasis has no cure, only therapies that may clear lesions for variable periods of time. Many patients prefer treatment only with emollients and the avoidance of provoking factors. Local symptoms (pain, itching, or the reduction of manual dexterity due to hand involvement) or cosmetic concerns (prominent hand, leg or facial lesions) may lead the patient to seek therapy. The purpose of treatment is to minimize the severity of psoriasis so that it no longer interferes substantially with the patient's life. We encourage patients to accept some limited disease to minimize adverse effects from overly aggressive treatment.

## Topical treatment

The initial treatment for limited psoriasis (less than 15–20% of the body surface affected) should be topical. The recognized methods of topical treatment are shown in Table 5.1.

## Emollients

Emollients may provide a weak but active treatment for psoriasis. These

**Table 5.1 Topical therapy for chronic plaque psoriasis**

Emollients
Keratolytic agents
Coal tar
Anthralin
Corticosteroids
Calcipotriene (calcipotriol)
Tazarotene

agents hydrate the hyperkeratotic surface of psoriatic plaques and may reverse the inflammatory consequences of a damaged stratum corneum. The most effective emollients such as petrolatum or aquaphor cream are greasy and sometimes disliked by patients.

## Keratolytic agents

Keratolytic agents such as 2–10% salicylic acid may be used either alone or in combination with topical corticosteroids or coal tar. They soften the scale of psoriatic plaques facilitating their removal and increase the efficacy of combination treatments. Side-effects of salicylic acid include eye and skin irritation. No studies have documented the efficacy of keratolytics as single treatment agents for psoriasis and at best they are adjunctive forms of therapy.

## Coal tar

Coal tar preparations infrequently clear psoriatic plaques when used alone. They are effective when used in combination with ultraviolet (UV) B phototherapy and their addition to shampoo preparations helps diminish psoriatic scaling of the scalp. Coal tar can cause an acneiform eruption or skin irritation and rarely, skin cancer induction has been reported.

## Anthralin

Anthralin is used widely throughout Europe but only occasionally in the US. The Ingram regimen incorporates the 24-hour application of an anthralin paste, a daily coal tar bath and UVB phototherapy. The value of anthralin use remains to be proven as studies have shown that coal tar-UVB and coal tar-UVB-anthralin regimens are similar in terms of treatment speed, efficacy and cost.[6]

Anthralin irritates perilesional skin through the formation of free radicals and it is oxidized to colored products that may stain skin and fabrics. These side-effects can be limited by incorporating free-radical scavengers and antioxidants into the preparations.[7]

The current preferred method of anthralin use is a short-contact regimen in which anthralin is applied for 0.5 to 1 hour before removal. This allows penetration of only lesional skin,[8] limiting side-effects while maintaining efficacy. This is a moderately effective treatment but not as good as potent topical corticosteroids. When effective, anthralin may provide a longer disease-free period than topical steroids.

## Corticosteroids

Topical corticosteroids are easy to use and have short-term efficacy. The more potent topical corticosteroids are consistently effective and are the initial choice of therapy by two-thirds of dermatologists in the United States.[9]

The many available corticosteroids differ in efficacy and are ranked by a potency class system. Once-daily topical corticosteroid use may be as effective as traditional twice-daily treatment with fewer side-effects.

Short term use provides minimal risk but prolonged therapy may result in thinning and pigmentary change of the skin, striae, and tachyphylaxis (tolerance to the action of the treatment). By 3–6 months after steroid-induced clearing, 50% or more of patients have relapsed with or without continuing use of steroids.[9] Steroids may also render the psoriasis unstable and occasionally a severe pustular variant may result. Topical corticosteroid efficacy can be improved by occlusion under a plastic film, but this increases the risk of side-effects. Pituitary–adrenal suppression can be induced in adults with daily use of 30 g or more of 0.025% betamethasone valerate cream under occlusion[10] and in infants even 1% hydrocortisone cream may result in a similar effect.[11]

## Calcipotriene

Calcipotriene (in some countries, calcipotriol) is a topically applied vitamin D derivative. Studies have shown that the efficacy of calcipotriene ointment is similar to that of a mid-potency topical steroid, 0.1% betamethasone valerate.[12] Long-term continuous therapy with calcipotriene for up to 12 months has been shown to result in consistent improvement.[13] This ointment causes appreciable irritation in some patients, especially on the face or genital area.

## Topical retinoids

Recent research has show that a unique retinoid molecule, tazarotene, can work topically with an acceptable minimal toxicity. Tazarotene used as a 0.05% or 0.1% gel can produce 50–100% improvement in approximately 70% of patients.[14,15] Burning, irritation and redness occur in 10–20% of patients but can be mitigated by emollients or topical steroids. Adjunctive use with mid- or high-potency steroids or calcipotriene may enhance the efficacy of tazarotene treatment.[16] There are reports of a treatment response remaining up to 3 months after active treatment with tazarotene has been discontinued.[17] The drug was approved in the US and many European countries in 1997–1998.

# Phototherapy and systemic treatments for moderate to severe psoriasis

Indications for more aggressive treatment include the involvement of large areas (more than 20% of the body surface) where topical treatment is impractical, a poor response to topical therapy, or psoriasis that is psychologically limiting or occupationally disabling. The choices are phototherapy, systemic drug therapy or a combination of these modalities (Table 5.2). All these modalities have potential toxicity, and the benefit/risk ratio of each must be periodically evaluated to avoid excessive toxicity.

## Phototherapy (UVB radiation)

UVB radiation utilizes wavelengths of 280 to 320 nm and, in combination with coal tar preparations (the Goeckerman regimen), is the safest option for

---

**Table 5.2 Phototherapy and systemic therapies for moderate to severe psoriasis**

Phototherapy (UVB +/– Tar)
Photochemotherapy (PUVA)
Methotrexate
Retinoids
Cyclosporin

people with moderate-to-severe disease as the risks are limited to a very small increase in skin cancer induction.

Crude coal tar 1% in a hydrophilic ointment is applied for 2–10 hours then washed off prior to UVB treatments which are given up to two times each day. If the tar is not washed off, it can act as a UVB blocker. This treatment leads to substantial improvement in psoriasis in at least 80% of patients.[18] Approximately 30 treatments are needed to obtain a reasonable response. Intensive treatment with UVB phototherapy and coal tar in an inpatient setting is rapidly effective within 2 to 3 weeks. Remission can be maintained by intermittent UVB phototherapy. Outpatient treatment is also effective although generally less rapid. UVB phototherapy without coal tar is used regularly only in patients with guttate psoriasis but in this situation it can achieve a rapid response.

Recently, several UVB phototherapy variations have been studied including narrow-band UVB (311 nm)[19] and individual psoriasis plaque irradiation with a 308 nm excimer laser.[20] It has been proposed that these modifications may make this modality even safer by limiting UV exposure. However, the efficacy of these modalities remains to be proven.

## Photochemotherapy (PUVA)

The second form of UV therapy, photochemotherapy, combines methoxsalen, a photosensitizing drug, with UVA phototherapy in the range of 320–400 nm.[21] Methoxsalen is administered 1–2 hours prior to light exposure in a dosage of 0.4–0.6 mg/kg body weight. The dosage of UVA is determined by the patient's skin type. Peak erythema occurs at approximately 48 hours post-treatment and thus treatments may be repeated up to two or three times weekly (more frequent treatments would increase the risk of burning). The mechanisms of action of PUVA have not been definitively elucidated but theories include: (a) a suppressive action on cell-mediated immune responses in the skin and (b) the intercalation of methoxsalen into DNA, resulting in crosslinks that interfere with DNA synthesis and block cell proliferation.[21,22]

PUVA is a highly effective treatment, which provides resolution of skin lesions after 20 to 30 treatments in over 85% of patients.[19,23] Maintenance can often be achieved with treatment as little as once every 2 to 4 weeks, which can be tapered to eventual discontinuation of treatment. The duration of remission ranges from 6 to 12 months. Topical or bath applications of methoxsalen have been utilized, but there is an increased risk of skin burning.

PUVA patients may report nausea, burning, and pruritus. Long-term risks include an increase in skin cancer and photodamage. The frequency of squamous cell carcinomas of the skin is increased in PUVA patients, most significantly after 160 treatments. There is an increased risk of genital cancer if this area is not shielded. A small incidence of melanomas was found in a population of patients treated with PUVA for over 20 years.[24] This finding raises a concern about the amount of PUVA patients can safely receive and the importance of following these patients carefully. Benign and premalignant keratoses, irregular pigmentation and wrinkling can also be induced with intensive PUVA therapy.

If treatment is limited to less than 160 treatments, the risk of skin cancer or photodamage is limited and the therapeutic index of this treatment is high.[25] PUVA can be combined with an oral retinoid to minimize radiation exposure but it is uncertain whether this decreases the incidence of photodamage or skin cancers.

## Methotrexate

Methotrexate is a folic acid antagonist and the gold standard for effective therapy of patients with moderate-to-severe psoriasis. Methotrexate may be the next choice in severe psoriatics if phototherapy or PUVA is discontinued because of long-term usage, intolerable side-effects, a limited response or inconvenience. Methotrexate blocks DNA synthesis resulting in the inhibition of cell proliferation in rapidly dividing tissues such as the hyperproliferative psoriatic epidermis and normal gastrointestinal and germinative epithelium.[26] It is also thought to have an immunosuppressive effect on mononuclear cells in the skin, blood, and lymphatic tissues.[27]

Methotrexate is most commonly administered orally in three doses (usually 2.5 to 5 mg each) at 12-hour intervals.[28] This regimen is repeated once weekly and can inhibit the replication of hyperproliferative cells with minimal side-effects. This dosing regimen is preferred by 70% of dermatologists.[29] An alternative is an oral or parenteral dose of methotrexate given once weekly. For this regimen, the usual dosage in a 70 kg adult is 10 to 25 mg/week.

The guidelines for methotrexate use were updated in 1998.[30] Patients must have normal renal function, blood cell counts, and liver function. Since 85% of methotrexate is excreted through the kidneys, patients with poor renal function may have sustained increases in plasma drug concentrations resulting in side-effects similar to a drug overdose, including cutaneous or gastrointestinal erosions and leukopenia.

The development of hepatic fibrosis or cirrhosis is the major long-term side-effect of methotrexate and thus this medication should not be used in patients with a history of abnormal liver function or excessive alcohol intake. In studies of psoriatic patients with a cumulative methotrexate dose of 1.5 g or less, approximately 3% develop cirrhosis. The proportion increases to 20 to 25% among patients who have received 4 g or more of methotrexate.[30] We believe that methotrexate-related liver disease occurs less frequently than previously reported, possibly because of improved patient selection and the use of rotation of additional therapies for extensive psoriasis.

Standard tests of liver function and imaging procedures do not reliably identify cirrhosis. However, liver function tests should be done initially and at intervals of 2–3 months, as they are relatively inexpensive and may be helpful. The 1998 methotrexate guidelines[30] recommend that if there are no hepatic risk factors prior to therapy, a liver biopsy should be performed indefinitely after each 1.5 g of cumulative drug use. If liver risk factors are present when starting therapy, a liver biopsy should be done at or soon after the start of therapy. If fibrosis is found, the drug should be stopped even though methotrexate-related cirrhosis is of low aggressiveness and may not progress with continued treatment.[31] The drug can be re-started in the future with careful observation. Drug dosage should be constantly titrated so that the smallest effective amount is used, and the goal of improvement should not be complete clearance of skin lesions as this may require aggressive and thus, risky dosing.

## Retinoids

Retinoids alone have limited effectiveness in psoriatic patients except in specialized cases. Only half of patients with extensive plaque psoriasis will achieve a 75% reduction in skin lesional area with the use of retinoids.[32] Acitretin, which recently replaced the almost identical etretinate, is most useful in patients with erythrodermic and acral localized psoriasis and in HIV-positive patients in whom UV therapy may increase T-cell suppression or virus activation. For generalized pustular psoriasis, both acitretin and isotretinoin (a better choice in women with child-bearing potential because of a shorter half-life) can produce rapid improvement and are extremely valuable treatment options.[33]

The mechanism for psoriatic improvement with retinoids may derive from their ability to stimulate epithelial differentiation. Retinoids activate and repress genomic function resulting in altered protein expression, which in turn affects clinical disease. Further, they replete the diminished number of Langerhans cells in psoriatic lesions and increase delayed hypersensitivity.

Acitretin should be started at a low dose (i.e. 0.3 to 0.4 mg/kg per day) to minimize flares and side-effects.[34] If required, this can be gradually increased. Acitretin therapy may be associated with many side-effects including skin dryness and erythema. Liver function tests and triglyceride levels may become elevated with treatment and thus should be checked prior to therapy and then at intervals of 1–2 months.

Because these drugs are teratogenic, pregnancy must be avoided during treatment and for at least 3 years following cessation of treatment. Acitretin is a clinically active metabolite of etretinate and in combination with alcohol, is converted back to etretinate which has a longer elimination half-life[35] and prolonged teratogenic potential. Thus, alcohol must not be consumed by patients on acitretin during treatment or for 2 months following discontinuation of treatment.

After 1 to 2 years of systemic retinoid therapy in high dosage, skeletal abnormalities, including ligamentous ossification and periosteal new bone formation, may occur in some patients.[36] Acitretin can be combined with PUVA to limit the dosage and thus the side-effects of both these therapeutic options.

## Cyclosporin

Cyclosporin is a relatively new treatment for extensive psoriasis and may be used in patients refractory to all other treatments.[37] Cyclosporin blocks production of a calcineurin-dependent factor essential for transcription of the interleukin-2 gene which in turn blocks the proliferation of activated T-cells and the production of their cytokines[38,39] thought to induce the psoriatic phenotype.

About 90% of patients respond to low doses of cyclosporin (Sandimmune or Neoral, 2 to 5 mg/kg per day, depending on which preparation is used) within 1 to 3 months. Once optimal improvement is reached, maintenance therapy is usually required although lower doses may be utilized.[40] It is recommended that cyclosporin should be given for no more than 1 year. Most patients relapse in 2 to 4 months if the dosage is decreased too low.

Cyclosporin may find great value in the initial treatment of acute, severe disease minimizing the need for hospitalization.[41] However, it may be associated with significant side-effects including hypertension and potentially irreversible impairment of renal function. Because cyclosporin is an immunosuppressive agent, there is an unproven possibility of an increased risk of cancer. Thus, it is wise to avoid combining cyclosporin treatment with phototherapy or other potentially mutagenic treatments. In the author's opinion, it will be important to find ways to rotate patients from cyclosporin after a few months to safe long-term treatments such as methotrexate or PUVA.

## Systemic corticosteroids

Oral corticosteroid therapy is effective, but is associated with many side-effects. Psoriasis may worsen significantly after corticosteroid therapy is stopped, and occasionally a severe, treatment-resistant pustular form may develop. This treatment should be reserved for acutely ill patients with erythrodermic psoriasis and should be given for only a short period.

# Therapeutic strategies

Several variables must be considered when selecting therapy for a patient with moderate-to-severe psoriasis including the patient's health and need for aggressive therapy, the patient's response to previous treatment, the therapeutic options available to the physician, and the patient's preferences. All treatments have side-effects, which must be suited to the patient, and certain variants of psoriasis require specialized treatment. The best strategy for long-term safety in treating psoriasis may be to rotate therapeutic regimens periodically before toxicity from any one modality becomes evident.[42]

## Future treatments

Recent research has revealed a likely etiologic role for T cells in psoriasis and thus immunotherapy has been of interest. Anti-CD4 monoclonal antibodies have been used with limited success to treat a small number of patients and many immunomodulating drugs are being tested.[43,44] Attempts to identify the gene alterations responsible for psoriasis may soon be successful and gene therapy may be available in the future.

## References

1. Lomholt G, Psoriasis: prevalence, spontaneous course and genetics: a census study on the prevalence of skin diseases on the Faroe Islands. Copenhagen, Denmark: GEC GAD, 1963.

2. Tomfohrde J, Silverman A, Barnes R et al, Gene for familial psoriasis, susceptibility mapped to the distal end of human chromosome 17q. *Science* 1994: 264; 1141–5.

3. Weinstein GD, McCullough JL. Ross PA. Cell kinetic basis for pathophysiology of psoriasis. *J Invest Dermatol* 1985: 85; 579–83.

4. Baker BS, Swain AF, Valdimarsson H, Fry L, T-cell subpopulations in the blood and skin of patients with psoriasis. *Br J Dermatol* 1984: 110; 37–44.

5. Cooper KD, Skin-infiltrating lymphocytes in normal and disordered skin activation signals and functional roles in psoriasis and mycosis fungoides type cutaneous T cell lymphoma. *J Dermatol* 1992: 19; 731–7.

6. Ashton RE, Andre P, Lowe NJ, Whitefield M, Anthralin: historical and current perspectives. *J Am Acad Dermatol* 1983: 9; 173–92.

7. Finnen MJ, Lawrence CM, Shuster S, Inhibition of dithranol inflammation by free-radical scavengers. *Lancet* 1984: 2; 1129–30.

8. Lowe NJ, Ashton RE, Koudsi H et al, Anthralin for psoriasis: short-contact anthralin therapy compared with topical steroid and conventional anthralin. *J Am Acad Dermatol* 1984: 10; 69–72.

9. Liem W, McCullough JL, Weinstein GD, Effectiveness of topical therapy for psoriasis: results of a national survey. *Cutis* 1995: 55; 306–10.

10. James VH, Munro DD, Feiwel M, Pituitary-adrenal function after occlusive topical therapy with betamethasone-17-valerate. *Lancet* 1967: 2; 1059–61.

11. Turpeinen M, Absorption of hydrocortisone from the skin reservoir in atopic dermatitis. *Br J Dermatol* 1991: 124: 358–60.

12. Kragballe K, Gjertsen BT, De Hoop D et al, Double-blind, right/left comparison of

calcipotriol and betamethasone valerate in treatment of psoriasis vulgaris. *Lancet* 1991: 337; 193–6.

13.   Ramsay CA, Berth-Jones J, Brandin G et al, Long term use of topical calcipotriol in chronic plaque psoriasis. *Dermatology* 1994; 189; 260–4.

14.   Weinstein GD, Tazarotene gel: efficacy and safety in plaque psoriasis. *J Am Acad Dermatol* 1997: 37; S33–8.

15.   Weinstein GD, Krueger CG, Lowe NJ et al, Tazarotene gel, a new retinoid, for topical therapy of psoriasis; vehicle-controlled study of safety, efficacy and duration of therapeutic effect. *J Am Acad Dermatol* 1997: 37; 85–92.

16.   Guenther L, Tazarotene combination treatments in psoriasis. *J Am Acad Dermatol* 2000; 43; S36–42.

17.   Lebwohl M, Ast E, Callen JP, Once-daily tazarotene gel versus twice-daily fluocinonide cream in the treatment of plaque psoriasis. *J Am Acad Dermatol* 1998; 38: 705–11.

18.   Stern RS, Armstrong RB, Anderson TF et al, Effect of continued ultraviolet B phototherapy on the duration of remission of psoriasis: a randomized study. *J Am Acad Dermatol* 1986: 15; 546–52.

19.   Gordon PM, Diffey BL, Mathews JNS, Farr PM, A randomized comparison of narrow-band TL-01 phototherapy and PUVA photochemotherapy for psoriasis. *J Am Acad Dermatol* 1999: 41: 728–32.

20.   Asawonda P, Anderson RR, Chang Y, Taylor CR, 308-nm excimer laser for the treatment of psoriasis: a dose-response study. *Arch Dermatol* 2000: 136; 619–24.

21.   Pathak MA, Fitzpatrick TB, Parrish JA, Pharmacologic and molecular aspects of psoralen photochemotherapy. In: Farber E, Cox AJ, Jacobs PH, Nall ML (eds) *Psoriasis: proceedings of the Second International Symposium.* New York: Yorke Medical Books, 1977, pp. 262–71.

22.   Kripke ML, Morison WL, Parrish JA, Systemic suppression of contact hypersensitivity in mice by psoralen plus UVA radiation (PUVA). *J Invest Dermatol* 1983: 81; 87–92.

23.   Melski JW, Tanenbaum L. Parrish JA et al, Oral methoxsalen photochemotherapy for the treatment of psoriasis: a cooperative clinical trial. *J Invest Dermatol* 1977: 68; 328–35.

24.   Stern RS, Nichols KT, Vakeva LH, Malignant melanoma in patients treated for psoriasis with methoxsalen (psoralen) and ultraviolet A radiation (PUVA). The PUVA Follow-up Study. *New Engl J Med* 1997: 336; 1041–5.

25.   Stern RS, Laird N, Melski J et al, Cutaneous squamous-cell carcinoma in patients treated with PUVA. *N Engl J Med* 1984: 310; 1156–61.

26.   McCullough JL, Weinstein GD, The action of cytotoxic drugs on cell proliferation in psoriasis. In: Wright NA, Camplejohn RS (eds) *Psoriasis: cell proliferation.* Edinburgh: Churchill Livingstone, 1983, pp. 347–54.

27.   Jeffes EWB III, McCullough JL, Pittelkow MR et al, Methotrexate therapy of psoriasis: differential sensitivity of proliferating lymphoid and epithelial cells to the cytotoxic and growth-inhibitory effects of methotrexate. *J Invest Dermatol* 1995: 105; 183–8.

28.   Weinstein GD, Frost P, Methotrexate for psoriasis: a new therapeutic schedule. *Arch Dermatol* 1971: 103; 33–8.

29.  Peckham PE, Weinstein GD, McCullough JL, The treatment of severe psoriasis: a national survey. *Arch Dermatol* 1987: 123; 1303–7.

30.  Roenigk HH, Auerbach R, Maibach H et al, Methotrexate in psoriasis: consensus conference. *J Am Acad Dermatol* 1998: 38; 478–85.

31.  Zachariae H, Methotrexate side-effects. *Br J Dermatol* 1990: 122 (Suppl 36); 127–33.

32.  Gollnick HPM, Orfanos CE, Clinical efficacy of etretinate and acitretin: European experience. In: Roenigk HH Jr, Maibach HI (eds) *Psoriasis, 2nd edn*. New York: Marcel Dekker, 1991, pp. 725–48.

33.  Moy RL, Kingston TP, Lowe NJ, Isotretinoin vs etretinate therapy in generalized pustular and chronic psoriasis. *Arch Dermatol* 1985: 121; 1297–301.

34.  Ling MR, Acitretin: optimal dosing strategies. *J Am Acad Dermatol* 1999: 41; S13–17.

35.  Larsen FG, Jakobsen P, Knudsen J et al, Conversion of acitretin to etretinate in psoriatic patients is influenced by ethanol. *J Invest Dermatol* 1993: 100; 623–7.

36.  DiGiovanna JJ, Helfgott RK, Gerber LH, Peck GL, Extraspinal tendon and ligament calcification associated with long-term therapy with etretinate. *N Engl J Med* 1986: 315; 1177–82.

37.  Ellis CN, Fradin MS, Messana JM et al, Cyclosporine for plaque-type psoriasis: Results of a multidose, double-blind trial. *N Engl J Med* 1991: 324; 277–84.

38.  Wong RL, Winslow CM, Cooper KD, The mechanism of action of cyclosporin A in the treatment of psoriasis. *Immunol Today* 1993: 14; 69–74.

39.  O'Keefe SJ, Tamura J, Kincaid RL et al, FK-506- and CsA-sensitive activation of the interleukin-2 promoter by calcineurin. *Nature* 1992: 357; 692–4.

40.  Shupack J, Abel E, Bauer E et al, Cyclosporine as maintenance therapy in patients with severe psoriasis. *J Am Acad Dermatol* 1997: 36; 423–32.

41.  Koo J, Cyclosporine in dermatology. Fears and opportunities. *Arch Dermatol* 1995: 131; 842–5.

42.  Weinstein GD, White GM, An approach to the treatment of moderate to severe psoriasis with rotational therapy. *J Am Acad Dermatol* 1993: 28; 454–9.

43.  Owen CM, Harrison PV, Successful treatment of severe psoriasis with basiliximab, an interleukin-2 receptor monoclonal antibody. *Clin Exp Dermatol* 2000: 25; 195–7.

44.  Grundmann-Kollmann M, Mooser G, Schraeder P et al, Treatment of chronic plaque-stage psoriasis and psoriatic arthritis with mycophenolate mofetil. *J Am Acad Dermatol* 2000: 42; 835–7.

# 6

## Advances in the treatment of rosacea

*Ronald Marks*

## Introduction

Rosacea is a common and cosmetically disabling disease which remains almost as mysterious aetiologically now as when the disorder was first described. Despite its frequency and disfiguring nature it has provoked a surprisingly small amount of serious investigation. It is in fact a fascinating disorder comprising many diverse elements and processes which defy rational explanation and demands thought and vigorous research activity. It is best defined as a chronic degenerative and inflammatory disorder of facial skin particularly affecting facial convexities including the cheeks, nose, forehead and chin, and is characterized by flushing, erythema and telangiectasia punctuated by episodes of papules, pustules and swelling.

For the most part treatment has been inadequate because, although it has been possible to control the inflammatory episodes of papules and pustules in most patients, we have until recently been near powerless to do very much about the distressing persistent redness suffered by most patients. We are equally impotent at controlling the telangiectasia and diffuse puffy swelling often seen. A major reason for our inability to design better treatments has been our lack of understanding of the nature of the disease and its causation. For this reason we have included a brief overview of the aetiopathogenesis of the condition.

## Aetiopathogenesis

Rosacea has been clinically recognized as a distinct entity for hundreds of years, and indeed there are descriptions in the literature of both Shakespeare and Chaucer of rumbustious and larger than life characters who would appear to have rosacea. Their reddened faces, swollen noses and blemished pimpled skin were thought to indicate intemperance and a debauched riotous lifestyle. There can be no doubt that alcohol is capable of causing facial flushing but apart from this there is no evidence that drinking alcohol regularly and/or to excess results in rosacea. Our own studies many years ago could not identify any special dietary factors in patients with rosacea compared to matched controls.[1] The same is true for both gastrointestinal dysfunction and associations with particular gastrointestinal diseases. Recent interest in the role of *Helicobacter pylori*[2,3] stems from historical views as to the 'gut origin' of rosacea but as yet there is no real evidence that this interesting microbial species has anything to do with the cause of rosacea.

Other myths that have accumulated over the years include the view that rosacea has a psychological cause. It seems likely that this is the result of confusing effect with cause. It would be very surprising if patients with a persistently reddened 'clown-like' face didn't become anxious and depressed about their appearance. When investigated, rosacea patients were found to be more depressed than a control group[4] but then so are patients with other chronic facial rashes – including acne. Regrettably public attitudes to skin disease vary from indifference to distaste and when the skin disorder in question is highly visible and on the face, instead of sympathy, the patient is often avoided and disdained. Whatever the basis for this primitive response it leads to social isolation, despair and depression.

The pustules and episodes of inflammation as well as a response to systemic antibiotics have suggested an infective cause for rosacea but qualitative and quantitative studies of the bacterial flora do not support this view.[4] Similarly, detailed histological investigations have not identified any hint of a causative microorganism. The normally present follicle mite, *Demodex folliculorum*, is undoubtedly increased in numbers in the facial skin of patients with papular rosacea[5,6] and has been indicated as a pathogenetic villain by some authors.[7,8] It is true that on very rare occasions bits of this odd mite seem to have found their way into the centre of foci of inflammatory cells,[9] but the significance of this is uncertain as the great majority of inflammatory foci do not have a trace of *Demodex* in them even after serial sectioning.[10] Even more destructive to the possibility of a pathogenetic role for the *Demodex* mite is the occasional finding of *Demodex* lying free in the dermis unaccompanied by inflammation (Fig. 6.1).

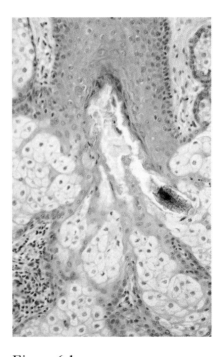

Figure 6.1

Photomicrograph showing *Demodex* mite in a sebaceous gland. There is no inflammation (H&E, ×90).

More recently it has become recognized that solar damage to the facial skin probably plays some role in the development of the disease. There certainly seem to be increased amounts of solar elastotic degenerative change in histological sections from biopsies of rosacea patients.[10] The disorder occurs on the maximally insolated areas of the cheeks, chin, nose and forehead while sparing the comparatively shaded parts (underside of chin, nasolabial folds and hairy scalp). Interestingly, it is only when baldness develops that rosacea develops on the scalp.[11] The disorder is certainly considerably more frequently seen in fair-skinned North West Europeans or those descended from this group and those of Celtic origin but is uncommon in pigmented Asiatic subjects and rare in black individuals.

A suggested sequence for the pathogenesis is set out in Fig. 6.2. It is clear that we cannot be certain as to the initiating cause of rosacea. Damage to upper dermal connective tissue with consequent small vessel dilatation does, however, appear to be an important component and it seems that climatic stimuli are likely to induce these changes. If this is indeed the case, the best chance we have of making a significant impact on the natural history of the disease is to stimulate dermal connective tissue repair in order to provide some support for the capillary vasculature in the upper dermis.

# Topical treatments

## Corticosteroids

Non-dermatologists when confronted by a patient with a red rash tend to prescribe topical corticosteroids without

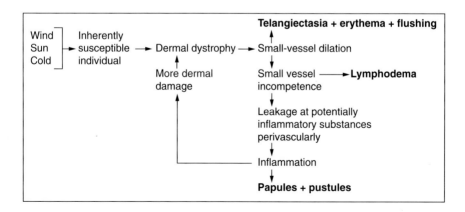

## Figure 6.2

An algorithm demonstrating the possible sequence of events in the pathogenesis of rosacea.

recourse to a diagnosis. When the red rash in question is rosacea a cutaneous catastrophe is just around the corner. The corticosteroids, especially the more potent members of this group of agents, cause dermal thinning and connective tissue atrophy which in the face allows even greater dilatation of the dermal vasculature thus aggravating the already dilated state of the vasculature. Patients mistreated in this way develop a characteristic and readily identifiable clinical appearance with a bright red complexion and marked telangiectasia but few inflammatory papules[12] (Fig. 6.3). Regrettably, this iatrogenic complication is only very slowly reversible. After stopping the use of the topical corticosteroid the odd facial appearance persists for many months or even years. The best advice with regard to topical corticosteroids, especially the potent ones, is just not to use them in facial skin problems, particularly rosacea.

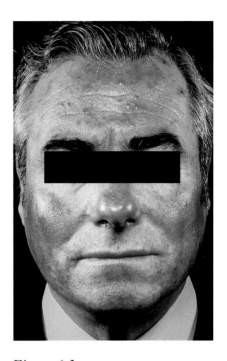

## Figure 6.3

Photograph of a man with rosacea who had been treated for more than 1 year with betamethasone valerate ointment.

## *Supportive and adjunctive treatments*

Affected facial skin often feels sore in rosacea and patients appreciate using some sort of soothing emollient cream. Use of this type of harmless preparation may also divert patients from using any of the more dangerous topical corticosteroid preparations that they may have to hand. It should be noted that the best emollient to use is the one that the patient prefers – several may have to be tried before the 'right one' is found.

Many rosacea patients claim that the sun aggravates their facial disorder. This taken with the climatically induced dermal dystrophy in this condition would suggest that it is completely logical to protect the skin from further UV injury by prescribing sunscreens. Although it would seem sensible to recommend the use of sunscreens, it has to be said that there is no positive evidence to support their use in rosacea.

Patients and their family often ask about diet as they almost certainly have heard from one source or another that hot spicy foods, hot drinks and alcoholic drinks cause rosacea or at least make the disorder worse. It must be said that there is no evidence of this, although there is no doubt that rosacea patients flush more than controls to any stimulus, including food and beverages. If such flushing is particularly marked in some patients it is probably sensible to ask them to desist from indulging in the foods that they say are responsible as any reduction in the flushing can only be beneficial.

The question of camouflage often arises, especially in women with bright red cheeks, nose and forehead. This group need considerable sympathy and reassurance as well as a formal treatment plan which now may well include laser therapy (see later in this chapter). In the short term advice on the best way of hiding the problem is appreciated. Green tinted cosmetics are quite helpful or if available the advice of a consultant in cosmetic camouflage should be sought.

## Metronidazole

Preparations of metronidazole (0.75% or 1.0%) have been available for the topical treatment of rosacea for nearly 15 years and cannot now be described as a novel approach.[13,14] Nonetheless, it is worth stating that they have become an established way of managing mild to moderate papular rosacea. It is uncertain how metronidazole works. It does not appear to have antidemodex activity and, as has

been said previously, no bacterial involvement has been found in rosacea.

The gel preparations in use are usually well tolerated although they can cause some mild burning and irritation when applied to the face. In trials in which topical metronidazole preparations have been compared with oral tetracyclines they have been shown to produce an equal degree of improvement.[15,16]

## Azelaic acid

This agent is formulated as a 20% gel and is designed for use in acne but it has been submitted to clinical trial in patients with rosacea.[17] The clinical trial was placebo controlled and had a randomized double-blind design. The azelaic acid preparation was shown to reduce both the numbers of inflammatory lesions and the degree of erythema. Other trials[18] also support the use of this agent in rosacea and it is likely that it will become licensed for use in the near future.

## Sulphacetamide and sulphur topical preparations

The past few years has seen the rebirth of an old generic preparation containing sulphacetamide 10% and sulphur 5%. It is claimed that it is useful for rosacea, acne and seborrhoeic dermatitis. Anecdotal reports attest as to its efficacy, but there is little clinical trial data available.

## *Retinoids*

If the observation that patients with rosacea show more solar elastotic degeneration then it might be expected that measures to reduce this tissue change would improve rosacea at the same time. If chronic photodamage plays an important role in the pathogenesis of rosacea then it is reasonable to suggest that manoeuvres to reduce this will improve the disease. Interestingly, the few studies there have been suggest that this may be the case. Kligman reported the successful use of topical tretinoin in rosacea in an open study[19] in a limited number of patients and the writer has also obtained good results in two patients with recalcitrant erythematotelangiectatic disease. Most patients with rosacea have a fair and sensitive skin which is easily irritated by tretinoin. Considerable explanation and persuasion is necessary to ensure that these patients use the topical retinoid for the several months that it takes before any improvement is seen.

# Systemic treatments

## *Antibiotics*

It has been known for many years that the oral tetracyclines improve the inflammation in rosacea. In a double-blind placebo-controlled study oral tetracycline (250 mg 6-hourly) greatly reduced the number of inflammatory papules present after 6 weeks.[20] Interestingly, ampicillin (250 mg 6-hourly)

which was used in a third group of patients in the same study was also found to result in improvement in patients although not to the same degree. The tetracyclines do not seem to improve the erythema and telangiectasia. The swelling that sometimes accompanies the papules and pustules is helped by the tetracyclines but the persistent oedema is not changed much.

If the treatment is suddenly withdrawn the papules may well recur within a few days and it is best to slowly 'tail off' the tetracyclines over a few weeks until the tendency for the papules to recur stops.

All the tetracyclines seem equally effective, although it has to be admitted there are no studies which compare efficacy of different tetracycline analogues in rosacea. It is the prejudice of the author to use either minocycline or doxycycline and in view of the rare, serious, adverse reactions to the former[21] to mainly prescribe the latter drug.

A reasonable question to ask is 'why do the tetracyclines work?' Unfortunately there is no categoric answer to this question. The therapeutic action does not seem to be due to an antibacterial effect and the assumption is that their anti-inflammatory action is responsible.[22]

Erythromycin and ampicillin are also helpful, although they are not as therapeutically active as the tetracyclines. Oral metronidazole was shown by Pye and Burton[23] to reduce inflammatory rosacea with a similar degree of efficacy as the tetracyclines. It is not often used because of its unpleasant side-effects and the restrictions on alcohol ingestion. It was suggested that the therapeutic efficacy of metronidazole in rosacea may be due to a toxic action of the drug on *Demodex folliculorum*, but this has not been supported by experimental evidence.

## Isotretinoin

There are some patients whose rosacea stubbornly refuses to improve with any of the topical agents or systemic antibiotics discussed above. They are often a despondent and desperate group of patients prepared to try almost anything offered to them. Isotretinoin has been used in such patients and has been found helpful in some. We noted that it reduced the size of the rhinophymatous nose as judged by an image analysis technique and a volumetric assessment derived from the amount of water in a plaster cast of the nose.[24] Isotretinoin was found to reduce the number of inflammatory papules within 6 weeks at a dose of 0.5 mg/kg in a group of eight patients.[25] The Munich group have also studied the efficacy of isotretinoin in patients with severe rosacea and have obtained impressive results.[26] The various adverse side-effects as well as the cost dictate that only those with the most severe and recalcitrant disease are treated cautiously with this drug.

## Anti-flushing agents

Regardless as to whether rosacea is caused by some form of cutaneous 'vasomotor instability' or whether the vascular component is entirely due to a passive vasodilatation consequent on dermal dystrophy, most would agree that reduction in the frequency and intensity of flushing is likely to be beneficial. The simplest therapy is to advise the patient to avoid those stimuli that he or she knows precipitate flushing. Unfortunately, this is not always possible because either the stimuli are not known or because they are so trivial they cannot be avoided. To help reduce flushing some clinicians have tried a pharmacological approach employing clonidine, a combination of aspirin and H1 blocking antihistamines or amitriptyline.[27] Some patients are said to be improved by this type of regimen, but the writer's experience is that such reduction in flushing is unimpressive.

# Miscellaneous novel treatments

Oral terbinafine had been noted as improving patients with rosacea and the results of definitive studies are awaited.[28] Treatment of rosacea with miticidal agents has been reported – for example oral ivermectin and topical permethrin cream[29] – once again the results of formal clinical trials are awaited.

# Surgical and laser therapy

Patients with rhinophyma are greatly improved by surgical manoeuvres to

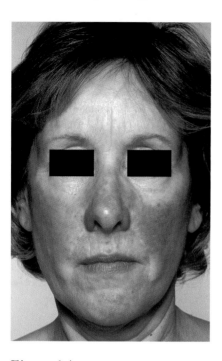

## Figure 6.4

Woman with rosacea treated with pulsed dye laser everywhere except her left cheek.

reduce and refashion the nose. A variety of techniques have been used including cold steel paring, electrosurgical paring, dermabrasion and laser resurfacing. Healing is usually extremely rapid because re-epithelialization takes place from the follicular remnants left after the surface has been removed.

A recently introduced laser technique has addressed a previously intractable problem – the distressing and persistent erythema of the cheeks. Using either the tunable pulsed dye laser or the ruby laser, the redness and telangiectasia can be eliminated after two or three sessions only.[30] In our studies using the pulsed dye laser, it was shown using objective measurement methods that the erythema and the telangiectasia could be rapidly eliminated in the treated sites compared to untreated areas[31] (Fig. 6.4). The results are excellent and it is unfortunate that this treatment is not universally available. Of great interest is the fact that areas treated by lasers in this way tend not to develop further inflammatory lesions. The treatment is slightly uncomfortable and may cause cosmetic disability for up to 3–4 weeks, but all the patients the author has encountered who have been treated in this way have thought any discomfort very much worthwhile.

## Conclusion

Although we are still groping in the dark when it comes to understanding the sequence of tissue events in rosacea as well as its ultimate cause, we are able to assist most patients with the disease. There are enough treatment modalities around for virtually all patients to be helped. To finish on an 'upnote' the advent of laser treatment has meant that those unfortunate few with persistent red clown-like cheeks can look forward to regaining normal facial skin.

# References

1. Marks R, Beard RJ, Clark ML et al, Gastrointestinal observations in rosacea. *Lancet* 1967: i; 739–43.

2. Utas S, Ozbakir O, Turasan A, Utas C, Helicobacter pylori eradication treatment reduces the severity of rosacea. *J Am Acad Dermatol* 1999: 40; 483–5.

3. Hirschmann JV, Does Helicobacter pylori have a role in the pathogenesis of rosacea? *J Am Acad Dermatol* 2000: 42; 537–9.

4. Marks R, Rosacea: hopeless hypothesis, marvellous myths and dermal disorganization. In: Marks R, Plewig G (eds) *Acne and related disorders*. London: Martin Dunitz, 1989, pp. 293–9.

5. Forton F, Seys N, Density of *Demodex folliculorum* in rosacea: a case control study using standardised skin surface biopsy. *Br J Dermatol* 1993: 128; 650–9.

6. Erbagci Z, Ozgoztasi O, The significance of *Demodex folliculorum* density in rosacea. *Int J Dermatol* 1998: 37; 421–5.

7. Rufli T, Büchner SA, T-cell subsets in acne rosacea lesions and the possible role of *Demodex folliculorum*. *Dermatologica* 1984: 169; 1–5.

8. Shelley WB, Shelley ED, Burmeister V, Unilateral demodectic rosacea. *J Am Acad Dermatol* 1989: 20(5 part 2); 915–7.

9. Ecker BI, Winkelmann RK, *Demodex* granuloma. *Arch Dermatol* 1979: 115; 343–4.

10. Jimenez-Acosta F, Planas L, Penneys N, *Demodex* mites contain immunoreactive lipase. *Arch Dermatol* 1989: 125; 1436.

11. Gojewska M, Rosacea on common male baldness. *Br J Dermatol* 1975: 93; 63–6.

12. Leyden JJ, Kligman AM, Steroid rosacea. *Arch Dermatol* 1974: 110; 619–22.

13. Lowe NJ, Henderson T, Millikan LE, Parker F, Topical metronidazole for severe/recalcitrant rosacea: a prospective, open trial. In: Marks R, Plewig G (eds) *Acne and related disorders*. London: Martin Dunitz, 1989, pp. 327–30.

14. Jorizzo JL, Lebwohl M, Tobey RE, The efficacy of metronidazole 1% cream once daily compared with metronidazole 1% cream twice daily and their vehicles in rosacea: a double-blind clinical trial. *J Am Acad Dermatol* 1998: 39; 502–4.

15. Neilsen PG, A double-blind study of 1% metronidazole cream versus systemic oxytetracycline therapy for rosacea. *Br J Dermatol* 1983: 109; 63–5.

16. Monk BE, Logan RA, Cook J et al, Topical metronidazole in the treatment of rosacea. *J Dermatol Treat* 1991: 2; 91–3.

17. Carmichael AJ, Marks R, Graupe KA, Zaumseil RP, Topical azelaic acid in the treatment of rosacea. *J Dermatol Treat* 1993: 4(Suppl 1); S19–22.

18. Bjerke R, Fyrand O, Graupe K, Double-blind comparison of azeliac acid 20% cream and its vehicle in treatment of papulo-pustular rosacea. *Acta Derm Venerol* 1999: 79; 456–9.

19. Kligman AM, Topical tretinoin for rosacea: a preliminary report. *J Dermatol Treat* 1993: 4; 71–3.

20. Marks R, Ellis J, Comparative effectiveness of tetracycline and ampicillin in rosacea. *Lancet* 1971: ii; 1049–52.

21. Gough A, Chapman S, Wagstaff K et al, Minocycline induced autoimmune hepatitis and systemic lupus erythematosus-like syndrome. *Br Med J* 1996: 312; 169–72.

22. Marks R, Davies MJ, The distribution in the skin of systemically administered tetracycline. *Br J Dermatol* 1969: 81; 448–51.

23. Pye RJ, Burton JL, Treatment of rosacea by metronidazole. *Lancet* 1976: i; 1211–2.

24. Irvine C, Kumar P, Marks R, Isotretinoin in the treatment of rosacea and rhinophyma. In: Marks R, Plewig G (eds) *Acne and related disorders*. London: Martin Dunitz, 1989, pp. 301–6.

25. Fulton RA, Dick DC, Mackie RM, The use of isotretinoin in rosacea. In: *Retinoid therapy*. MTP Press, 1984, pp. 315–19.

26. Hoting E, Paul E, Plewig G, Treatment of rosacea with isotretinoin. *Int J Dermatol* 1986: 25; 660–3.

27. Wilkin JK, The red face: flushing disorders. *Clin Dermatol* 1993: 11(2); 211–23.

28. Rashid A, Williams TG, Oral terbinafine in the treatment of rosacea. Poster shown at the annual meeting of the AAD 2001.

29. Forstinger C, Kittler H, Binder M, Treatment of rosacea-like dermodicidosis with oral ivermectin and topical permethrin cream. *J Am Acad Dermatol* 1999: 41; 775–7.

30. Duffy DM, Weiss R, Tanghetti E, Narurkar V, Lasers for the treatment of facial telangiectasia: a comparison of modalities and techniques. *Skin Aging* 1999: March; 57–66.

31. Clark SM, Lanigan SW, Marks R, Laser treatment of erythema-telangiectate rosacea. 1998: unpublished data.

# 7

## Advances in the management of urticaria

*Anne Kobza Black and Clive EH Grattan*

## Introduction

Urticarial weals in the skin and deeper angioedema swellings of the subcutis and submucosa result from leakage of plasma and recruitment of inflammatory cells through undamaged small blood vessels made temporarily permeable by vasoactive mediators. Histamine released from mast cell granules in response to a range of stimuli is the most important mediator of urticaria and associated angioedema. Physical stimuli, including cold, sweating, pressure and light stroking of the skin may cause degranulation of the mast cells in some people and this is the basis for defining subgroups of patients with physical urticaria. The term ordinary urticaria is used for all other patients after those with urticarial vasculitis and C1 esterase deficiency have been excluded.

Urticaria may last for days or years. By convention it is called chronic if disease activity continues on most days beyond 6 weeks, and acute if it remits sooner. Acute urticaria may be linked with upper respiratory infections[1] or to environmental allergens, such as nuts or shellfish, whereas chronic urticaria is more likely to be due to physical causes or endogenous serum factors, including autoantibodies. When a cause cannot be identified it is called 'idiopathic'. After exclusion of chronic urticaria patients with predominantly physical urticarias, about 50% have a histamine-releasing factor in their serum as demonstrated by the development of a weal and flare reaction at the site of intradermal testing with their own serum (the autologous serum skin test).[2] In some of these patients the releasing histamine factor is an IgG autoantibody directed against the high-affinity IgE receptor (FcεRI)[3] on mast cells and basophils, or less frequently against IgE bound to the receptor.[4] In others, the nature of the serum factor remains to be identified.[5,6]

The majority of chronic urticaria patients show some response to antihistamines, even though the mast cell degranulating stimulus remains elusive. Other proinflammatory mediators including eicosanoids, neuropeptides and platelet activating factor may be important in the disease pathogenesis of those patients unresponsive to antihistamines. A small but important group of patients with recurrent angioedema can be identified by low levels of functional C1 esterase inhibitor and the C4 component of complement. Kinin-like peptides generated by complement pathway activation cause capillary permeability without histamine release so treatment with antihistamines is ineffective and inappropriate. The management of C1 esterase inhibitor deficiency is not covered in this chapter. However, it should be noted that the angioedema occasionally seen with angiotensin-converting enzyme (ACE) inhibitors may also be kinin-mediated since bradykinin is usually inactivated by ACE.

It should be recognized that urticaria and angioedema are distressing conditions which can affect the quality of life severely. In studies of patients attending an urticaria clinic, the quality of life was comparable to those of patients awaiting triple coronary bypass surgery[7] or attending as outpatients with psoriasis.[8] Assessment of the quality of life as well as reduction in itching and wealing should be included in future trials of therapy for urticaria.

## Management

The rational management of urticaria should take account of likely causes and mediators involved. Explanation and attention to general measures may be as important as drug therapy. An outline of management is shown in Fig. 7.1. Minimizing stress, overheating and alcohol may be helpful. Some patients obtain relief from pruritus by taking a cool shower or applying cooling lotions or ice-packs during acute attacks.

Aspirin, nonsteroidal anti-inflammatory drugs and opiates may have a nonspecific aggravating effect on ordinary urticaria and should be avoided if possible. Paracetamol is usually a satisfactory alternative. Diets excluding, for example, food colourings and additives may be of some value to a limited number of patients. Addition of an $H_2$ antagonist or a mast cell-stabilizing drug may provide additional benefit for a few. Second-line therapies carry more risk but may be essential for the effective control of particular situations such as angioedema of the mouth or disabling delayed pressure urticaria. Third-line therapies involving immunosuppressive agents are only appropriate for patients with chronic recurrent autoimmune urticaria refractory to other measures and should be administered under the supervision of a specialist clinician.

## First-line treatment of urticaria

### Antihistamines

Histamine is the main mediator of urticaria. In the skin $H_1$ receptor activation induces itching, flare and wealing while $H_2$ activation plays a lesser role in the wealing response. Thus $H_1$ antihistamines are the mainstay of symptomatic treatment of urticaria. Antihistamines compete with histamine for its receptors and block its action. Generally, $H_1$ antihistamines are rapidly absorbed usually reaching

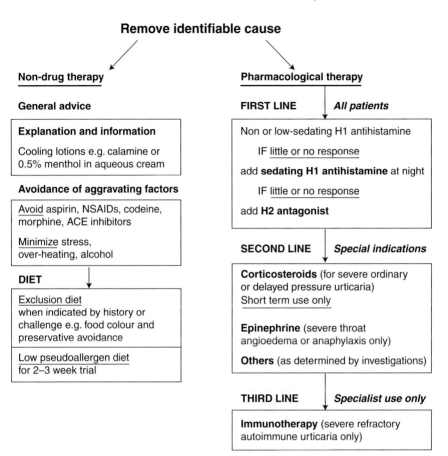

**Remove identifiable cause**

**Non-drug therapy**

**General advice**

| Explanation and information |
| --- |
| Cooling lotions e.g. calamine or 0.5% menthol in aqueous cream |

**Avoidance of aggravating factors**

| Avoid aspirin, NSAIDs, codeine, morphine, ACE inhibitors |
| --- |
| Minimize stress, over-heating, alcohol |

**DIET**

| Exclusion diet when indicated by history or challenge e.g. food colour and preservative avoidance |
| --- |
| Low pseudoallergen diet for 2–3 week trial |

**Pharmacological therapy**

**FIRST LINE** | *All patients*

| Non or low-sedating H1 antihistamine |
| --- |
| IF little or no response |
| add **sedating H1 antihistamine** at night |
| IF little or no response |
| add **H2 antagonist** |

**SECOND LINE** | *Special indications*

| **Corticosteroids** (for severe ordinary or delayed pressure urticaria) Short term use only |
| --- |
| **Epinephrine** (severe throat angioedema or anaphylaxis only) |
| **Others** (as determined by investigations) |

**THIRD LINE** | *Specialist use only*

| **Immunotherapy** (severe refractory autoimmune urticaria only) |
| --- |

Figure 7.1

Management of chronic ordinary urticaria.

peak serum concentrations within 2 hours. Many are metabolized by the liver, and some of their active metabolites have a longer half-life than the parent compound and determine the activity profile of the medication.

The use of classic, traditional antihistamines is limited by their sedative and anticholinergic side-effects, paradoxical excitation in children and possible induction of tolerance with sustained use. Except for hydroxyzine they are less potent than the second generation of antihistamines, but are useful if night-time sedation is required. Doxepin is a tricyclic antidepressant with potent $H_1$ antihistamine activity, and is useful for the anxious patient at night at a dose of 25–50 mg. It also reacts with α adrenergic receptors. It should not be used concurrently with monoamine oxidase inhibitors, tricyclic antidepressants or epinephrine (adrenaline). Cimetidine has been reported to produce clinically important fluctuations of steady-state levels of doxepin.

A major advance was the introduction of the second generation of potent specific $H_1$ receptor antagonists in the 1980s, which are now the treatment of choice[9] (Table 7.1). Their main advantage is low sedation at doses recommended by the manufacturer and lack of anticholinergic side-effects. Reduction in sedation is partially due to their lipophobic property which limits their passage across the blood–brain barrier. Most low sedation antihistamines can be administered without the need to stop alcohol intake, although excessive intake should be avoided. In a few patients low sedation antihistamines may affect skilled tasks, and patients should be warned of this possibility.

In most trials hydroxyzine and second generation antihistamines have generally improved the itching and wealing of chronic urticaria by approximately two-thirds. Thus these newer antihistamines are as effective as each other and hydroxyzine. There is no evidence that tolerance occurs. Many are available without a prescription.

Terfenadine and astemizole were the first second-generation, low-sedation antihistamines available. Rarely they are capable of inducing cardiac QTc prolongation leading to ventricular tachycardias including an irregular tachycardia (torsade de pointes). This is more likely if the recommended dose is exceeded or if they are taken in circumstances where cytochrome P450 (isoenzyme CYP3A) in the liver, the main enzyme that metabolizes these drugs, is reduced. This can occur with liver disease or concurrent use of medication inhibiting cytochrome P450 (e.g. erythromycin, clarithromycin) or with imidazole antifungal agents (e.g. ketoconazole and itraconazole). Because of these potential problems, astemizole has been withdrawn by the manufacturer and terfenadine is not available in many countries. An active metabolite of terfenadine, fexofenadine, which does not have the potential cardiac side-effects of the parent compound terfenadine, is now available and is licensed for urticaria at a dose of 180 mg/day.

Loratadine is a derivative of azatadine, and does not prolong QTc. Although it is also metabolized in the liver by cytochrome P450, so far no clinically relevant drug interactions have been reported. Cetirizine, a derivative of hydroxyzine, is poorly metabolized and is excreted predominantly in the urine unchanged, and its dose should be reduced in renal disease. It has been shown to be more sedative than placebo in some studies and is best taken at night. It may cause headache, dry mouth and gastrointestinal upset. Cetirizine reduces dermal eosinophil accumulation and is theoretically more useful in urticarias such as delayed pressure urticaria and urticarial vasculitis where this may be a significant feature. However, in practice such an additional benefit is clinically not obvious.

Acrivastine, a derivative of triprolidine, has a rapid onset and short duration of action. It is also not metabolized significantly in the liver and is excreted unchanged predominantly in the urine. It can be taken on demand 1 hour before a known precipitant of urticaria, such as cold or cholinergic urticaria.

Mizolastine has recently become available as a second-generation antihistamine.[10] The main metabolic pathway is hepatic glucuronidation. Although there is no increase of QTc with mizolastine alone, there is some QTc prolongation when mizolastine is used in conjunction with ketoconazole. Therefore concurrent administration with any drug which inhibits hepatic cytochromes such as erythromycin and ketoconazole and any class I and class III antiarrhythmic agent, or in patients with cardiac or hepatic impairment, is contraindicated.

The general strategy is to reduce urticarial activity with minimal side-effects. Itching and wealing respond better than erythema. It is important that regular antihistamine treatment is used for chronic urticaria, and studies in allergic rhinitis support the value of uninterrupted antihistamine administration. Patients vary in their response to different antihistamines, but a self-assessment schedule will demonstrate the most suitable for patients.[11] All should be taken in adequate doses timed in relationship to maximal urticarial activity, for example itching is most severe in the evening and at night.[12]

Different classes of antihistamine such as a low-sedating one in the morning, and a sedating one such as hydroxyzine 10–25 mg or doxepin 10–25 mg at night can be combined. The patient, however, needs to be warned that cognitive function and reflexes may be impaired in the morning. Low-sedation antihistamines such as cetirizine and loratadine also can be used together. A combination of $H_1$ and $H_2$ antihistamines may be more effective in individual patients than $H_1$ antihistamines alone. This can be tried for a limited period (4–6 weeks), with newer ones such as ranitidine 150 mg twice a day being preferable to cimetidine which has more drug interactions and antiandrogenic effects.

Tolerance is frequently claimed to develop after continuous use of antihistamines. With the older classical ones, the most likely cause of a reduction in efficacy is poor compliance. However no tolerance has been reported to second-generation antihistamines. Antihistamines cross the placenta. Although there is no reliable evidence that they are teratogenic, they should be avoided during pregnancy, if possible. If not, chlorpheniramine appears to be the least risky to use. Triprellenamine is recommended by some in the USA.[13] The recommendation is that loratadine should be avoided in pregnancy (as large doses in animals

## Table 7.1 Some second-generation antihistamines

| Generic name | Proprietary name | Form/strength | Recommended dose | Dosage in children | Onset of action (h) |
|---|---|---|---|---|---|
| Cetirizine | Zirtek; Reactine | 10 mg tablets; 5 mg per 5 ml solution | 10 mg daily | 6–12 years, 10 mg daily; 3–6 years, 5 mg daily; not for urticaria under 6 years | 0.5 |
| Loratadine | Clarityn | 10 mg tablets; 5 mg per 5 ml syrup | 10 mg daily | 6–12 years, 10 mg daily; 2–5 years, 5 mg daily | 2 |
| Acrivastine | Semprex; Benadryl Allergy Relief | 8 mg capsules | 8 mg three times daily | Not recommended under 12 years | 0.5 |
| Fexofenadine | Telfast 180 | 180 mg tablets | 180 mg daily | Not recommended under 12 years | 1–3 |
| Mizolastine | Mizollen | 10 mg tablets | 10 mg daily | Not recommended under 12 years | <0.5 |

[a]Avoid all in pregnancy if possible

cause congenital malformations), as should mizolastine which is a recently developed antihistamine. There is no specific contraindication for the other newer antihistamines during pregnancy, but they should only be used if the benefit to the mother outweighs the potential risk to the fetus.

The so-called third-generation of antihistamines which are active metabolites of second-generation antihistamines, e.g. fexofenadine a derivative of terfenadine which causes even less sedation, may become the treatment of choice.[14] Norastemizole, a metabolite of astemizole is now in development for human use, and descarboethoxy loratadine, a metabolite of loratadine, has recently become available.

First-line therapies used in combination with antihistamine therapy are mast cell stabilizers, the β-agonist terbutaline[15] and the calcium channel blocker nifedipine. These have been studied in small numbers of patients and additional benefit remains to be

| Duration of action (h) | Precautions[a] | Drug interactions | Some side-effects | Other effects |
|---|---|---|---|---|
| 24 | Renal insufficiency | | May cause sedation | Inhibits leucocyte migration, inhibits vascular adhesion molecule expression |
| 12–24 | | | | |
| <12 | Renal impairment | | | |
| 24 | | | | |
| 24 | Hepatic impairment; QT prolongation; Electrolyte disturbance | Macrolide antibiotics, imidazole antibiotics, neuroleptics, tricyclic antidepressants, SSRIs, protease inhibitors, grapefruit | Weight gain, QTc prolongation with cytochrome P450 inhibitors | |

confirmed. Double-blind randomized studies have shown benefit when compared with chlorpheniramine[16] and placebo while on antihistamines.[17]

## Second-line agents

### Corticosteroids

No controlled studies have been undertaken of the use of corticosteroids but they are effective in most patients with severe chronic urticaria when given orally usually at higher doses in the region of 0.5 mg/kg per day. Though short courses are useful for acute exacerbations prolonged use should be avoided because of the risk of unacceptable side-effects. Potent topical steroids under occlusion for 2 weeks in 23 patients with chronic urticaria induced improvement for 3 weeks with side-effects in 50%,[18] but are not recommended for standard clinical use.

## Table 7.2 Emergency treatment of nonhereditary angioedema

| Severity | Clinical signs | Drug | Proprietary preparations | Dose | Route of administration | Comments |
|---|---|---|---|---|---|---|
| Moderate | Some swelling of tongue | Ephedrine spray 2% | | Two to four puffs into oropharynx[a] | | Unlicensed non-proprietary preparation prepared in pharmacy |
| | | Adrenaline aerosol | Primatene Mist (Whitehall Laboratories, USA) | Two to four puffs into oropharynx[a] | | Unlicensed in UK; prescribed on named-patient basis; ordered from IDIS World Medicines |
| Severe | Respiratory embarrassment, generalized swelling or loss of consciousness | Adrenaline 1/1000 (1 mg/ml) | Mini-I-Jet (Medeva, UK); Epipen (ALK, UK); Anapen (Allerayde, UK) | Adult 0.5 ml | Subcutaneous or intramuscular injection | Preloaded syringes (0.3 ml adult, 0.15 ml child); prescribed on named-patient basis; injects automatically on skin contact (beware of injecting a digit) |
| | | Chlorpheniramine | | Adult 10–20 mg (max 40 mg in 24 h) | Intravenous | |
| | | Hydrocortisone succinate | | Adult 100–300 mg | Intravenous | Continued for at least 24 h to prevent relapse |

[a]Local vasoconstrictor effect rather than systemic absorption

There are also uncontrolled studies reporting the benefit of anabolic steroids in refractory urticaria[19] and anecdotal reports of leukotriene receptor antagonists in aspirin-sensitive chronic urticaria.[20]

The emergency treatment of non-hereditary angioedema causing respiratory embarrassment from swelling of the larynx is epinephrine (adrenaline) (Table 7.2). It acts rapidly by vasoconstriction and decreasing vasopermeability, and also binds to the mast cell β-receptors inhibiting further mediator release. For moderately severe swellings in the oropharyngeal mucosa it can be inhaled for its predominantly local vasoconstrictor effect, but there is no licensed adrenaline aerosol in the UK at present. For severe reactions especially of anaphylactic type where there may be associated widespread urticaria, wheezing and loss of consciousness, epinephrine (adrenaline) must be injected either intramuscularly or subcutaneously by a medical attendant, a colleague or self-administration. Side-effects include palpitations, dry mouth, nervousness and gastric pain. Arrangements should be made for the patients to be taken to the nearest hospital emergency department, and treatment should be repeated after 10–15 minutes if there is no improvement. Patients who have had severe reactions should be shown how to self-administer adrenaline and keep two unexpired epinephrine pens available. Details of the treatment of anaphylaxis can be obtained elsewhere.[21]

## Third-line treatments

Immunosuppressive treatments have been used in patients with severe unremitting urticaria in whom endogenous histamine-releasing factors have been demonstrated by a positive autologous serum skin test.

An uncontrolled trial of plasmapheresis in eight patients with severe chronic urticaria refractory to antihistamines and histamine-releasing activity in the serum demonstrated temporary symptomatic improvement in six and clearance of urticaria in two of these for 3 and 8 weeks.[22] The patient who relapsed after 8 weeks was treated subsequently with prednisolone tapering from 30 to 0 mg over 2 months and azathioprine between 150 and 100 mg daily. Her urticaria remitted and then remained clear on azathioprine alone, suggesting that it may have potential in the management of this group of patients.

Methotrexate at a dose of 15 mg/ week was thought to induce remission in a patient with urticaria uncontrolled on prednisolone 20 mg/day.[23]

Of 12 patients with severe chronic urticaria treated with cyclosporin at 2.5–3.5 mg/kg per day for 4 weeks in an open study, 9 improved or cleared.[24] Some of the effect may have been due to inhibition of mast cell histamine release in addition to immunosuppression. Seven of the responders were still improved over a month after stopping treatment and two remained clear at 12 weeks. Eight experienced reversible tremor, nausea or parasthesia, but none developed hypertension or abnormal renal function, unlike the three patients treated by Fradin et al.[25] Their patients responded rapidly to 6 mg/kg per day cyclosporin but treatment had to be withdrawn because of toxicity. The efficacy of cyclosporin at a dose of 4 mg/kg per day for 1–2 months has recently been confirmed in a double-blind randomized placebo-controlled study of 30 patients with severe chronic urticaria and a positive autologous serum test.[26]

Ten patients with severe chronic urticaria and a positive autologous serum test were treated with intravenous immunoglobulin infusions (IVIG) at 0.4 g/kg per day for 5 days in a regimen used for autoimmune disease. Clinical benefit was noted in nine.[27] Of these, three remained in remission after 3 years, one following an initial relapse and a further course of IVIG. The encouraging results of immunosuppressive treatment need to be confirmed in placebo-controlled trials, and in patients with or without demonstrable histamine-releasing activity in the serum.

The results of subcutaneous interferon-alpha at 3 MIU three times per week for chronic urticaria was disappointing, although some patients appeared to show an early partial response.[28,29]

## Physical urticarias

Severe cases of physical urticaria remain difficult to treat.

In symptomatic dermographism, potent topical steroids under occlusion for 6 weeks reduce itching and wealing,[30] but potential use is limited. Treatment with photochemotherapy has been useful for some patients.[31]

For cold urticaria, low-sedation antihistamines rather than cyproheptadine are the treatment of choice. The use of 'desensitization' or induction of tolerance with frequent exposures to cold has been re-emphasized.[32] Combination therapy with terbutaline (3 × 2.5 mg daily) and aminophylline (3 × 150 mg daily) for at least 6 weeks improved lesions in 37/42 patients.[33] In a family with familial cold urticaria, stanozolol 5 mg daily to twice a day improved four patients.[34] The anabolic steroid danazol at a dose of 200 mg three times a day has been used to treat severe cholinergic urticaria.[35]

Uncontrolled observations in small numbers of patients with delayed pressure urticaria, have suggested that dapsone 50 mg daily[36] and sulphasalazine[37] may be a useful therapy.

Plasmapheresis is a potential therapy for the most severely affected patients with solar urticaria.[38]

## Conclusion

The unpredictability and lack of an identifiable cause of the urticaria for many patients can be frustrating, but attention to detail in therapeutic manoeuvres can be rewarding for patients and physicians alike.

Immunotherapy may be of value for those not responding to conventional therapy in the future once its usefulness and safety have been established in placebo-controlled studies.

# References

1.  Zuberbier T, Ifflander J, Semmler C, Henz BM, Acute urticaria: clinical aspects and therapeutic responsiveness. *Acta Derm Venereol* 1996: 76; 295–7.

2.  Grattan CEH, Pathogenesis of chronic 'idiopathic' urticaria. *Allergy* 1995: 3; 3–11.

3.  Hide M, Francis DM, Grattan CEH et al, Autoantibodies against the high-affinity IgE receptor as a cause of histamine release in chronic urticaria. *N Engl J Med* 1993: 328; 1599–601.

4.  Grattan CEH, Francis DM, Hide M, Greaves MW, Detection of circulating histamine releasing autoantibodies with functional properties of anti-IgE in chronic urticaria. *Clin Exp Allergy* 1991: 21; 659–704.

5.  Niimi N, Francis DM, Kermani F et al, Dermal mast cell activation by autoantibodies against the high affinity IgE receptor in chronic urticaria. *J Invest Dermatol* 1996: 106; 1001–6.

6.  Kermani F, Niimi N, Francis DM, O'Donnell BF et al, Characterization of a novel mast cell-specific histamine releasing activity in chronic idiopathic urticaria. *J Invest Dermatol* 1995: 105; 452.

7.  O'Donnell BF, Lawlor F, Simpson J et al, The impact of chronic urticaria on the quality of life. *Br J Dermatol* 1997: 136; 197–201.

8.  Poon E, Seed PT, Greaves MW, Kobza Black A, The extent and nature of disability in different urticarial conditions. *Br J Dermatol* 1999: 140; 667–71.

9.  Simons FER, Simons KJ, The pharmacology and use of H₁-receptor antagonist drugs. *New Engl J Med* 1994: 330; 1663–70.

10.  Prakash A, Lamb HM, Mizolastine. A review of its use in allergic rhinitis and chronic urticaria. *Biodrugs* 1998: 10; 41–63.

11.  Greaves ME, Antihistamine treatment: a patient self-assessment method in chronic urticaria. *BMJ* 1981: 283; 1435–7.

12.  Sabroe RA, Seed PT, Stat C et al, Chronic idiopathic urticaria: comparison of the clinical features of patients with and without anti-Fcε RI or anti-IgE autoantibodies. *J Am Acad Dermatol* 1999: 40; 443–50.

13.  Simons FER, H₁-receptor antagonists. Comparative tolerability and safety. *Drug Safety* 1994: 10; 350–80.

14.  Handley DA, Magnetti A, Higgins AJ, Therapeutic advantages of third generation antihistamines. *Exp Opin Drugs* 1998: 7; 1045–54.

15.  Spangler DL, Vanderpool GE, Carrol MS, Tinkelman DG, Terbutaline in the treatment of chronic urticaria. *Ann Allergy* 1980: 45; 246–7.

16.  Liu H-N, Pan L-M, Chu T-L, Nifedipine treatment of chronic urticaria: a double-blind cross-over study. *J Dermatol Treat* 1990: 1; 187–9.

17.  Bressler RB, Sowell K, Huston DP, Therapy of chronic idiopathic urticaria with nifedipine: demonstration of beneficial effect in a doule-blinded, placebo-controlled, cross over study. *J Allergy Clin Immunol* 1989: 83; 756–63.

92    Dermatologic Therapy in Current Practice

18. Ellingsen AR, Thestrup-Pedersen K, Treatment of chronic idiopathic urticaria with topical steroids. An open trial. *Acta Derm Venereol* 1996: 76; 43–4.

19. Brestel EP, Thrush LB, The treatment of chronic glucocorticoid dependent chronic urticaria with stanozolol. *J Allergy Clin Immunol* 1988: 82; 265–9.

20. Ellis MH, Successful treatment of chronic urticaria with leukotriene antagonists. *J Allergy Clin Immunol* 1988: 102; 876–7.

21. Bochner BS, Lichtenstein LM, Anaphylaxis. *New Engl J Med* 1992: 324; 1785–90.

22. Grattan CEH, Francis DM, Slater NGP et al, Plasmapheresis for severe, unremitting, chronic urticaria. *Lancet* 1992: 339; 1078–80.

23. Weiner MJ, Methotrexate in corticosteroid resistant urticaria. *Ann Int Med* 1989: 110; 848.

24. Barlow RJ, Kobza Black A, Greaves MW, Treatment of severe chronic urticaria with cyclosporin. *Eur J Dermatol* 1993: 3; 273–5.

25. Fradin MS, Ellis CN, Goldfarb MT, Vorhees JJ, Oral cyclosporine for severe chronic idiopathic urticaria and angio-oedema. *J Am Acad Dermatol* 1991: 25; 1065–7.

26. Grattan CEH, OiDonnell BF, Francis DM et al, Randomized double-blind study of cyclosporin in chronic 'idiopathic' urticaria. *Br J Dermatol* 2000: 143; 365–72.

27. O'Donnell BF, Barlow RJ, Kobza Black A, Greaves MW, Intravenous immunoglobulin in autoimmune chronic urticaria. *Br J Dermatol* 1998: 138; 101–6.

28. Torrelo A, Harto A, Ledo A, Interferon therapy for chronic urticaria. *J Am Acad Dermatol* 1995: 32; 684–5.

29. Czarnetzki B, Algermissen B, Jeep S et al, Interferon treatment of patients with chronic urticaria and mastocytosis. *J Am Acad Dermatol* 1994: 30; 500–1.

30. Lawlor F, Kobza Black A, Murdoch FD, Greaves MW, Symptomatic dermographism, wealing, mast cells and histamine are decreased in skin following application of a potent topical steroid. *Br J Dermatol* 1989: 121; 629–34.

31. Logan RA, O'Brien TJ, Greaves MW, The effect of psoralen phototherapy (PUVA) on symptomatic dermographism. *Clin Exp Dermatol* 1989: 14; 25–8.

32. Henquet CJM, Martens BPM, Van Vloten WA, Cold urticaria: a clinico-therapeutic study in 30 patients; with special emphasis on cold desensitization. *Eur J Dermatol* 1992: 2; 75–7.

33. Husz S, Toth-Kasa I, Kiss M, Dobozy A, Treatment of cold urticaria. *Int J Dermatol* 1994: 33; 210–3.

34. Ormerod AD, Smart I, Reid TMS, Milford-Ward A, Familial cold urticaria. Investigation of a family and response to stanozolol. *Arch Dermatol* 1993: 129; 343–6.

35. Wong E, Eftekhari N, Greaves MW, Milford Ward A, Beneficial effects of danazol on symptoms and laboratory changes in cholinergic urticaria. *Br J Dermatol* 1987: 116; 553–6.

36. Gould DJ, Campbell D, Dayani A, Delayed pressure urticaria. Successful treatment of 5 cases with dapsone. *Br J Dermatol* 1991: 125(Suppl 38); 25.

37.  Spangler RJM, Squire E, Benson P, Chronic sulfasalazine therapy in the treatment of delayed pressure urticaria and angioedema. *Ann Allergy Asthma Immunol* 1995: 74; 155–9.

38.  Duschet P, Leyen P, Schwarz T et al, Solar urticaria – effective treatment by plasmapheresis. *Clin Exp Dermatol* 1987: 12; 185–8.

# 8

# The management of the photodermatoses

*James Ferguson*

## Introduction

The photodermatoses, as a diagnostic group, can be usefully subdivided into distinct disorders (Table 8.1) each of which has an individual management programme.

The therapeutic pitfall with this group of disorders is to see the clinical problem as purely light avoidance. The majority of these complaints have abnormal sensitivity which may extend from the UVB into the UVA and even the visible wavebands. When severe, difficulties may arise even during the winter months, when light avoidance is difficult and topical sunscreen use may only be of limited benefit. Other stratagems have had to be developed to maintain any sort of quality of life. Unfortunately, systemic sunscreens are not yet a reality and numerous other systemic agents, each of which has a putative mechanistic basis, have been assessed, albeit with limited study, and have been found wanting.

| Table 8.1 The photodermatoses | |
|---|---|
| Idiopathic | Polymorphic light eruption (PLE) <br> Actinic prurigo (AP) <br> Chronic actinic dermatitis (CAD) <br> Solar urticaria (SU) <br> Hydroa vaccineforme (HV) <br> Juvenile spring eruption (JSE) |
| Drug/chemical-induced | Photocontact/systemic |
| Cutaneous porphyrias | Erythropoietic protoporphyria (EPP) <br> Porphyria cutanea tarda (PCT) <br> Variegate porphyria (VP) and others |
| Genophotodermatoses | Xeroderma pigmentosum <br> Rothmund Thomson and others |
| Photoaggravated | Psoriasis, atopic dermatitis, lupus erythematosus |

# Individual disease management

## Polymorphic light eruption (PLE)

The management programme for PLE is outlined in Table 8.2.[1] As in all disease management, therapy is proportional to disease severity and the degree of disruption to normal life.

For the great majority who are mildly affected when exposed to holiday sunshine, control of sunlight exposure coupled with the careful use of a broad waveband (UVB/A) photoprotective sunblock[2,3] may allow a gradual increase in natural protection, i.e. tanning (hardening) with relative freedom over the vacation and subsequent summer. Such a process, although easy to suggest in the clinic, is

not always so easy to follow for the patient. The dose per unit time of UV experienced by a patient varies greatly with latitude, time of day/year, and such factors as pollution and cloud cover. Patients naturally find it difficult to 'judge' their exposure to achieve their 'hardened skin' required. In time the development of an electronic dosimeter should enable a more accurate and therefore safer approach.

For those more severely affected PLE patients who have problems in UK sunlight, a different photoprotective approach is required. Artificial induction of hardening (often termed desensitization) has been used successfully in a range of photodermatoses[4,5] and is considered the treatment of choice for those patients unsuccessfully managed with the basic approach. The

### Table 8.2 Polymorphic light eruption management programme

| | |
|---|---|
| Investigation | If diagnostic doubt phototest (exclude solar urticaria) Consider sunscreen allergy/photoallergy: patch/photopatch test Exclude PLE-like variant of LE |
| Provide | Patient information |
| Discuss | Nature and sources of UV radiation Avoidance of allergens/photoallergens |
| Demonstrate | Use of appropriate broad spectrum sunblock. Topical steroid-reducing regimen |
| Consider | UVB (broad or narrowband) or PUVA desensitization |

N.B. Although a wide range of systemic agents, including antimalarials, nicotinamide, E. coli extract and beta carotene have been used, controlled study data are required to convince clinicians disappointed with their results. Sample information sheets are available at http://www.dundee.ac.uk/dermatology

principle of such treatment is simple. Early on in the sunshine season (i.e. springtime in regions furthest from the equator), a course of phototherapy (UVB) or photochemotherapy (PUVA) is administered to those sites normally exposed to sunlight. Careful increments between treatments allows a build-up of skin thickening and pigmentation with subsequent photoprotection which, if topped up with natural sunlight, will provide an 'in-built' sunscreen for the rest of the summer. There are, however, problems, so great care must be taken to tailor the procedure to each patient's requirements.[6-8]

Although a range of successful methodologies have been used, they generally follow a similar pattern (Table 8.3). The minimal erythema dose (MED), or the minimal phototoxic dose (MPD) in the case of PUVA, is determined. The starting dose is taken as 70% of the MED, increments are controlled at 20% or 10% with a downward adjustment according to the severity of the skin response during previous treatment. Different centres will have different regimens which will depend on the different skin type populations as well as local factors such as distance to travel, etc.

As artificially induced photoprotection is a localized skin effect, a decision must be made at the start of therapy whether to treat limited areas or the whole body. One policy has been to

## Table 8.3 Narrow-band UVB phototherapy desensitization regimen

1. Determination of minimal erythema dose (MED)

2. First exposure – 70% of MED

3. Subsequent exposures

| | | |
|---|---|---|
| (a) | if no erythema | Increase by 20% at each visit |
| (b) | minimal erythema | Same dose |
| (c) | asymptomatic, well-defined erythema | Postpone exposure until next visit. Then same dose, and thereafter 10% increments at each visit |
| (d) | painful erythema ± oedema or bullae | Omit further exposures until recovery. Reduce exposure dose by half; thereafter 10% increments at each visit |

Outpatients: 15 exposures; Monday, Wednesday, Friday × 5 weeks

Inpatients: 10 exposures; Monday–Friday × 2 weeks

treat the whole body in milder cases and limited areas in those severely affected, i.e. only exposing those areas considered essential to expose. The latter group are asked to choose clothing items of thick cotton which will be worn in exactly the same fashion during desensitization treatment (Fig. 8.1).

Prior to starting therapy, it is important to emphasize that each patient is different and that the first desensitization course is exploratory, usually providing information on increments that can be tolerated without PLE induction for future course planning. Often the second and subsequent courses are less hazardous as the individual's programme has been established. In addition, it is important that patients are advised how to 'top up' with natural sunlight, so that the artificially induced photoprotection is not lost. This can be a problem if desensitization is conducted too early in the year or if the weather, post-treatment, is poor. Clearly little can be done about the latter.

Patients usually value an information sheet not only about their photodermatosis but also what to expect and what is expected of them during and after a desensitization course.

Occasionally treatment with potent topical or even systemic steroid may be required for those patients experiencing a disease flare during desensitization.

The preferred choice of desensitization source continues to be debated. PUVA does seem to have some long-

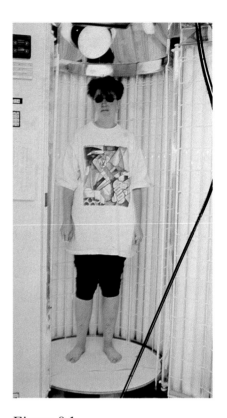

## Figure 8.1

Young (PLE) patient undergoing limited skin site desensitization in a UVB light cubicle.

term disadvantage when compared with broadband UVB.[9] More recently, the TL-01 narrow-band source has become generally available and has proved an effective alternative in the management of PLE.[10] It has also been shown to be of value in other photodermatoses.[11]

## Actinic prurigo (AP)

Although similar to the management of
PLE, AP is usually of greater severity
and desensitization may require
patience. As the age of onset of AP is
frequently in the first decade, UVB
seems a better approach for those
considered too young for PUVA.[12-14]
The management programme is essentially as for PLE. One important option
for therapy-resistant cases is to
consider the use of thalidomide. This
oral hypnotic and immunosuppressive
agent has been frequently reported to
be effective in AP.[15] Unfortunately,
sedation, dizziness, teratogenic effects
and a high incidence of peripheral
neuropathy have greatly restricted its
use. In addition, it is very difficult to
obtain supplies.

## Chronic actinic dermatitis (CAD)

Also known as photosensitivity
dermatitis and actinic reticuloid
syndrome (PD/AR), this condition can
present in a variety of ways.[16] The
diagnosis can be difficult for broad-
spectrum UV sensitivity which extends
into the visible region is accompanied
by multiple contact allergy to a wide
range of agents.[16] The key to management is through phototest, patch and
photopatch test investigations (Table
8.4). Management of an acute flare
requires steroid therapy.

### Table 8.4 Chronic actinic dermatitis management programme

| | |
|---|---|
| Define | Wavelength dependency of abnormal responses |
| | Contact and photoallergens |
| Discuss | Nature and sources of UV and visible radiation |
| | Relevance of occupation and other environmental factors |
| | Role and avoidance of contact allergens |
| Demonstrate use of | Appropriate sunscreens usually of a broad spectrum, non-fragrant sunblock type |
| | Emulsifying ointment as a soap substitute |
| | Reducing-strength topical steroid regimen for flares |

If severe and fails to respond to the above:

| | |
|---|---|
| Consider | Extending patch test series (missed allergens) |
| | Use of Museum film[18] |
| | Phototherapy (UVB) |
| | Photochemotherapy (PUVA) |
| | Azathioprine, cyclosporin |

CAD can be managed in the majority of cases with simple photoprotective measures[17,18] and contact allergen avoidance. There is, however, need for awareness of new allergen development. Although most patients can avoid the need for long-term systemic immunosuppression, cyclosporin and/or azathioprine is required for those who fail to achieve a satisfactory result with simpler measures.[19,20]

## Solar urticaria (SU)

This uncommon photodermatosis although often arising spontaneously may also rarely be due to heat, drugs and the cutaneous porphyrias. For many, complete or partial suppression with non-sedative antihistamines ($H_1$ or $H_1+H_2$) produces a satisfactory outcome[21] (Fig. 8.2). For others (Table 8.5), topical photoprotection tailored to the SU wavelength dependency is

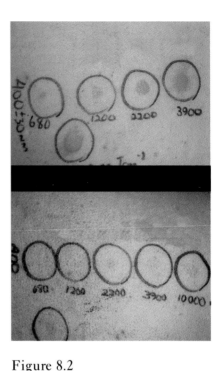

### Figure 8.2

Two hours after cetirizine (10 mg) the repeat monochromator provocation test reveals complete urticarial suppression.

| Table 8.5 Solar urticaria management programme | |
| --- | --- |
| Define | Wavelength dependency by phototesting |
| Discuss | Sources of causal wavelengths |
| | Appropriate sunscreen use |
| Consider | Non-sedative antihistamine use ($H_1 + H_2$) |
| | Phototherapy/photochemotherapy |
| | Hydroxychloroquine |
| | Plasmapheresis |

adequate. In those who fail with topical prevention, careful desensitizing phototherapy or photochemotherapy should be considered. In the most severe cases unresponsive to the above, plasmapheresis (in those with a positive intradermal test) has been shown to be successful in some cases.[22,23]

## Hydroa vacciniforme (HV)

Conventional sunscreens appear rarely to help in this uncommon condition. Desensitization with UVA has been reported to be effective.[24] PUVA, although tried, has been associated with vesicle provocation, a finding to be expected for UVA wavelengths are known to provoke HV. The most recent development is the finding that narrow-band UVB is an effective prophylaxis.[7,11]

## Juvenile spring eruption (JSE)

This underdiagnosed condition, which particularly affects males, is best treated with sunscreen or encouragement to grow hair over the ears. The condition is usually mild and self limiting.

## Drug/chemical-induced photosensitivity

The simple identification and the removal of a topical drug/chemical or the systemic therapeutic agent responsible will result in improvement. Unfortunately, some agents[25] can persist in the skin for many months. In these, knowledge of the causal wavelength will enable correct photoprotection to be chosen. Occasionally, a systemic agent such as amiodarone cannot (for medical reasons) be stopped. UVB phototherapy or PUVA desensitization can be considered in such cases.[11] Although phototoxicity is the commonest mechanism, occasionally drug-induced lupus erythematosus, pellagra and pseudoporphyria are diagnostic pitfalls.

## Cutaneous porphyrias

Management of this disease group is covered elsewhere.[26,27] Visible wavelength sunscreen protection may be of partial assistance (Table 8.6). In erythropoietic protoporphyria (but not the rarer, more severe porphyrias) desensitization may be of help.[11]

## Genophotodermatoses (xeroderma pigmentosum, XP)

The management of patients with XP is based on early diagnosis by cell mutation studies, lifelong protection from UV exposure by modifications in behaviour, the use of appropriate clothing and the use of broad spectrum photoprotection. Clinical monitoring to enable early diagnosis and treatment of skin cancer is essential.

## Table 8.6 Erythropoietic protoporphyria/ porphyria cutanea tarda management programme

Erythropoietic protoporphyria
| | |
|---|---|
| Try | Titanium, zinc (pigmentary grade), visible wavelength topical photoprotection |
| Consider | Beta-carotene 60–300 mg/day[27] Phototherapy desensitization |

Porphyria cutanea tarda
| | |
|---|---|
| Consider | Hydroxychloroquine, low dose Venesection Avoid hepatotoxins |

## Conclusion

As the photodermatoses are a diverse group of conditions, it is not surprising that their management is quite different from disease to disease. Nevertheless, common factors do exist. To be precise, to avoid UV radiation it is necessary to have a clear understanding of the nature of sunlight and artificial sources. It is also important to know not only how but also which sunscreens to use for individual diseases. Perhaps the most important recent development, which is relevant for the majority of the diseases, is desensitization. We have improved our knowledge regarding which type of light source, and when and how this form of treatment should be used.

## References

1. Ferguson J, Polymorphic light eruption and actinic prurigo. *Curr Probl Dermatol* 1990: 11; 127–47.

2. Holzle E, Plewig G, Hofmann C et al, Polymorphous light eruption. Experimental reproduction of skin lesions. *J Am Acad Dermatol* 1982: 7; 111–25.

3. Nordlund JJ, Klaus SN, Mathews-Roth MM et al, New therapy for polymorphous light eruption. *Arch Dermatol* 1973: 108; 710–12.

4. Ortel B, Tanew A, Wolff K et al, Polymorphous light eruption: Action spectrum and photoprotection. *J Am Acad Dermatol* 1986: 14; 748–53.

5. Addo HA, Sharma SC, UVB phototherapy and photochemotherapy (PUVA) in the treatment of polymorphic

light eruption and solar urticaria. *Br J Dermatol* 1987: 116; 539–47.

6. Bilsland D, Ferguson J, The management of polymorphic light eruption. *J Dermatol Treat* 1992: 3; 99–101.

7. Ferguson J, The management of the photodermatoses with phototherapy. In: Honigsmann H, Jori G, Young AR (eds) *The fundamental bases of phototherapy.* Milano: OEMF Spa, 1996, pp. 171–9.

8. Man I, Dawe RS, Ferguson J, Artificial hardening for polymorphic light eruption: practical points from ten years' experience. *Photodermatol Photoimmunol Photomed* 1999: 15; 96–9.

9. de Gruijl FR, Long-term side effects and carcinogenesis risk in UVB therapy. In: Honigsmann H, Jori G, Young AR (eds) *The fundamental bases of phototherapy.* Milano: OEMF Spa, 1996, pp. 153–70.

10. Bilsland D, George SA, Gibbs NK et al, A comparison of narrow band phototherapy (TL-01) and photochemotherapy (PUVA) in the management of polymorphic light eruption. *Br J Dermatol* 1993: 129; 708–12.

11. Collins P, Ferguson J, Narrow-band UVB (TL-01) phototherapy: an effective preventative treatment for the photodermatoses. *Br J Dermatol* 1995: 132; 956–63.

12. Orr PH, Birt AR, Hereditary polymorphic light eruption in Canadian Inuit. *Int J Dermatol* 1984: 23; 472–5.

13. Birt AR, Hogg GR, The actinic cheilitis of hereditary polymorphic light eruption. *Arch Dermatol* 1979: 115; 699–702.

14. Farr PM, Diffey BL, Treatment of actinic prurigo with PUVA: mechanism of action. *Br J Dermatol* 1989: 120; 411–18.

15. Lovell CR, Hawk JLM, Calnan CD et al, Thalidomide in actinic prurigo. *Br J Dermatol* 1983: 108; 467–71.

16. Ferguson J, Photosensitivity dermatitis and actinic reticuloid syndrome (chronic actinic dermatitis). *Semin Dermatol* 1990: 9; 47–54.

17. Ferguson J, The management of the photosensitivity dermatitis and actinic reticuloid (PD/AR) syndrome. *J Dermatol Treat* 1990: 1; 143–5.

18. Dawe R, Russell S, Ferguson J, Borrowing from museums and industry: two photoprotective devices. *Br J Dermatol* 1996: 135; 1016–17.

19. Murphy GM, Maurice PDL, Norris PG et al, Azathioprine treatment in chronic actinic dermatitis: a double-blind controlled trial with monitoring of exposure to ultraviolet radiation. *Br J Dermatol* 1989: 121; 639–46.

20. Norris PG, Camp RDR, Hawk JLM, Actinic reticuloid: response to cyclosporine. *J Am Acad Dermatol* 1989: 21; 307–9.

21. Bilsland D, Ferguson J, The management of idiopathic solar urticaria. *J Dermatol Treat* 1991: 1; 321–3.

22. Duschet P, Leyen P, Schwarz T et al, Solar urticaria – effective treatment by plasmapheresis. *Clin Exp Dermatol* 1987: 12; 185–8.

23. Leenutaphong V, Holzle E, Plewig G et al, Plasmapheresis in solar urticaria. *Photodermatology* 1987: 4; 308–9.

24. Sonnex TS, Hawk JLM, Hydroa vacciniforme: a review of ten cases. *Br J Dermatol* 1988: 118; 101–8.

25. Johnson BE, Ferguson J, Drug and chemical photosensitivity. *Semin Dermatol* 1990: 9; 39–46.

26.  Bickers DR, Merk H, The treatment of the porphyrias. *Semin Dermatol* 1986: 5; 186–97.

27.  Todd DJ, Erythropoietic protoporphyria. *Br J Dermatol* 1994: 131; 751–66.

# 9

# The management of ichthyotic disorders

*Peter CM van de Kerkhof and Peter M Steijlen*

The following ichthyotic skin disorders of cornification are presented in this chapter: Ichthyoses (ichthyosis vulgaris, X-linked recessive ichthyosis, congenital ichthyoses), palmoplantar keratoderma (orthokeratotic disorders, acanthokeratolytic disorders), erythrokeratoderma variabilis of Mendes da Costa, Darier's disease, and pityriasis rubra pilaris. The presentation of these classes of disorders of cornification is by no means complete. For a more comprehensive review of the literature the reader is referred to a recent monograph.[4]

## Introduction

Ichthyotic disorders comprise both acquired and hereditary skin disorders which are clinically characterized by excessive scaling covering a substantial part of the body. In this chapter the term 'ichthyotic disorders' will be used as a designation for the large repertoire of disorders of cornification. Keratinocytes are generated in the basal layer of the epidermis and move to the surface through successive stages of differentiation. This process of differentiation and cornification involves complex metabolic changes, including programmed alterations in cell proteins, membrane glycosylation and lipid biosynthesis.[1-3] Ichthyotic disorders comprise a large and heterogeneous group of skin diseases. In general, the ichthyotic disorders are monogenic with a Mendelian inheritance. A few have a polygenic inheritance or are acquired.

## General treatment approaches

The treatment of ichthyotic skin disorders is, until now, non-specific. In general the following approaches are used.

### Bland emollients

Bland emollients smooth the skin and improve the appearance. Indeed in mildly affected patients, applications of emollients may be the sole approach.

### Keratolytics

Where there are hyperkeratotic lesions, the application of keratolytics may be indicated. Salicylic acid (5–20%) in an ointment base may result in substantial improvements. Propylene glycol 50% in water, applied under plastic occlusion, is another approach which may help considerably where there is hyperkeratosis. Urea as a 10% o/w cream is helpful in ichthyosis and dry skin condition, but its mode of action is not known.

## Topical retinoids

The use of all-*trans*-retinoic acid and 13-*cis*-retinoic acid is well established in acne,[5] and these preparations have also proved to be helpful in several ichthyotic disorders.[6-10]

## Vitamin D₃ analogues

The effect of calcipotriol in disorders of keratinization is well established.[11,12] The value of the analogues and calcitriol and tacalcitol in the treatment of disorders of keratinization has not been investigated so far.

## Systemic retinoids

Acitretin is the systemic retinoid of choice in various ichthyotic disorders.[13,14] Its use, however, is not restricted to the more severe manifestations.

# Ichthyosis

The ichthyosis group of disorders comprises different aetiological entities with a more or less similar clinical phenotype, characterized by a variable degree of generalized scaling.

## *Autosomal dominant ichthyosis*

The prevalence of autosomal dominant ichthyosis (ADI, sometimes known as ichthyosis vulgaris) is estimated at about 1%. Usually ADI starts during infancy. In general it is characterized by a fine white scaling.

The flexures are spared and there is marked follicular hyperkeratosis. Exaggerated skin markings on the palms and soles are also characteristic hallmarks. Filaggrin, a structural protein of the corneocytes, causing aggregation of keratin filaments, and its precursor profilaggrin are reduced in ADI.[15] The expression of ichthyosis vulgaris usually is mild and seldom causes social embarrassment.

Bland emollients are usually sufficient to control the condition. There are no controlled studies available on the efficacy of topical retinoids. A marked improvement or clearing was reported in four out of nine patients treated with calcipotriol. However, no significant difference as compared to placebo was observed.[11]

## *X-linked recessive ichthyosis*

X-linked recessive ichthyosis (XRI) has an estimated prevalence of 1:2000–1:6000 males. Like ADI, XRI has its onset in the first year of life.

Brown-coloured scales are found covering the extremities which as in ADI, leave the flexures unaffected. The trunk may be involved to a variable extent. The underlying defect is a deficiency of the enzyme steroid sulphatase which catalyses the breakdown of cholesterol sulphate.[16] Accumulation of cholesterol sulphate in the cornified cell layer causes increased cohesion between keratinocytes, and therefore retention hyperkeratosis. Two other associated features of steroid sulphatase deficiency are cryptorchidism and insufficient cervical dilatation causing premature delivery.

Although patients may respond sufficiently to emollients, many patients require a more effective treatment. 13-*cis*-Retinoic acid (0.1% in a cream) proved to be effective in three out of seven patients with XRI.[17] Patients applied treatments twice daily.

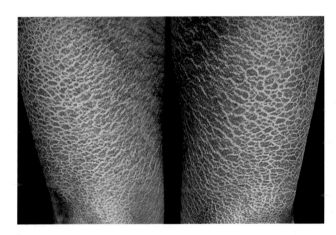

a

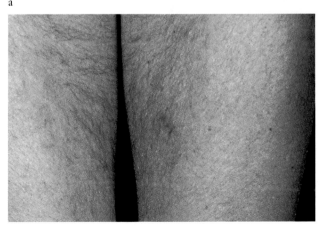

b

## Figure 9.1

A patient with X-linked-recessive ichthyosis treated with acitretin. The effect of 8 weeks treatment with acitretin (35 mg/day during 12 weeks). (a) Before treatment. (b) After 12 weeks of treatment.

Recently, we treated a group of six patients with XRI with the cytochrome P-450 inhibitor liarozole. This compound inhibits the 4-hydroxylation of all-*trans*-retinoic acid and hence has a retinoid effect. This experimental 'retinoid-like' compound caused a substantial improvement in XRI.[18]

Calcipotriol ointment has proved to be effective in XRI.[11] Out of eight patients suffering from XRI, four experienced a marked improvement following a 12-week treatment period. This improvement was much better compared to placebo treatment ($P$ = 0.03).[11]

Oral retinoid treatment with acitretin may be indicated in XRI in severely affected patients. The efficacy of acitretin in XRI is illustrated in Fig. 9.1.

# Congenital ichthyosis

## Lamellar ichthyosis

Lamellar ichthyosis is a group of very rare ichthyoses. These disorders are characterized by scaling covering the entire body surface. These disorders appear immediately after birth. In contrast to ADI and XRI, the scaling is also observed on the flexures. At the clinical level lamellar ichthyosis can be accompanied by erythroderma.

Although some authors have suggested that erythrodermic autosomal lamellar ichthyosis and non-erythrodermic autosomal recessive lamellar ichthyosis might represent different entities, no consensus has been reached on that issue so far. In some patients transglutaminase has been shown to be markedly deficient, whereas in other patients transglutaminase activity is normal.[19] From a genetic point of view two modes of inheritance have been reported: an autosomal recessive trait (most frequently) and an autosomal dominant trait (rare).

In general lamellar ichthyosis requires active treatment. Topical treatment with all-*trans*-retinoic acid[7–10] has been reported to have some therapeutic effect. However, irritation of the skin is a serious limitation. Using a bilateral paired double-blind comparison, 13-*cis*-retinoic acid (0.1% in cream) proved to be effective in seven out of nine patients with non-erythrodermic autosomal recessive lamellar ichthyosis.[17,20] Patients were instructed to apply the creams twice daily for 4 weeks. In another study, two of seven patients showed a marked improvement following treatment with 13-*cis*-retinoic acid. Irritation was observed in 33% of the patients.[17,19] The cytochrome P-450 inhibitor liarozole in a cream base proved to be effective in a group of three patients.[18]

Calcipotriol ointment proved to be highly effective in four patients.[11] The clinical response to a 12-week treatment with calcipotriol ointment was impressive.[21] Figure 9.2 illustrates this. No irritation was observed in these patients. Acitretin at doses between 10 and 60 mg per day is very effective in most cases of lamellar ichthyosis (Fig. 9.3). Out of a group of seven patients suffering from

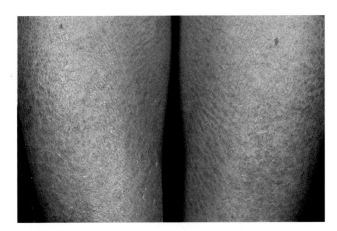

a

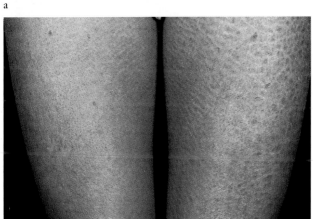

b

## Figure 9.2

A patient treated with calcipotriol ointment and its vehicle. (a) Before treatment. (b) Side treated with calcipotriol ointment (left) and side treated with the vehicle only (right).

lamellar ichthyosis, four required doses of 25 mg or lower.[22] Patients with the erythrodermic variant may respond with aggravation to doses higher than 25 mg per day. Also from a therapeutic point of view, lamellar ichthyoses are a heterogeneous group of disorders.

## Bullous ichthyosiform erythroderma and ichthyosis bullosa Siemens

Both disorders are very rare. In both conditions patients suffer from blistering and scaling from birth.

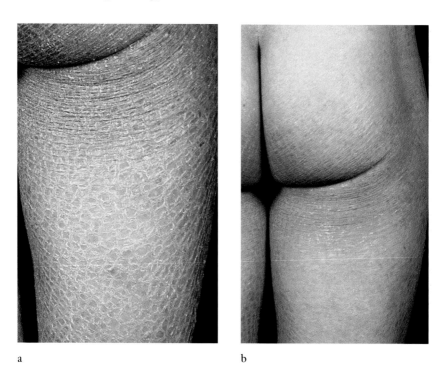

a                                          b

## Figure 9.3

A patient suffering from lamellar ichthyosis treated with acitretin (35 mg/day). (a) Before treatment. (b) After 1 month of treatment.

In bullous ichthyosiform erythroderma of Brocq (CBIE) (also known as epidermolytic hyperkeratosis) the underlying gene defect has been found in the genes coding for keratin 1 or keratin 10.[23] At first the clinical picture is characterized by bullae and erythroderma. Later in life, hyperkeratoses dominate the clinical picture.

The underlying gene defect in ichthyosis bullosa of siemens (IBS) has been found in the keratin $2^e$ cluster.[24]

The patients suffer from blistering that is more superficial than in CBIE.

Calcipotriol ointment has been reported to be successful in CBIE.[21] Topical treatment with liarozole proved to be effective in two patients with CBIE.[18] In general, patients with CBIE or IBS are treated with acitretin (lower than 25 mg/day). The clinical efficacy of low-dose acitretin in CBIE is remarkable (Fig. 9.4). If higher doses are used, blistering will occur. IBS can

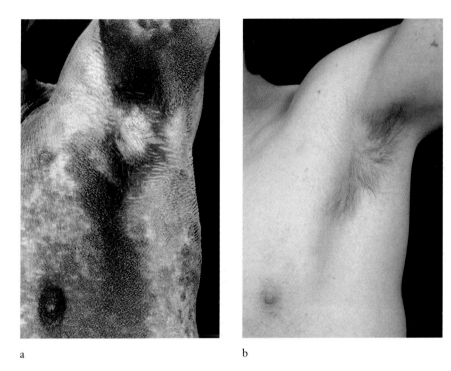

a                                    b

## Figure 9.4

A patient suffering from congenital bullous ichthyosiform erythroderma treated with etretinate (25 mg/day). (a) Before treatment. (b) After 1 month of treatment.

be treated with acitretin at doses of 25–60 mg/day. Recently, we reported the efficacy of etretinate and acitretin in IBS.[25] Figure 9.5 illustrates the response of IBS to acitretin.

## Palmoplantar keratoderm a

Palmoplantar keratoderma comprises a large collection of different disease entities.[26] The different entities can be identified by careful clinical and histological description. Of importance for the diagnosis are (i) localization of the hyperkeratosis, whether confined to the palms and soles, or transgreding; whether diffuse or confined to a linear or patchy distribution pattern; (ii) the presence or absence of associated features; (iii) the presence or absence of erythema; and (iv) histological characteristics of the hyperkeratosis. For a

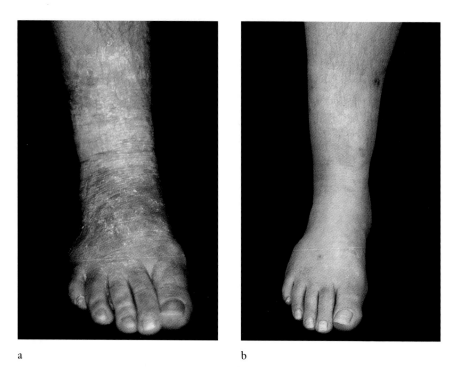

a                                        b

## Figure 9.5

A patient suffering from ichthyosis bullosa siemens (IBS) treated with acitretin
(35 mg/day). (a) Before treatment. (b) After 1 month of treatment.

detailed account the reader is referred
to a recent review.[26] In this chapter on
therapeutic management diagnostic
aspects which have a therapeutic
relevance are highlighted.

Bland emollients, keratolytics and
hydrocolloid occlusive dressings are of
relevance for all patients with palmoplantar keratoderma. Keratolytics may
be painful in the fissuring hyperkeratoses. Hydrocolloid occlusive dressings may be very helpful in cases of

painful fissuring. So far, topical
retinoids have not been shown to be
helpful in palmoplantar keratoderma.
In a placebo-controlled study, calcipotriol ointment did not prove to be
helpful.[11]

One hallmark which is crucial for the
selection of the right treatment is the
histological type of hyperkeratosis.
Patients may suffer from an orthokeratosis which is characterized by a thick
epidermis with a thickened granular

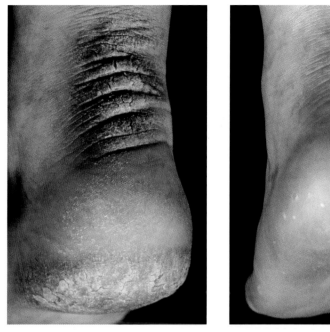
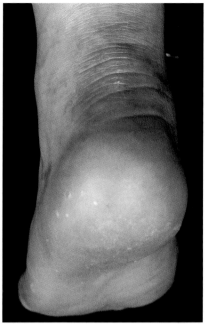

a                                                        b

## Figure 9.6

A patient with palmoplantar keratoderma Greither treated with acitretin (35 mg/day).
(a) Before treatment. (b) After 9 weeks of treatment with acitretin.

layer. However, in some cases epidermolytic change is the main histological feature of the hyperkeratosis. Palmoplantar keratoderma with epidermolytic change is also designated as Vörner's disease. Recently a case of Vörner's disease was reported in which the patient responded very well to topical calcipotriol.[27]

Acitretin at doses in the range 25–60 mg/day is indicated in the treatment of palmoplantar keratoderma with orthokeratosis. The results of this treatment are satisfactory (Fig. 9.6).[28] However, in cases of palmoplantar keratoderma with a substantial erythema, such as 'Mal de Meleda', the dosage of acitretin should be relatively low as a total elimination of the hyperkeratosis may result in tenderness.[29] In cases of epidemolytic change, acitretin treatment may result in severe fissuring, erythema and sometimes blistering; in these patients

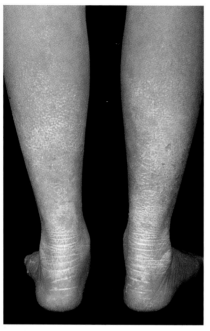
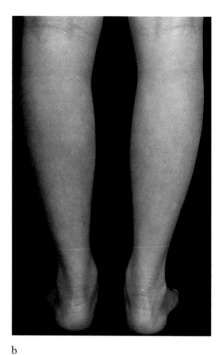

a                                          b

## Figure 9.7

A patient with erythrokeratodermia variabilis Mendes da Costa (35 mg/day). (a) Before treatment. (b) After 1 month of treatment with acitretin.

acitretin treatment is contraindicated. In palmoplantar keratoderma clinical and histological investigations are required before an adequate treatment can be selected.

## Erythroderma variabilis Mendes da Costa

Erythrokeratoderma variabilis (EKV) was described by Mendes da Costa in 1925.[30] It is a rare genodermatosis with an autosomal dominant mode of inheritance. The skin manifestations are highly characteristic. Sharply defined figurated patches of erythema that vary in size and localization are observed. In addition, sharply demarcated yellow–brown hyperkeratotic plaques of geographic outline are seen, which show a more consistent appearance. EKV usually becomes manifest during the first years of life and has a chronic course. In general, the skin manifestations are rather extensive.

In EKV acitretin treatment is indicated. So far, topical retinoids or calcipotriol have not been reported to have substantial therapeutic value. A patient with EKV was treated in the Nijmegen centre with acitretin and had a substantial improvement after only 1 month of treatment using a dose of 35 mg/day (Fig. 9.7).[31]

# Darier's disease

Darier's disease is inherited as an auto-somal dominant trait. The estimated prevalence ranges from 1:55,000 in England to 1:100,000 in Denmark. For detailed information the reader is referred to a review.[32] Skin-coloured to red-brownish papules are found on the predilection sites such as the chest, back, hairline, neck, scalp and ears. Usually, the bodyfolds such as armpits, inguinal folds, and the skin below the breasts are affected mildly. Lesions on hands and feet consist of small pits, spiky hyperkeratoses, verruca plana-like papules and nail changes. The disease usually starts between the ages of 6 and 10 years. Exacerbations occur after exposure to heat, sunlight and stress and after the use of lithium.

On histological examination acan-tholysis is found due to disruption of the desmosome-keratin-filament complexes, as observed by electron microscopy. The underlying genetic defect has recently been localized on chromosome 12.[33]

Topical treatment remains the first line of treatment and aims at keratolysis and rehydration of the stratum corneum. In most cases, however, a more active therapeutic approach is required. Topical treatment with all-*trans*-retinoic acid is effective to some extent. However irritation with aggravation of erythema and tenderness is a serious limitation. A marked improvement in topical retinoid treatment is provided by 13-*cis*-retinoic acid (0.1% cream).[20,34] Indeed, efficacy has been reported to be comparable with that of all-*trans*-retinoic acid, whereas irritation is less severe. After a 3–10-week treatment period, four of seven patients showed a clear-cut improvement compared to placebo treatment. Topical treatment with calcipotriol ointment was not successful.[11] In all patients, aggravation was observed.[35] However, some efficacy was reported by another group.[12]

Acitretin[36,37] is indicated if topical treatments cannot control the condition. However, the response to acitretin is variable. In many patients dosages of 35 mg/day or higher will cause severe aggravation. Some patients, however, need dosages of 60 mg/day. The best approach (Fig. 9.8) is to start treatment with acitretin at 10 mg/day and to increase the dosage gradually in order to find the optimal dose in the individual patient.

# Pityriasis rubra pilaris

Pityriasis rubra pilaris is relatively rare. The disorder may occur during the

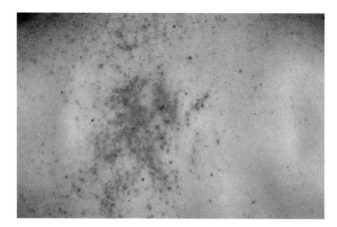

### Figure 9.8

A patient with Darier's disease treated with acitretin (35 mg/day). (a) Before treatment. (b) After 5 months of treatment.

a

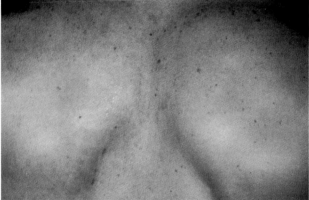

b

first decade of life, but usually the disorder manifests itself between the 40th and the 60th year of life. Several forms of pityriasis rubra pilaris exist:[38]

1. *Classical adult form (type I)* is characterized by follicular erythematous hyperkeratotic papules localized on the trunk and extremities. Erythematous areas may expand up to erythroderma. Sharply demarcated areas of symptomless skin within involved areas may be seen. Palmoplantar keratoderma and nail changes with splinter haemorrhages complete the picture. About 80% of the patients have a spontaneous remission after 1–3 years.

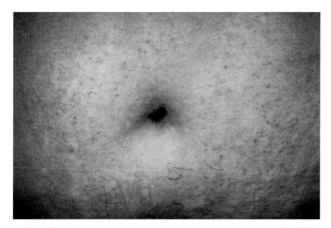

a

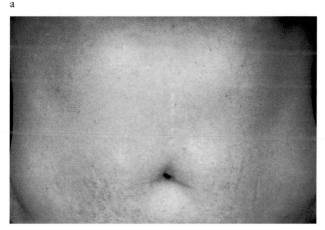

b

Figure 9.9

A patient suffering from pityriasis rubra pilaris treated with acitretin (60 mg/day).
(a) Before treatment.
(b) After treatment.

2. *Atypical adult form (type II)* comprises about 5% of patients with pityriasis rubra pilaris. The changes are less typical and are confined to some follicular hyperkeratoses and some areas with eczematous changes and lamellar scaling.

3. *Classical juvenile form (type III)* has the same hallmarks as type I.

The disorder manifests itself between the 5th and 10th year of life. Within 1–2 years spontaneous remissions may occur.

4. *Circumscribed juvenile form (type IV)* is a relatively rare form. It is characterized by sharply demarcated erythematosquamous plaques with follicular hyperkeratoses.

5. *Atypical juvenile form (type V)* is a relatively rare but severe expression of pityriasis rubra pilaris. Erythroderma and follicular plugging are the clinical hallmarks. This form may be confused with ichthyosis.

The histopathological appearance of pityriasis rubra pilaris is characterized by follicular plugging with parakeratotic foci adjacent to the plugs. Acanthosis of the epidermis and a lymphohistiocytic infiltrate are other features, but are non-specific.

Bland emollients are of some help, but in general a more active approach is required. So far, topical retinoids have not been demonstrated to be of therapeutic value in pityriasis rubra pilaris. Calcipotriol ointment has been shown to be effective in four patients suffering from pityriasis rubra pilaris.[39] It is the experience of the author that calcipotriol also contributes to the efficacy of acitretin. Acitretin is indicated in severe manifestations of pityriasis rubra pilaris.[40,41] Although the results are unpredictable, most patients show a substantial improvement (Fig. 9.9).[42] If acitretin is contraindicated or ineffective, methotrexate may be tried. The results of methotrexate in pityriasis rubra pilaris are disappointing in general.[39] Cyclosporin is not effective in pityriasis rubra pilaris.[43]

## Conclusion

Ichthyotic disorders comprise a large repertoire of distinct disease entities. In these disorders some common therapeutic principles exist. Bland emollients and keratolytics are usually indicated as a first step. Topical retinoids should be tried as an effective principle. In fact, retinoid preparations with less irritancy make this a real opportunity (13-*cis*-retinoic acid cream and adapalene cream are currently available formulations with a low irritancy potential). Calcipotriol ointment or cream is a new opportunity. However, in widespread disease it should be kept in mind that the patient may not use more than 100 g of the preparation per week.

Acitretin is a highly effective systemic treatment. Guidelines for use of acitretin should be adhered to strictly. It is of importance to realize that most patients will use acitretin over many years, if not decades. On the other hand, the management of ichthyotic disorders is to a large extent also disease specific. For example, in epidermolytic disorders acitretin is contraindicated or should be prescribed in very low doses only. In Darier's disease aggravation by irritation is frequently observed during treatment. In palmoplantar keratodermas with substantial erythema, acitretin treatment should be used in low doses.

Important new developments have appeared on the horizon. New retinoids with very low irritancy, developed for the treatment of acne and psoriasis, will certainly have a major impact on ichthyotic disorders. Cytochrome P-450 inhibitors are two enzymes of major importance for keratinization: 4-hydroxylase inhibitors and 24-hydroxylase inhibitors. 4-Hydroxylase inhibitors prevent the inactivation of active all-*trans*-retinoic acid and 24-hydroxylase inhibitors prevent the inactivation of active all-*trans*-retinoic acid and 24-hydroxylase inhibitors prevent the inactivation of active vitamin D$_3$. Therefore, the development of these compounds will have a major impact on the treatment of ichthyotic skin disorders.

# References

1. Watt FM, Terminal differentiation of epidermal keratinocytes. *Cell Biol* 1989: 1; 1107–15.

2. Eckert RL, Structure, function and differentiation of the keratinocyte. *Physiol Rev* 1989: 69; 1316–46.

3. Phillips Smack O, Korge BP, James WO, Keratin and keratinization. *J Am Acad Dermatol* 1994: 30; 85–102.

4. Traupe H, *The ichthyioses. a guide to clinical diagnosis, genetic counseling and therapy*. Berlin: Springer-Verlag, 1989.

5. Elbaum OJ, Comparison of stability of topical isotretinoin and topical tretinoin and their efficacy in acne. *J Am Acad Dermatol* 1988: 19; 486–91.

6. Fulton JE, Gross PR, Cornelius CE, Kligman AM, Darier's disease. treatment with topical vitamin D3 acid. *Arch Dermatol* 1968: 98; 396–9.

7. Stüttgen G, Zur lokalbehandlung von Keratosen mit Vitamin-A-säure. *Dermatologica* 1962: 124; 65–80.

8. Beer P, Untersuchungen über die wirkung der Vitamin-A-säure. *Dermatologica* 1962: 124; 192–5.

9. Plewig G, Wolff HH, Braun Falco O, Lokalbehandlung normaler und pathologischer menschlicher Haut mit Vitamin-A-säure. Klinische, histologische und elektronmikroskopische Untersuchungen. *Arch Klin Exp Dermatol* 1971: 239; 390–413.

10. Muller SA, Belcher RW, Esterly NB et al, Keratinizing dermatoses, combined data from four centres on short-term topical treatment with tretinoin. *Arch Dermatol* 1977: 113; 1052–4.

11. Kragballe K, Steijlen PM, Ibsen HH et al, Efficacy tolerability and safety of calcipotriol ointment in disorders of keratinization: results of a randomized, double blind, vesicle controlled, right/left comparative study. *Arch Dermatol* 1995: 131; 556–60.

12. Simonart T, Peny MO, Noel JC, De Dobbeleer G, Topical calcipotriol in the treatment of Darier's disease. *Eur J Dermatol* 1996: 6; 36–8.

13. Happle R, Van de Kerkhof PCM, Traupe H, Retinoids in disorders of keratinization: their use in adults. *Dermatologica* 1987: 175(Suppl 1); 107–24.

14. Van de Kerkhof PCM, Retinoids – prospects of new applications in dermatology. *Retinoids Tomorrow Today* 1996: 45; 2–4.

15. Nirunsuksimi W, Presland RB, Brunbaugh SG, Decreased profilaggrin expression in ichthyosis vulgaris is a result of selectively impaired posttranscriptional control. *J Biol Chem* 1995: 270; 871–6.

16. Shapiro LJ, Weiss R, Webster O, France JT, X-linked ichthyosis due to steroid sulphatase deficiency. *Lancet* 1978: 1; 70–2.

17. Lucker GPH, Van de Kerkhof PCM, Castelijns FACM et al, Topical treatment

of ichthyosis with 13-*cis*-retinoid acid. A clinical and immunohistochemical study. *Eur J Dermatol* 1995: 5; 566–71.

18.   Lucker GPH, Heremans AMC, Boegheim PJ, Steijlen PM, Topical liarozole treatment of hereditary ichthyosis: a double blind, bilaterally paired, clinical and immunohistochemical study *J Invest Dermatol* 1999: 105; 496 (Abstract).

19.   Huber M, Rettler I, Bernasconi K et al, Mutations of keratinocyte transglutaminase in lamellar ichthyosis. *Science* 1995: 267; 525–8.

20.   Steijlen PM, Reifenschweiler DOH, Happle R et al, Topical treatment of ichthyosis and Darier's disease with 13-cis-retinoic acid. A clinical and immunohistological study. *Arch Dermatol* 1993: 285; 221–6.

21.   Lucker GPH, van de Kerkhof PCM, van Dijk MR, Steijlen PM, Effect of topical calcipotriol on congenital ichthyosis. *Br J Dermatol* 1994: 131; 546–50.

22.   Steijlen PM, van Dooren-Greebe RJ, van de Kerkhof PCM, Acitretin in the treatment of lamellar ichthyosis. *Br J Dermatol* 1994: 130; 211–4.

23.   Digiovanna JJ, Ball SJ, Clinical heterogeneity in epidermolytic hyperkeratoses. *Arch Dermatol* 1994: 130; 1026–35.

24.   Kremer H, Zeeuwen P, McLean WHI et al, Ichthyosis bullosa of Siemens is caused by mutation in the keratin 2e gene. *J Invest Dermatol* 1994: 103; 286–9.

25.   Steijlen PM, Van Dooren-Greebe RJ, Happle R, van de Kerkhof PCM, Ichthyosis bullosa of Siemens responds well to low-dosage oral retinoids. *Br J Dermatol* 1991: 125; 469–71.

26.   Lucker GPH, van de Kerkhof PCM, Steijlen PM, The hereditary palmoplantar keratoses: an updated review and classification. *Br J Dermatol* 1994: 131; 1–14.

27.   Lucker GPH, van de Kerkhof PCM, Steijlen PM, Topical calcipotriol in the treatment of epidermolytic palmoplantar keratoderma of Vörner. *Br J Dermatol* 1992: 2; 503–5.

28.   van de Kerkhof PCM, van Dooren-Greebe RJ, Steijlen PM, On the efficacy of acitretin in keratodermia palmaris et plantaris transgrediens et progrediens Greither. *Eur J Dermatol* 1992: 2; 503–5.

29.   van de Kerkhof PCM, van Dooren-Greebe RJ, Steijlen PM, Acitretin in the treatment of mal de Meleda. *Br J Dermatol* 1992: 127; 191–2.

30.   Mendes da Costa S, Erythro-keratodermia variabilis in mother and a daughter. *Acta Derm Venereol* 1925: 6; 225–61.

31.   van de Kerkhof PCM, Steijlen PM, van Dooren-Greebe RJ et al, Acitretin in the treatment of erythrokeratodermia variabilis. *Dermatologica* 1990: 181; 330–3.

32.   Burge SM, Wilkinson WD, Darier-White disease: a review of the clinical features in 163 patients. *J Am Acad Dermatol* 1992: 27; 40–50.

33.   Richard G, Wright AR, Harris S et al, Fine mapping of the Darier's disease locus on chromosome 12q. *J Invest Dermatol* 1994: 103; 665–8.

34.   Steijlen PM, Happle R, van Muyen GNP, van de Kerkhof PCM, Topical treatment with 13-*cis*-retinoic acid improves Darier's disease and induces the expression of a unique keratin pattern. *Dermatologica* 1991: 182; 178–83.

35.   Lucker GPH, van de Kerkhof PCM, Castelijns FACM, Steijlen PM, Topical treatment of Darier's disease with

13-cis-retinoic acid. A clinical and immunohistological study. *J Dermatol Treat* 1997: 7; 227–30.

36. Lauharanta J, Kanerva L, Turjamaa K, Geiger JM, Clinical and ultrastructural effects of acitretin in Darier's disease. *Acta Derm Venereol* 1988: 68; 492–8.

37. van Dooren-Greebe RJ, van de Kerkhof PCM, Happle R, Acitretin monotherapy in Darier's disease. *Br J Dermatol* 1989: 121; 375–9.

38. Griffiths WA, Pityriasis rubra pilaris. *Clin Exp Dermatol* 1980: 38; 105–12.

39. van de Kerkhof PCM, Steijlen PM, Topical treatment of pityriasis rubra pilaris with calcipotriol. *Br J Dermatol* 1994: 130; 675–8.

40. Chapalain V, Beylot-Barry M, Doutre MS, Beylot C, Treatment of pityriasis rubra pilaris a retrospective study of 14 patients. *J Dermatol Treat* 1999: 10; 113–7.

41. Kirby B, Watson R, Pityriasis rubra pilaris treated with acitretin and narrow band ultraviolet B (Re-TL-01). *Br J Dermatol* 2000: 142; 370–93.

42. Knowles WR, Chernosky ME, Pityriasis rubra pilaris. Prolonged treatment with methotrexate. *Arch Dermatol* 1970: 102; 603–12.

43. Meyer P, van Voorst PC, Lack of effect of cyclosporin A in pityriasis rubra pilaris. *Acta Derm Venereol* 1989: 69; 272.

# 10

## The treatment of fungal infections

*David T Roberts*

## Introduction

Fewer than 200 of the many thousands of species of fungi are recognized as human pathogens and many of these are only pathogenic in the presence of diminished host defence. The advent of new diseases such as acquired immune deficiency syndrome (AIDS) has allowed fungi which were previously considered non-pathogenic to cause significant and sometimes fatal disease. Fungi may cause disease in various ways. They may directly invade the skin and mucous membranes but spread no further; such diseases are known as superficial mycoses. Subcutaneous mycoses can invade tissues just deep to the skin, which in some circumstances can include bone; these conditions are known as subcutaneous mycoses. Deep or systemic mycoses may involve any of the internal organs. In all of these circumstances symptoms and signs are caused by proliferation of the fungus and the resultant tissue reaction. Some fungi, notably certain species of mushrooms, are poisonous and their ingestion is sometimes fatal, whilst others can produce toxins which are capable of causing disease. These toxins include aflatoxins, ochratoxins and trichothecenes, most of which are found in contaminated grain. Some fungal toxins are useful and well known in medicine and these include the ergot alkaloids and muscarine. Airborne fungi may produce allergic reactions and asthma may be related to the inhalation of fungal spores. Contact allergy, notably to lichens also occurs. Contamination of foodstuffs by fungi, thus rendering the food inedible, may also be significantly detrimental to human health. Many deaths from starvation occurred in the mid 19th century because of the potato famine caused by the fungus *Phytophthora infestans*.

The majority of fungal infections are exogenous, in that they originate in the environment and can be inhaled, ingested or implanted in some way into the skin. However, the commonest fungal infection in humans is caused by those species of dermatophytes which only inhabit the keratin layer of the epidermis, the hair or the nail, and spread occurs from human to human. Such infections are known as anthropophilic. The majority of these infections affect the feet and, in some countries, around 15% of the population have a fungal infection of the toeclefts[1] and about one-third of these spread to involve the toenails. Anthropophilic fungi are well adapted to life on the human host and produce little in the way of an inflammatory response which would, of course, be detrimental to the organism. *Trichophyton rubrum*, which is responsible for most chronic infection of humans is notably well adapted and can survive in small pieces of keratin, for example deposited on the floors of changing rooms, for a considerable period of time. It remains all the while capable of infecting another human.[2]

The ubiquitous nature of fungi and their resilience is responsible for the high prevalence of fungal infections of the skin. The increasing use of communal bathing facilities for sport and leisure suggests that the incidence of such infections will continue to rise and it is difficult to eradicate the organisms from the environment because they are protected in small pieces of keratin. Disinfectants which are active against fungi and able to penetrate keratin cannot be used in bathing facilities because of their adverse effects on the skin of the users. It is likely, therefore, that only effective treatment will produce a major impact on disease prevalence.

## Antifungal therapy

Before antifungal antibiotics became available, therapy concentrated on removal of infected keratin. Scalp infection required epilation, often induced by radioactive substances.

Regrowth of healthy hair sometimes but not always occurred and patients required isolation during the infectious period. Topical preparations containing salicylic acid, still widely used as a keratolytic, were introduced for the treatment of foot infection and the best known preparation, Whitfield's ointment, is still occasionally used and is effective, providing it is applied for long enough for the keratin to turn over at the site involved. This is at least 4 weeks on glabrous skin and sometimes longer in areas such as the palms and soles where the keratin layer is much thicker.

Griseofulvin, a weakly fungistatic agent active only against dermatophytes, was originally isolated in 1939 as a metabolite of the mould *Penicillium griseofulvum*.[3] It was originally developed as a plant fungicide but was reported in 1958 to be effective when given orally to animals infected experimentally with dermatophytes.[4] Soon after it was shown to be safe for human use and undoubtedly revolutionized the treatment of tinea capitis in that it rendered epilation unnecessary. It also proved very effective in the treatment of tinea corporis but was less effective in the thick keratin of the palms and soles. Although it produced satisfactory cure rates in fingernail infection, slower growing toenails responded very poorly even when the drug was given for very long periods of 12–18 months.[5]

Amphotericin B was the next antifungal agent to be introduced but it is not absorbed from the gastrointestinal tract and is therefore only available for parenteral use. It is also significantly nephrotoxic and is mainly used in life-threatening systemic disease and in some severe subcutaneous mycoses. It has no place in the therapy of superficial infection. Flucytosine is orally absorbed but is active only against yeasts, and resistance develops so rapidly to flucytosine that it only has a place in the short-term treatment of systemic yeast infections, nearly always in conjunction with amphotericin B.

The last 25 years have seen the discovery of a number of synthetic antifungal compounds which are available for both oral and sometimes topical use. The introduction of these drugs has rendered antifungal therapy much safer and more effective than previously and now antifungal preparations of various sorts are the most widely prescribed group of medicaments in dermatological therapy. The majority of these drugs belong to the azole or allylamine group of compounds. The topical azoles clotrimazole and miconazole were introduced in the 1970s and are now widely prescribed as topical preparations and are available over the counter. Ketoconazole, itraconazole and fluconazole are azoles that are orally absorbed and are active against yeasts and a variety of different moulds. The allylamine terbinafine is also a broad-spectrum antifungal agent which is orally absorbed. It is the most potent antidermatophyte agent but is relatively inactive against some *Candida* species notably *C. albicans*. The broad spectrum morpholine amorolfine is not

available for systemic use but is marketed both as a cream and as a nail lacquer.

# Mechanism of action and pharmacokinetics of antifungal drugs

## Griseofulvin

Griseofulvin inhibits fungal microtubules which are essential for mitosis and therefore inhibits cell replication. It is poorly absorbed orally and must be taken with a meal which preferably has a reasonably high fat content. More recently micronized and ultramicronized preparations have been introduced which are better absorbed when dispersed in polyethylene glycol.[6] The bioavailability of griseofulvin is very variable and ranges from as low as 25% up to a high of 70%.[7] The drug appears to be transported to the skin via the sweat and through transepidermal fluid loss.[8] This high concentration in sweat is responsible for the drug having its highest concentration in the stratum corneum. The drug is eliminated from the skin quite rapidly and this, combined with its fungistatic nature, means that the drug requires to be given for the whole of the keratin turnover time at the diseased site. This means that a minimum of 4 weeks therapy is necessary in glabrous skin, at least 6 to 8 weeks for scalp infection, 6 to 12 months for fingernail infection and 12 to 18 months for toenail disease.[9] Griseofulvin rarely results in serious toxicity, but headaches and gastrointestinal effects such as nausea and vomiting and dyspepsia are common in up to 20% of cases. The drug sometimes results in photosensitivity and can precipitate lupus erythematosus. Other effects such as arthralgia, serum sickness, blurred vision, vertigo, paraesthesia and syncope are much less common.

## Azoles and triazoles

These drugs act on the biosynthetic pathway of ergosterol which is an essential component of the fungal cell membrane. The drugs inhibit the enzyme 14α-demethylase which is responsible for the conversion of lanosterol to ergosterol (Fig. 10.1). This results in ergosterol depletion which leads to cell wall leakage and eventual cell death. 14α-Demethylase is a cytochrome P450 enzyme that is similar to human cytochrome P450 3A4, and this gives rise to a number of adverse drug interactions in patients who take other drugs which utilize the same enzyme system.[10]

Ketoconazole, itraconazole and fluconazole all act similarly, as do topical azole preparations. Both itraconazole and fluconazole are safer drugs than ketoconazole. Minor side-effects occur in 7–12% of patients on itraconazole and in about 16% of patients who receive fluconazole for longer than 7 days. Most of these affect the gastrointestinal tract and consist of nausea and vomiting. Liver function abnormalities are occasionally found with both drugs but are nearly always reversible on cessation of therapy.

## Ketoconazole

Ketoconazole was the first oral azole to be introduced and it is active against both yeasts and dermatophytes.[11] The drug is hydrophilic and is well absorbed if gastric acidity is normal. It is widely distributed throughout body tissues and it is delivered to the skin via both blood circulation and sweat. It achieves concentrations well above the minimal inhibitory level in skin. Ketoconazole can cause nausea and vomiting but produces an idiosyncratic hepatitis reaction in about 1 in 10–15,000 cases.[12]

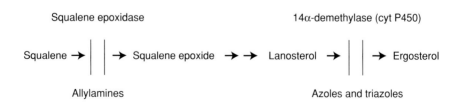

Figure 10.1

Mode of action of antifungal agents: effect on sterol biosynthesis.

This reaction usually occurs only after 8–10 weeks of treatment but may be very severe and slow to resolve. A number of fatalities have been reported and it is not prudent to prescribe ketoconazole for long-term use, e.g., in nail infections, unless there is absolutely no alternative.

## Itraconazole

Itraconazole is lipophilic and its bio-availability is therefore much improved when taken with a fatty meal. The highest concentrations are found in fat, vaginal cervical tissues and within the skin and nails.[13] Significant concentrations of the drug can persist in the skin for up to 4 weeks after cessation of treatment and for much longer periods in nails.

## Fluconazole

Fluconazole is hydrophilic and is highly bioavailable.[14] Its absorbtion is good and not influenced by food or acidity. The drug appears to be eliminated more slowly from skin than from plasma so it may continue to provide therapeutic benefit after discontinuation. It is less active against dermatophytes than itraconazole.

## *Allylamines*

The allylamines also inhibit ergosterol biosynthesis but affect the enzyme squalene epoxidase rather than 14α-demethylase as do the azoles. As well as producing ergosterol depletion the allylamines result in squalene accumulation because the conversion of the squalene to squalene epoxide is prevented. The intracellular accumulation of squalene appears to be toxic to the fungus at higher concentrations thus giving rise to a fungicidal effect in vitro.[15]

## Terbinafine

Terbinafine is the only allylamine available for oral use and it has a bioavailability of 70–80%. It is also lipophilic and this results in high concentrations in the skin and nails.[16] Concentrations well above those required to inhibit fungal growth have been identified for up to 2 months after depletion of plasma concentrations[17] and this results in terbinafine being effective over relatively short periods.

About 10% of patients on terbinafine exhibit adverse events and again gastrointestinal effects are most common. They generally occur during the first week of treatment and are caused by a relative delay in gastric emptying. Serous skin reactions and idiosyncratic liver reactions, mainly cholestasis have been described, but these reactions are generally reversible on cessation of therapy.[18]

## *Idiosyncratic reactions*

It is important to remember that all adverse reactions with antifungal drugs become much worse if the drug is continued and this occurs simply because the prescriber fails to relate the adverse event to the drug. Certainly some of the fatalities with ketoconazole were related to continued drug administration despite the occurrence of hepatitis. The relatively high incidence of hepatic effects with ketoconazole appears to have given rise to the suspicion that antifungal drugs are, in general, dangerous because of hepatotoxicity. Whilst this may well be the case with ketoconazole, it is not true of other systemic antifungals – their capacity to produce hepatotoxicity is no greater than many other commonly prescribed drugs. However, it must be remembered that these idiosyncratic reactions do occur and medical attendants should be vigilant.

## Relative efficacy of antifungal agents

This is the subject of much debate amongst competing pharmaceutical companies and the proponents of one or other drug. The answer to this apparently simple question is by no means clear cut and is dependent upon a number of different factors. The mode of action, minimum inhibitory concentration (MIC) (or minimum fungicidal concentration, MFC), spectrum of activity and pharmacokinetics all play a role in in vivo efficacy, and even if this four-piece jigsaw fits together, efficacy still must be proven in properly controlled clinical studies. Having established efficacy, cost effec-tiveness then becomes an important issue, having regard to acquisition cost, duration of treatment, cost of monitoring, cost of treating relapses and the potential costs of treating adverse events.

It is clear that a single drug is not the most effective for all types of infection. Dermatophytes respond differently than do other moulds and this difference is even more marked when comparing moulds and yeasts. Terbinafine is the most potent oral antidermatophyte agent in terms of its MIC against a variety of dermatophytes. It is about ten times more potent than itraconazole and about 100 times more potent than griseofulvin (Table 10.1). Furthermore, the MIC of terbinafine is equivalent to its MFC which renders it truly fungicidal in vitro. Itraconazole is the only other oral agent which achieves fungicidal levels but its MFC is around ten times higher again than its MIC and its MFC is thus, in turn, 100 times greater than the MFC of terbinafine (Table 10.2).[19] However, these levels must be related to concentrations achieved in diseased tissue to be in any way meaningful.

Much work has been carried out on nail concentrations of these newer agents given that onychomycosis presents the toughest therapeutic test for any drug because of the avascular nature of the target organ. Antifungal drugs have been identified at the distal end of the nail around 4 weeks after the start of therapy and it is presumed that they get there both via diffusion along the nail plate from the matrix and

## Table 10.1 In vitro MIC's (μg/ml)

| Terbinafine | Itraconazole | Fluconazole | Ketoconazole | Griseofulvin |
|---|---|---|---|---|
| 0.003–0.06 | 0.06–0.5 | 1–64 | 0.5–16 | 0.25–64 |

Organisms
*T. rubrum; T. interdigitale; T. tonsurans; T. violaceum; T. soudanense; M. canis; M. gypseum; E. floccosum*

Clayton YM, *Br J Dermatol* 1994: 130 (Suppl 43); 7–8.

## Table 10.2 Geometric mean MIC and MFC values (μg/ml) for dermatophyte isolates

| | MIC | MFC |
|---|---|---|
| Terbinafine | 0.004 | 0.004 |
| Itraconazole | 0.078 | 0.595 |

Clayton YM, *Br J Dermatol* 1994: 130 (Suppl 43); 7–8.

upwards via diffusion from the nail bed.[20] Fluconazole achieves the highest nail concentrations because of its high bioavailability. However, these concentrations are usually around the level of the MIC which is very variable. Itraconazole and terbinafine achieve similar concentrations in the nail and, in the case of itraconazole, these concentrations are considerably in excess of the MIC but only at or around the MFC. In the case of terbinafine nail concentrations are well in excess of the MIC which in turn is equivalent to the MFC. On this basis therefore it would appear that terbinafine is most likely to be the most effective antidermatophyte agent in vitro, especially in nail infection, but this still requires to be proven in clinical studies. The vigorous fungicidal/fungistatic debate which ensues depends upon information obtained from in vitro studies but also from comparative studies of efficacy and most importantly from comparative studies of relapse rates. It is logical to assume that fungicidal drugs have lower relapse rates than fungistatic agents.

Terbinafine is not used systemically in yeast infections because its action against *C. albicans* is fungistatic[21] and although its MIC against *Pityrosporum* yeasts is lower[22] it does not appear to be effective when given orally. However, topical terbinafine is useful in all forms of yeast infection because concentrations on the skin surface are much higher. Itraconazole and fluconazole are better drugs for yeast infections because of their lower MIC against both *Candida* and *Pityrosporum* yeasts and there appears to be little to choose between them. Fluconazole is better absorbed and therefore its effects may be more consistent but resistance has been described, almost entirely in immunocompromised patients in whom the drug is given either intermittently or continuously long term.[23] When such resistance does occur it appears to cross-resist with itraconazole but the same phenomenon does not seem to happen in reverse.[24] The relative effectiveness of these two drugs in yeast infection is therefore a matter of ongoing debate.

## Choice of therapy – topical or systemic?

The site and extent of infection dictates whether or not topical or systemic treatment should be chosen. It is generally accepted that those areas where the keratin is especially thick require systemic treatment. These include the scalp, the palms and soles and the nails. In addition, widespread infection of glabrous skin may also merit systemic treatment simply because compliance is likely to be better and the amount of topical treatment necessary is ultimately more costly. There are, however, theoretical exceptions to this general rule. Nail lacquers have been developed for onychomycosis and some topical preparations, notably topical terbinafine,

have been shown to be effective in infections of the palms and soles.[25] However, this does not mean that such treatment modalities are preferable to systemic treatment unless there are other contraindications to the use of an oral agent.

## Topical therapy

Topical therapy is widely used and is effective in dermatophyte infection of the toeclefts (athletes' foot) which is the commonest of all fungal infection together with small areas of tinea corporis and tinea cruris. Currently available evidence suggests that terbinafine cream is the treatment of choice. It has been shown to be more effective than clotrimazole cream over 1 week as compared to 4 weeks treatment duration.[26] In addition, relapses in 'cured' patients are lower than with clotrimazole.[27] This difference in efficacy has been revealed in clinical studies where compliance is closely monitored. In general use it is likely that compliance with a 1-week course of treatment twice daily to the toeclefts is likely to be much higher than with a treatment course of 4 weeks, and therefore the difference in efficacy may be, in reality, even more marked. Although there have been fewer comparative studies in patients with tinea cruris and tinea corporis, it is likely that the same results would obtain and terbinafine cream should be regarded as the treatment of choice. Topical azoles are a second option if terbinafine, currently a prescription only medicine, is not available.

Skin infections with *Candida* yeasts, notably *C. albicans* are almost always secondary to some other intercurrent disease. This may be a skin disease such as flexural eczema, flexural psoriasis or a napkin dermatitis. It is uncommon for yeast infections to occur outwith the flexures in otherwise healthy individuals. Diabetic patients are especially prone to yeast infections, and immunocompromised patients are also at risk. Patients on antibiotic therapy may develop candidosis but it nearly always affects the mouth. Cutaneous candidosis is rarely seen in this circumstance. There would appear to be little to choose between topical azoles and topical allylamines in cutaneous candidosis[28] but the yeast infection is either secondary to or results in such a significant inflammatory component that a combined antifungal/steroid preparation is regularly indicated. There is currently no preparation which combines terbinafine with a topical steroid but there are numerous preparations containing azoles and topical steroids and numerous others containing the polyene nystatin with topical steroids and sometimes an antibacterial or an antiseptic as well. These preparations are all useful in flexural candidosis and there are few studies to demonstrate any difference in efficacy. In general cutaneous candidosis does not present a major therapeutic problem, unless the intercurrent disease is difficult or impossible to control when the yeast infection would be both notably recalcitrant and recurrent.

*Pityrosporum* yeast infection exists in two forms. Pityriasis versicolor is generally accepted to occur when the yeast undergoes hyphal change and is then known as *Malassezia furfur*. Seborrhoeic dermatitis which affects the scalp, face, trunk and sometimes the flexures is thought to be the result of overgrowth of the yeast form without a yeast/mycelial shift. This is a controversial area and both theories on the aetiology and even on the nomenclature of the yeasts are constantly changing. However, such controversies do not materially affect treatment recommendations.

Pityriasis versicolor may be treated topically with various preparations ranging from propylene glycol in water through selenium sulphide shampoo to topical azoles or allylamines. There are various regimens in terms of treatment duration and all are effective if properly applied. However, pityriasis versicolor tends to show a 'vest and pants' distribution and treatment must be applied to all areas from the neck down to the elbows and knees, paying particular attention to the flexures. Such regimens are difficult to comply with and recurrence rates are consequently high. Systemic treatment may well be preferable and can be achieved over short treatment durations of 1 week or less. Even with successful treatment, the disease does recur in susceptible individuals. This may be because of a subtle diminution in host defence or it may be environmental, the disease being particularly prevalent in hot sweaty conditions.[29]

*Pityrosporum* yeasts are lipophilic and give rise to seborrhoeic dermatitis in patients with a relatively high sebum excretion rate. The disease may be confined to the scalp and produce classical dandruff. It can spread onto the face producing a typical pattern of dermatitis around the eyebrows, central forehead, and the nasolabial folds. Sometimes the disease spreads onto the central chest, particularly in men, and produces so-called petaloid lesions which are psoriasiform in appearance. Occasionally the flexures can be involved and sometimes a generalized dermatitis reaction occurs especially in elderly men. In younger men a widespread low-grade folliculitis occurs and has a typical appearance. Such a folliculitis becomes especially severe in AIDS patients and was formerly an early indicator of conversion from HIV seropositivity to AIDS. The advent of new therapeutic agents for AIDS has rendered classical seborrhoeic dermatitis and seborrhoeic folliculitis much less common.

Shampoos which have antiyeast activity are the mainstay of treatment. These products contain selenium sulphide, zinc pyrithione or ketoconazole. They should be used at least once weekly indefinitely although ordinary shampoos can be used in between. This serves to keep down the yeast population and is certainly helpful prophylactically. Despite this, outbreaks will occur from time to time and should be treated with a combination of an antifungal agent and a topical steroid. Clotrimazole with hydrocortisone or miconazole with hydrocortisone are useful for facial lesions although stronger steroids such as betamethasone with clotrimazole may be necessary for lesions on the trunk. The place for systemic therapy in seborrhoeic dermatitis is unknown simply because there are no well-conducted studies of efficacy.[29] This author believes that systemic treatment is rarely necessary in cases of classical seborrhoeic dermatitis but it is sometimes useful in cases of seborrhoeic folliculitis especially in the immunocompromised. Courses of treatment often require to be repeated on a regular basis.

# Systemic therapy

## Superficial infections

Dermatophyte infections of the scalp, palms and soles and nails require systemic treatment as do widespread infection of the glabrous skin of the trunk, limbs and groin (Figs 10.2–10.5). In addition pityriasis versicolor is probably best treated systemically (Fig. 10.6). An overall summary of the systemic treatment of superficial infections is presented in Table 10.3.

### Dermatophyte infection of the scalp (tinea capitis, scalp ringworm)

Scalp infection may be anthropophilic and spread from human to human.

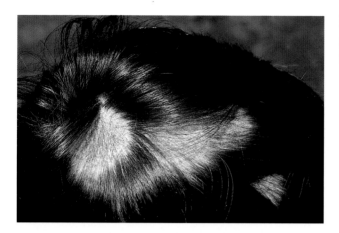

**Figure 10.2**

Scalp ringworm
(tinea capitis).

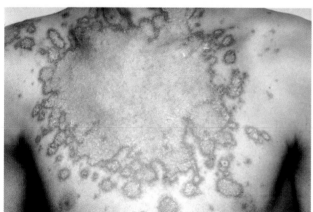

**Figure 10.3**

Body ringworm
(tinea corporis).

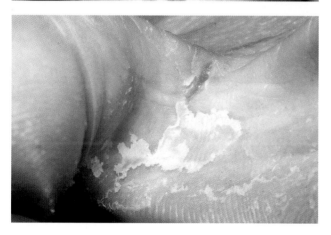

**Figure 10.4**

Athlete's foot.

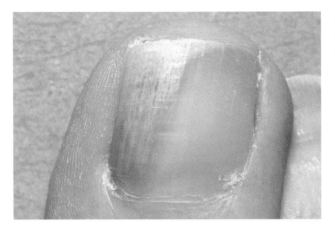

Figure 10.5

Onychomycosis
(tinea unguium).

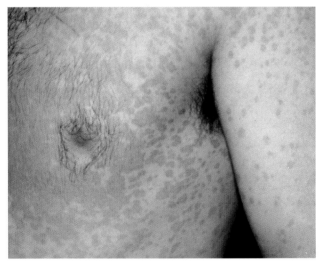

Figure 10.6

Pityriasis versicolor.

Different fungi have a different geographic distribution, and in some communities the disease reaches endemic proportions. Zoophilic infections are by their very nature much more sporadic and the appearance depends upon the fungus involved. In some cases both anthropophilic and more frequently zoophilic infections produce a brisk inflammatory response which sometimes appears as an abscess known as a kerion. All forms of dermatophyte infection of the scalp are much commoner in children than in adults.[30]

## Table 10.3 Systemic treatment of superficial infection

| Disease | Drug | Dose | Duration |
|---|---|---|---|
| T. capitis | Griseofulvin | 1–1.5 g daily (adults) | 8–12 weeks |
| | | 10–25 mg/kg (children) | 8–12 weeks |
| | Terbinafine | 250 mg daily (adults) | 2–4 weeks |
| | | 62.5 mg daily (<20 kg body weight) | 2–4 weeks |
| | | 125 mg daily (20–40 kg body weight) | 2–4 weeks |
| | | 250 mg daily (>40 kg body weight) | 2–4 weeks |
| T. corporis/cruris | Griseofulvin | 500 mg daily | 4 weeks |
| | Terbinafine | 250 mg daily | 1 week |
| | Itraconazole | 100 mg daily | 4 weeks |
| | | 200 mg daily | ? 2 weeks |
| T. pedis/manuum | Griseofulvin | 1 g daily | 8 weeks |
| | Terbinafine | 250 mg daily | 2 weeks |
| | Itraconazole | 400 mg daily | 1 week |
| T. unguium | Griseofulvin | 1 g daily | 6–9 months (fingernails) 12–18 months (toenails) |
| | Terbinafine | 250 mg daily | 6 weeks (fingernails) 12 weeks (toenails) |
| | Itraconazole | 200 mg daily | 12 weeks |
| | | 400 mg daily | 1 week × 3 (fingernails) |
| | | 400 mg daily | 1 week × 4 (toenails) |
| Pityriasis versicolor | Itraconazole | 200 mg daily | 5–7 days |

Infections caused by different dermatophytes require different treatment regimens. This may be because of relative differences in the MICs or it may be because of biological differences in the type of infection. Ectothrix infections are more recalcitrant to treatment than endothrix infections. It may be that this is due to the problem of drug distribution and penetration but there is no proof of this. Comparative studies of different drugs and different treatment regimens provide a guide as to which drugs are more effective.

However, certainly in the developed world, a cure must be achieved in all cases. Patients therefore have to be treated on an individual basis and treatment continued for as long as there are signs of viable infection which is bound to vary from individual to individual.

Because the disease mostly occurs in children, griseofulvin is the drug of choice in the majority of countries. New antifungal agents are inevitably licensed in adults long before a license is obtained for use in children, and terbinafine, itraconazole and fluconazole are still only licensed for children in a few countries. There are many clinical studies using newer agents which have now been carried out and there does not appear to be any significant safety issue regarding their use in children. However, such use is, in most countries, still off-label and many prescribers feel uncomfortable using drugs in such a fashion, especially in children. Griseofulvin in doses of 10 mg/kg body weight per day for 4–6 weeks is still considered adequate in theory but is rarely so in practice. Larger doses of 20–25 mg/kg body weight per day are regularly used with no perceived increase in adverse events.[31] Treatment durations of 6–12 weeks are often necessary to completely clear patients of infection and as stated above this should be done by careful individual follow up. General medical practitioners still tend to prescribe 'by the book' whereas specialists tend more to be guided by experience and thus use higher doses for longer periods. This results in a significant number of treatment failures being referred to a specialist. Although the acquisition cost of griseofulvin is low, these higher dosage, longer duration regimens result in newer more costly drugs being more cost effective because of their greater potency.

Ketoconazole is not considered appropriate for tinea capitis in children because of its safety concerns but such concerns do not appear to apply to itraconazole or fluconazole.[32] Clinical trials in tinea capitis have often been small and poorly controlled, largely because of the difficulty in carrying out such studies in children. Furthermore, some studies have used fixed dosages whereas others have varied the dosage according to body weight which is likely to be superior. The results of these therapeutic studies vary very markedly even though the same fungus was involved. The reasons for such variation are not entirely clear but treatment compliance is obviously a likely cause.

Itraconazole either given continuously for 4–6 weeks in a dose of 5 mg/kg body weight per day[33] or the same dose given for 1 week per month for 2–3 consecutive months[34] is efficacious in the optimum number of cases. There are few data regarding the efficacy of fluconazole in the treatment of tinea capitis. A study comparing 1.5, 3 and 6 mg/kg doses for 20 days was conducted and there was an 89% cure rate in the 6 mg/kg group.[35] Another study revealed good results using 5 mg/kg for 30 days. Finally a smaller study showed that a once-weekly dosing at 8 mg/kg for 4–6 weeks was also effective.[36]

Early studies in the use of terbinafine in tinea capitis were carried out in Pakistan where most patients were infected with *T. violaceum*. The dosage of terbinafine in children is well established: 62.5 mg daily for children below 20 kg body weight, 125 mg daily for children of 20–40 kg body weight, the full dose of 250 mg daily for patients over 40 kg.[37] The study compared terbinafine in the above dosages for 4 weeks with griseofulvin in a dose of 6–12 mg/kg per day for 8 weeks. The study found 93% of the terbinafine group completely cured as compared with 88% of the griseofulvin group.[38] A further study in Pakistan examined 1, 2 and 4 weeks of therapy with terbinafine in patients, again predominantly with *T. violaceum* infection, and the cure rates were, respectively, 34%, 80% and 86%.[39] Finally, the same authors conducted a study comparing terbinafine and itraconazole each given for 2 weeks and revealed cure rates at week 12 of follow-up of 78% in the terbinafine group and 86% in the itraconazole group.[40]

A study in ectothrix infections using terbinafine in an open fashion for 6 weeks showed only 32% cure rates at 8 weeks follow-up and this suggests that ectothrix infections require longer treatment periods, possibly similar in length to courses of griseofulvin.[41]

The incidence of adverse events in children is low and certainly acceptable for all three drugs with a similar profile to that in adults. There do not appear to be any reports of serious adverse liver reactions with any of the drugs in children.

## Dermatophyte infections of glabrous skin

Oral treatment is indicated in widespread infection where compliance with topical therapy may be suboptimal and may indeed be more cost effective because of the area involved. Oral terbinafine is very effective in a dose of 250 mg daily for a maximum of 2 weeks. There are some data from small studies suggesting that only 1 week's treatment is equally effective.[42] Griseofulvin and itraconazole in doses of 500 mg and 100 mg daily, respectively, probably require 4 weeks of treatment. The duration of itraconazole therapy can be reduced with increasing dosage through 200 mg daily for 2 weeks down to 400 mg daily for 1 week.

## Dermatophyte infection of the palms and soles

Griseofulvin appears to be less effective in the treatment of infections of plantar skin than it is in the scalp or in glabrous skin.[43] A study comparing terbinafine 250 mg daily with griseofulvin 1 g daily, both for 6 weeks, revealed mycological cure rates of 75% in the terbinafine group and only 45% in the griseofulvin group.[44] A placebo-controlled study using terbinafine 250 mg daily for only 2 weeks revealed similar cure rates at follow-up in the terbinafine group.[45]

A large study comparing terbinafine 250 mg daily with itraconazole 100 mg daily for 2 weeks showed terbinafine to be markedly superior at follow-up.[46] There was no significant difference between terbinafine 250 mg daily for 2 weeks and itraconazole 100 mg daily for 4 weeks suggesting that itraconazole in a dose of 100 mg daily is suboptimal.[47] It is likely that itraconazole in a dose of 200 mg daily is comparable with terbinafine over similar treatment durations and a dose of 400 mg daily may allow even shorter treatment durations of 1 week with itraconazole but is significantly more costly.

## Dermatophyte nail infection (onychomycosis)

Dermatophytes are a predominant cause of onychomycosis and various studies have revealed around 90% of cases of toenail infection to be secondary to dermatophytes.[48] Yeast infections are much commoner in fingernails but are generally not primary and are dealt with in the chapter on nail disease. A number of prevalence studies have been carried out in onychomycosis and some of these employed questionnaires and photographs whilst others were mycologically controlled. The studies employing questionnaires and photographs suggested a prevalence of around 3% in Europe[49] whereas those studies which were mycologically controlled, although much smaller, suggested higher prevalences of between 5% and 10% both in Europe[50] and north America. There is no doubt, therefore, that dermatophyte onychomycosis is one of the most common dermatological diseases, and for this reason the cost implications of therapy are significant. Indeed, it is perfectly

valid to ask whether or not the disease should be treated at all given the spiralling costs of health care and the necessity to fix priorities. There are those who believe that onychomycosis is only of cosmetic significance but this is far from the truth. It is a disease of insidious onset but relentless progression and is therefore much commoner in older age groups. These are the very patients who develop peripheral vascular disease or possibly diabetes and in such cases coexistence of a fungal infection of the nails can cause significant morbidity which arguably could be equally or even more costly than treatment of the fungal infection in the first place. Objective quality of life studies have shown that onychomycosis produces much more psychological stress than previously thought. The mechanical importance of fingernails gives rise to far less argument as to whether fingernail infection should be treated. There is therefore a strong case to be made for treating patients who present with onychomycosis.

In most countries griseofulvin, terbinafine and itraconazole are the three drugs licensed for use in onychomycosis. Ketoconazole is precluded on the grounds of toxicity and the use of fluconazole has concentrated on the therapy of yeast infections although there is some recent work in nail disease. It is now generally recognized that griseofulvin is a poor drug in toenail infections and, if used, requires to be given for very lengthy treatment periods of 12 months or more. Even then cure rates vary between a low of only 10% and a high of just under 50%[51] and it does not compare favourably with either itraconazole or terbinafine and can no longer be recommended, other than perhaps in children when it remains the only licensed preparation. However, the number of children requiring treatment for onychomycosis is relatively small. Both itraconazole and terbinafine have been extensively studied in onychomycosis in various treatment regimens. Terbinafine is recommended for use in a dose of 250 mg daily for 6 weeks in fingernails and 12 weeks in toenails. The initially used dose of itraconazole (100 mg daily) proved ineffective and the drug is now recommended for use in either a continuous regimen of 200 mg daily for 12 weeks in toenails or in a so-called pulsed regimen where the drug is given in a dose of 400 mg daily for 1 week repeated monthly for 2 months in fingernail infections and 3 or 4 months in toenail infections. This intermittent dosage regimen is based upon the theory that the drug remains in the nail for long periods after cessation of treatment. Indeed this is true and is likely to be a characteristic of the target organ rather than itraconazole in particular. Fluconazole also tends to be given intermittently but in a somewhat different fashion. In general the drug is given as a single weekly dosage in the range 150–600 mg/week for treatment durations of 12–24 weeks. Treatment costs therefore tend to vary widely with these quite significantly different treatment regimens.

A number of comparative studies have been carried out, mainly comparing terbinafine with itraconazole and it is clear that the results vary depending upon the design of the protocol. The primary cure rate must be assessed mycologically and based upon positive microscopy and culture at entry with mycological cure defined as negative microscopy and culture. Studies which have culture negativity only as a cure are invalid because it is impossible to tell whether or not nails which remain positive on microscopy contain viable fungus or simply dead hyphae, and the latter cannot be assumed. Follow-up must be long enough for the nail to grow out completely which can take up to 18 months. A follow up of 72 weeks is therefore optimum and certainly final follow-ups below 52 weeks are of little value.

There are few studies which fulfil these strict criteria and one which compared continuous terbinafine with continuous itraconazole with a final follow-up of 52 weeks has revealed terbinafine to be superior.[52] A study comparing terbinafine 250 mg daily for 3 and 4 months with three and four pulses with itraconazole at a dose of 400 mg daily for 1 week per pulse is the most important current comparative study, because itraconazole is mostly advocated for use in a pulsed regimen. This very large study included 120 patients in each of the four groups and mycological cure based on microscopy and culture negativity was the primary criterion of cure. Both the terbinafine regimens were found to be markedly superior to both the itraconazole regimens in this study and the difference was mirrored by the clinical cure rates and the patient and physician global assessment indices.[53] It would appear therefore that continuous terbinafine is superior to itraconazole in either a continuous or a pulsed regimen. A study comparing terbinafine with 150 mg of fluconazole given weekly for 12 and 24 weeks also revealed terbinafine to be superior.[54] Terbinafine should therefore be considered the treatment of choice in dermatophyte onychomycosis with pulsed itraconazole as an alternative.

There remains a consistent failure rate of 20–30% in toenail infection. The usual reasons such as poor compliance, immunosuppression or dermatophyte resistance are unlikely to explain this consistently and quite high failure rate and most cases probably relate to kinetic problems with the nail or the relatively 'dormant' state of the fungus. The space between the toenail and nailbed is by no means an ideal environment for the dermatophyte. It therefore develops arthroconidia during which time it takes up very little nutrient. In such cases it will probably take up very little drug as well and this explains at least the length of treatment necessary and may explain some of treatment failures. In some patients a linear or round dense white area can be seen clinically. If the nail is reflected in such cases a mass of keratin can be removed which histologically contains a dense clump of closely packed thick-walled hyphae.[55] This is known as either a linear or a round dermatophytoma and it is quite likely that drugs do not penetrate adequately into this area as is the case in an aspergilloma in the lung. It is probably best either to excise this area or indeed to avulse the toenail in such cases before prescribing treatment. This is likely to lead to much improved cure rates although there are no studies to conclusively show this as yet.

## Non-dermatophyte nail infection

*Scytalidium dimidiatum*, previously known as *Hendersonula toruloidea*, is the only mould which is a certain primary pathogen of nail and it is the only non-dermatophyte mould which has the capacity to produce interdigital infection or athletes' foot. A large number of saprophytic moulds are known to have the ability to invade damaged nail but it is unlikely that most, if any, have the capacity to invade healthy nail as do dermatophytes. However, the prevalence and treatment of choice of non-dermatophyte mould infections remains controversial. They are likely to be secondary to some other cause of nail dystrophy, very possibly a dermatophyte infection, and the best antidermatophyte agent is probably the treatment of choice. However, in cases of doubt the nail should be removed rather than treated with oral antifungal agents. An Australian study comparing terbinafine with a placebo carefully recorded the presence of all non-dermatophyte moulds and yeasts in nails which were all positive for dermatophytes. In this study only one-third of cases had a dermatophyte only and two-thirds revealed a 'mixed' culture. However, there was no difference in the cure rates between the dermatophyte-only nails and the 'mixed' nails, again suggesting that these were all primary dermatophyte infections with other moulds present as saprophytes.[56]

## Pityriasis versicolor

Itraconazole, ketoconazole and fluconazole can be used systemically in the treatment of pityriasis versicolor and there are various regimens available. Itraconazole in a dose of 200 mg daily for 1 week produces cure rates of over 90% and this is cheap, convenient and safe. However, it requires to be repeated from time to time in recurrent cases and all patients should be warned that the depigmentation which results in chronic cases will take some time to clear even after successful treatment.

## Subcutaneous fungal infection

The three most important diseases in this group are mycetoma, chromoblastomycosis and phaeohyphomycosis, and sporotrichosis. Less common infections include lobomycosis and zygomycosis.

## Mycetoma

This disease may be caused by fungi (eumycetoma) or filamentous bacteria (actinomycetoma). About half the cases of eumycetoma respond to ketoconazole in a dose of 200–400 mg daily. Ultimately itraconazole may prove to be the superior drug both in terms of efficacy and safety but there are few data available. Radical surgery is still the treatment of choice in most cases.[57]

Actinomycetomas respond to treatment with antibiotics such as dapsone, clotrimoxazole, rifampicin and streptomycin and generally do better than eumycetomata.

## Chromomycosis

Various therapeutic regimens have been tried and these include itraconazole 100–200 mg daily together with flucytosine 30–35 mg/kg four times daily. Others tried include a combination of amphotericin B together with flucytosine and sometimes thiabendazole. More recently a study in Madagascar, an endemic area for chromomycosis has revealed that terbinafine 500 mg daily is highly effective and this may ultimately become the treatment of choice.[58]

## Sporotrichosis

The traditional treatment for sporotrichosis is 1 ml of a saturated solution of potassium iodide three times daily increasing to 4–6 ml three times daily. Iodism will develop unless the dose is slowly increased to optimal levels. More recently studies have revealed that itraconazole and terbinafine can be effective and these may well ultimately supplant potassium iodide as first-line therapy.[59]

## Lobomycosis and zygomycosis

The organism responsible for lobomycosis cannot be cultured. Therefore drug efficacy cannot be examined in vitro and thus far no therapeutic regimen has produced satisfactory cure rates.[57] Zygomycosis does, however, respond well to potassium iodide in similar regimens to those used in sporotrichosis.

## Conclusion

The advent of a number of new antifungal agents has rendered the treatment of fungal infections much easier and more effective but the diagnosis should always be confirmed and treatment chosen carefully depending upon the specific type of infection.

## References

1. Howell SA, Clayton YM, Pham QC, Tinea pedis, the relationship between symptoms, organisms and host characteristics. *Microbiol Ecol Health Dis* 1998: 1; 131–5.

2. Gentles JC, Evans EGV, Foot infections in swimming baths. *BMJ* 1973: 3; 260–2.

3. Oxford AE, Raistrick H, Simonart P, Griseofulvin, C17H1706CI, a metabolic product of *Penicillium griseofulvum* Dierckx. *Biochem J* 1939: 33; 240–8.

4. Gentles JC, Experimental ringworm in guinea pigs: oral treatment with griseofulvin. *Nature* 1958: 182; 476–7.

5. Araujo OE, Flowers FP, King MM, Griseofulvin: a new look at an old drug. *An Pharmacother* 1990: 24; 851–4.

6. Becker LE, Griseofulvin. *Dermatol Clin* 1984: 2; 115–20.

7. Gupta AK, Sauder DN, Shear NH, Antifungal agents: an overview. Part 1. *J Am Acad Dermatol* 1994: 30; 677–98.

8. Shah VP, Epstein WL, Riegelman S, Role of sweat in accumulation of orally administered griseofulvin in skin. *J Clin Invest* 1974: 53; 1673–8.

9. Roberts DT, Evans EGV, Advances in the management of superficial fungal infection. *Practitioner* 1993: 237; 153–7.

10. Albengres E, Le Louet H, Tillement J-P, Systemic fungal agents: drug interactions of clinical significance. *Drug Saf* 1998: 18; 83–97.

11. Daneshmend TK, Warnock DW, Clinical pharmacokinetics of ketoconazole. *Clin Pharmacokinet* 1998: 14; 13–34.

12. Lewis JH, Zimmerman HJ, Beson GD, Ishak G, Hepatic injury associated with ketoconazole therapy; analysis of 33 cases. *Gastroenterology* 1994: 86; 503–13.

13. Haria M, Bryson HM, Goa KL, Itraconazole: a reappraisal of its pharmacological properties in therapeutic use in the management of superficial fungal infection. *Drugs* 1996: 51; 585–620.

14. De Greef HJ, De Doncker PRG, Current therapy of dermatophytoses. *J Am Acad Dermatol* 1994: 31 (Suppl); S25–30.

15. Clayton YM, Relevance of broad spectrum and fungicidal activity of

antifungals in the treatment of dermatomycoses. *Br J Dermatol* 1994: 130 (Suppl 43); 7–8.

16.  Faergermann J, Zehender H, Jones T, Maibach I, Terbinafine levels in serum, stratum corneum, dermis-epidermis (without stratum corneum), hair, sebum and eccrine sweat. *Acta Derm Venereol* 1990: 71; 322-6.

17.  Faergermann J, Zehender H, Denouel J, Millerioux L, Terbinafine levels in serum, stratum corneum, dermis-epidermis (without stratum corneum) sebum, hair and nails during and after 250 mg terbinafine orally once per day for four weeks. *Acta Derm Venereol* 1993: 73; 305–9.

18.  Hall M, Monka C, Krupp P et al, Safety of oral terbinafine. Results of a post marketing surveillance in 25,884 patients. *Arch Dermatol* 1997: 133; 1213–19.

19.  Ryder NS, Favre B, Antifungal activity and mechanism and action of terbinafine. *Rev Contemp Pharmacother* 1997: 8; 275–87.

20.  Faergermann J, Pharmacokinetics of terbinafine. *Rev Contemp Pharmacother* 1997: 8; 289–97.

21.  Ryder NS, Wagner S, Leitner I, In vitro activity of terbinafine against Candida and other yeasts by the NCCLS method. 36th Interscience Conference of Antimicrobial Agents in Chemotherapy. American Society of Microbiology, Washington DC, 15–18 September. Abstract E55, 1996, p. 91.

22.  Uchida K, Yamagouchi H, In vitro anti malassezia activity of terbinafine. *Jpn J Med Mycol* 1991: 32; 343–6.

23.  Boken DJ, Swindells S, Rinaldi MG, Fluconazole-resistant *Candida albicans*. *Clin Infect Dis* 1993: 17; 1018–21.

24.  Johnson EM, Davey KG, Szekely A, Warnock DW, Itraconazole susceptibilities of fluconazole susceptible and resistant isolates of five Candida species. *J Antimicrob Chemother* 1995: 36; 787–93.

25.  Savin R, Atton AV, Bergstresser PR et al, Efficacy of terbinafine 1% cream in the treatment of moccasin type tinea pedis; results of a placebo controlled multicentre study. *J Am Acad Dermatol* 1994: 30; 663-7.

26.  Evans EGV, Dodman B, Williamson DM et al, Comparison of terbinafine and clotrimazole in treating tinea pedis. *BMJ* 1993: 307; 645-7.

27.  Bergstresser PR, Elewski B, Hanifin J et al, Topical terbinafine and clotrimazole in interdigital tinea pedis: a multicentre comparison of cure and relapse rates with one and four week treatment regimens. *J Am Acad Dermatol* 1993: 28; 648–51.

28.  Evans EGV, The clinical efficacy of terbinafine in the treatment of fungal infection of the skin. *Rev Contemp Pharmacother* 1997: 8; 325–41.

29.  Faergermann J, Pityrosporum infections. In: Elewski BE (ed) *Cutaneous fungal infections*. Tokyo, Igaqu-Shoin, 1992, pp. 69–83.

30.  Dostrovsky A, Kallaner G, Raubitschek F, Sagher F, Tinea capitis: an epidemiologic, therapeutic and laboratory investigating of 6390 cases. *J Invest Dermatol* 1955: 24; 195–200.

31.  Krafchick B, The clinical efficacy of terbinafine in the treatment of tinea capitis. *Rev Contemp Pharmacother* 1997: 8; 313–24.

32.  Elewski BE, Tinea capitis: a current perspective. *J Am Acad Dermatol* 2000: 42; 1–20.

33. Elewski BE, Treatment of tinea capitis with itraconazole. *Int J Dermatol* 1997: 36; 537–41.

34. Gupta AK, Adam P, De Donker P, Itraconazole pulse therapy for tinea capitis: a novel treatment schedule. *Pediatr Dermatol* 1998: 15; 225–8.

35. Solomon BA, Colin R, Sharma R et al, Fluconazole for treatment of tinea capitis in children. *J Am Acad Dermatol* 1997: 37; 274–5.

36. Montero GF, Fluconazole for the treatment of tinea capitis. *Int J Dermatol* 1998: 37; 870–1.

37. Nejjam F, Zagula M, Carbiac MD et al, Pilot study of terbinafine in children suffering from tinea capitis: an evaluation of efficacy, safety and pharmacokinetics. *Br J Dermatol* 1995: 132; 98–105.

38. Alvi KH, Iqbal N, Khan KA et al, A randomised double blind trial of the efficacy and tolerability of terbinafine once daily compared to griseofulvin once daily in the treatment of tinea capitis. In: Shuster S, Jafary MH (eds) *Terbinafine in the treatment of superficial fungal infections*. London: Royal Society of Medicine Services, International Congress Series no. 205, 1993: pp. 35–40.

39. Haroon TS, Hussain I, Aman S et al, A randomised double blind comparative study of terbinafine for one, two and four weeks in tinea capitis. *Br J Dermatol* 1996: 135; 86–8.

40. Jahangir M, Hussain I, Hassan MUL, Haroon TS, A double blind randomised comparative trial of itraconazole versus terbinafine for two weeks in tinea capitis. *Br J Dermatol* 1998: 139; 672–4.

41. Dragos V, Lunder M, Lack of efficacy of six weeks treatment with oral terbinafine for tinea capitis due to *Microsporum canis* in children. *Pediatr Dermatol* 1997: 14; 46–8.

42. Farag A, Taha M, Halim S, One week therapy with oral terbinafine in cases of tinea cruris/corporis. *Br J Dermatol* 1994: 131; 684–6.

43. Roberts DT, Evans EGV, Advances in the management of superficial fungal infection. *Practitioner* 1993: 237; 153–7.

44. Savin RC, Oral terbinafine versus griseofulvin in the treatment of moccasin/type tinea pedis. *J Am Acad Dermatol* 1998: 23 (Suppl): 807–9.

45. White JE, Perkins PJ, Evans EGV, Successful two week treatment with terbinafine (Lamisil) for moccasin tinea pedis and tinea manuum. *Br J Dermatol* 199: 125; 260–2.

46. De Keyser P, De Backer M, Massart DL, Westelinck KJ, Two week oral treatment of tinea pedis comparing terbinafine 250 mg per day with itraconazole 100 mg per day: a double blind multicentre study. *Br J Dermatol* 1994: 130 (Suppl 43); 22–5.

47. Hay RJ, MacGregor JM, Wuite J et al, A comparison of two weeks terbinafine 250 mg per day with four weeks of itraconazole 100 mg per day in plantar type tinea pedis. *Br J Dermatol* 1995: 132; 604–8.

48. Summerbell RC, Kane J, Crajaden S, Onychomycosis, tinea pedis and tinea manuum caused by non dermatophyte filamentous fungi. *Mycoses* 1989: 32; 609–19.

49. Roberts DT, The prevalence of dermatophyte onychomycosis in the United Kingdom; results of an omnibus survey. *Br J Dermatol* 1992: 126 (Suppl 39); 23–7.

50. Heikkila H, Stubb S, The prevalence of onychomycosis in Finland. *Br J Dermatol* 1995: 133; 699–703.

51.  Davies RR, Everall JD, Hamilton E, Mycological and clinical evaluation of griseofulvin for chronic onychomycosis. *BMJ* 1957: 3; 464–8.

52.  Brautigam M, Nolting S, Schopf RE et al, Randomised double blind comparison of terbinafine and itraconazole in the treatment of toenail tinea infection. *BMJ* 1995: 311; 919–22 (see also published erratum. *BMJ* 1995: 311; 1350).

53.  Evans EGV, Sigurgeirsson B, Double blind randomised study of continuous terbinafine compared with intermittent itraconazole in treatment of toenail onychomycosis. *BMJ* 1999: 318; 1031–4.

54.  Havu V, Heikkila H, Kuokkanen K et al, A double-blind, randomized study to compare the efficacy and saftey of terbinafine (Lamisil) with fluconazole (Diflucan) in the treatment of onychomycosis. *Br J Dermatol* 2000: 142; 97–102.

55.  Roberts DT, Evans EGV, Subungual dermatophytoma complicating dermatophyte onychomycosis. *Br J Dermatol* 1998: 138(1); 189–90.

56.  Watson AB, Marley JE, Ellis DH et al, Terbinafine in onychomycosis of the toenail: a normal treatment protocol. *J Am Acad Dermatol* 1995: 33; 775–9.

57.  Lavall P, Goncalves AP, Jerdim ML et al, Tropical deep fungal infections. In: Canizares O, Harman R (eds) *Clinical tropical dermatology*. Oxford: Blackwell Scientific Publications, 1992, pp. 41–87.

58.  Esterre P, Inzan CK, Ratsioharana M et al, A multicentre trial of terbinafine in patients with chromoblastomycosis: effect of clinical and biological criteria. *J Dermatol Treat* 1998: 9 (Suppl 1); s29–34.

59.  Hull PR, Vismer HF, Treatment of subcutaneous sporotrichosis with terbinafine. *Br J Dermatol* 1992: 126 (Suppl 39); 51–5.

# 11

## Nail disease – advances in treatment

*Antonella Tosti, Robert Baran and Bianca Maria Piraccini*

## Introduction

There are several reasons for difficulties in treating nail disease. Before discussing the optimal treatment of the most common nail diseases, we briefly review some physiological characteristics of the nail that are very important in understanding nails and their treatment needs:

1. The nails grow very slowly and therefore we often have to wait for several months before seeing the results of our treatment. It is very important to make this clear to the patient who may otherwise discontinue the treatment because he/she feels it to be ineffective. Complete cure of a fingernail disorder usually requires several months, whereas the cure of a toenail disorder may require more than a year.

2. Vehicles utilized for enhancing penetration of drugs through the skin are not effective in the nail. Most topical drugs are therefore ineffective in the treatment of inflammatory disorders such as nail lichen planus and nail psoriasis.

3. Since the nails are largely exposed to environmental hazards, nail disorders are commonly precipitated or worsened by physical trauma. Moreover, there are a large number of nail disorders, such as nail brittleness, chronic paronychia or idiopathic onycholysis, that are directly due to environmental factors.

## Brittle nails

Since environmental and occupational factors that produce a progressive dehydration of the nail plate play a major role in the development of idiopathic nail brittleness, the management of brittle nails includes protective measures that prevent nail plate dehydration.

Patients should be advised to comply with the following guidelines:

1. Avoid repeated immersion of the hands in soap and water.
2. Avoid dehydrating chemicals, including nail polish removers.
3. Keep the nails short.
4. Protect hands with rubber gloves worn over light cotton gloves during household chores.

Topical treatment

Topical moisturizers after hand washing.

Systemic treatment

Biotin 2.5 mg/day for 6 months.[1]

# Acute paronychia

This is usually caused by *Staphylococcus aureus*, although other bacteria and *Herpes simplex* may be responsible.

Topical treatment

Local medication with antiseptics.

Systemic treatment

Whenever possible cultures should be taken. Administration of penicillinase-resistant antibiotics or antiviral agents depending on the causative organism.

Surgical treatment (except for *Herpes simplex*)

Drainage of the abscess by removing the base of the nail plate may be required. The nail is cut transversally with a nail splitter to accomplish this.

# Chronic paronychia

Chronic paronychia represents an inflammatory reaction of the proximal nail fold to irritants or allergens. Secondary colonization with *Candida albicans* and/or bacteria occurs in most cases.[2–3]

Management of chronic paronychia requires avoidance of a wet environment, chronic microtrauma and contact with irritants or allergens.

Patients should be advised to follow the same guidelines described for brittle nails.

Topical treatment

Application of a mild-potency topical steroid at bed time and topical preparations containing a steroid and an imidazole derivative in the morning.

Intralesional treatment

Injections of triamcinolone acetonide suspension (2.5 mg/ml) into the proximal nail fold facilitates resolution of the paronychia.

Systemic treatment

1. Systemic steroids (methylprednisone 20 mg/day for a few days) can be prescribed in severe cases with several nails involved to obtain fast relief of inflammation and pain.
2. Systemic antifungals are useless.

Surgical treatment

Paronychia not responding to medical therapy (e.g. due to a foreign body in hairdressers) should be treated by the excision of a crescent-shaped, full-thickness piece of the proximal nail fold, including its swollen portion. Complete healing by granulation takes about 4 weeks.

# Onycholysis

Onycholysis may be idiopathic or may be a symptom of numerous diseases that affect the nail bed such as psoriasis, onychomycosis, contact dermatitis etc. Since idiopathic onycholysis is favoured in a wet environment, its management requires the same guidelines prescribed for nail brittleness.[4]

## Topical treatment

1. The detached nail should be cut away and this should be repeated at 2-week intervals until the nail plate grows attached.
2. Application of a topical antiseptic solution and/or a topical antifungal to the exposed nail bed.
3. Treatment of the causative condition is required in all cases of onycholysis secondary to nail bed disease.

# Psoriasis

Nail psoriasis is poorly responsive to both topical and systemic treatments.[5] It is also scarcely influenced by sunlight exposure and other factors that improve skin psoriasis.[6-7]

## Topical treatment (applicable only in nail bed psoriasis)

1. Daily application of topical steroids or combinations of topical steroids with salicylic acid and/or retinoic acid. Although the efficacy of topical steroids can be enhanced by overnight occlusion, this technique should be used only for limited periods. A transungual delivery system (nail lacquer) containing steroids has recently been developed to optimize nail penetration. Preliminary studies indicate that this formulation is effective for treating nail psoriasis.[8]
2. Application of topical calcipotriol twice a day.[9]
3. In patients with pustular psoriasis topical antimetabolites (mechlorethamine, 5% 5-fluorouracil) can be useful.

## Intralesional treatment (applicable in nail matrix and nail bed psoriasis)

Intralesional steroid injections (triamcinolone acetonide 2.5 mg/ml) at a dose of 0.2 to 0.5 ml per nail. In patients with nail plate surface abnormalities the steroids should be injected into the nail matrix, whereas in patients with subungual hyperkeratosis the site of injection should be the nail bed.[10] Injections should be repeated monthly for 6 months, then every 6 weeks for the next 6 months and finally every 2 months for 6 to 12 months. A digital block is useful to make the treatment less painful, but when several digits are involved, a wrist block may be the appropriate anaesthesia.

## Systemic treatment (applicable in nail matrix and nail bed psoriasis)

1. Steroids, methotrexate or cyclosporin can clear the nail changes,

but they should be used only when nail psoriasis is associated with widespread disease or psoriatic arthritis.

2. Oral retinoids are useful in patients with thick nails, but not in onycholysis and pitting, since the latter two symptoms can be worsened by the treatment.

3. In pustular psoriasis, oral retinoids can arrest the development of pustular lesions and avoid permanent scarring of the nail apparatus (Fig. 11.1).[11]

4. Oral nimesulide (200 mg/day) is often successful in Hallopeau's acrodermatitis (Fig. 11.2).

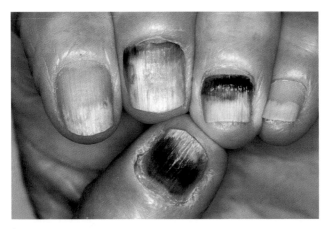

a

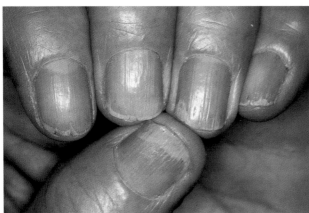

b

## Figure 11.1

Pustular psoriasis of the nails before (a) and after (b) treatment with etretinate 0.5 mg/kg per day for 3 months.

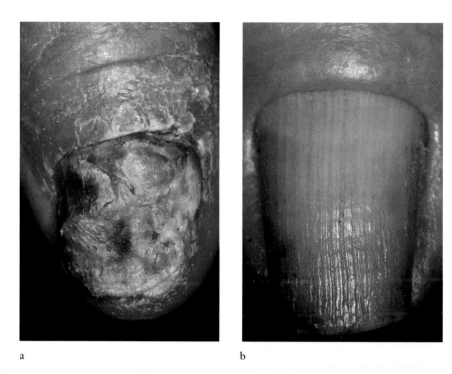

a                              b

## Figure 11.2

Hallopeau's acrodermatitis before (a) and after (b) treatment with oral nimesulide.

## Parakeratosis pustulosa

Whether parakeratosis pustulosa is a limited form of nail psoriasis or a clinical manifestation of other conditions such as atopic dermatitis is still being discussed.

### Topical treatment

Application of mild steroid and/or retinoic acid may induce partial remission of the nail changes. In most cases,

parakeratosis pustulosa resolves spontaneously as the child grows up.[12]

### Systemic treatment

Not applicable.

## Lichen planus

Lichen planus of the nail matrix requires aggressive treatment to prevent the definitive destruction of the nail. Pterygium and nail atrophy are not reversible and should not be treated.[13]

**Topical treatment (applicable only in nail bed lichen planus)**

Daily application of topical steroids to the nail bed after removal of the onycholytic nail plate.

**Intralesional treatment (applicable in nail matrix and/or nail bed lichen planus when few nails are affected)**

Intralesional steroid injections (triamcinolone acetonide 2.5 mg/ml) at a dose of 0.2 to 0.5 ml per nail. Injections should be repeated monthly for 3 to 6 months.

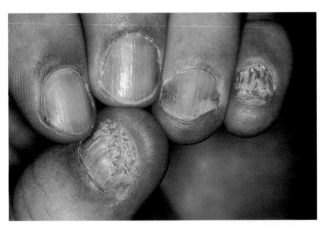

a

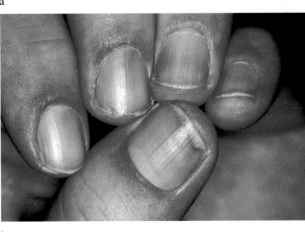

b

## Figure 11.3

Nail lichen planus before (a) and after (b) treatment with systemic steroids.

## Systemic treatment
### (nail matrix lichen planus involving several nails)

Oral methylprednisolone 0.5 mg/kg every other day for 2 to 6 weeks or intramuscular triamcinolone acetonide 0.5 mg/kg every month for 2 to 3 months (Fig. 11.3).[14] Most patients recover within 6 months after treatment, even though a certain degree of nail thinning and slight longitudinal striations frequently persist. Mild relapses are commonly observed, but recurrences are usually responsive to therapy. Oral retinoids such as etretinate or acitretin are a good alternative and should be used in the same manner as for treating psoriasis.

# Twenty nail dystrophy

This condition, characterized by nail roughness, can be idiopathic or associated with alopecia areata. The nail changes usually regress spontaneously in a few years. No treatment is required.[15]

# Yellow nail syndrome

The nail changes may improve spontaneously or after resolution of the associated systemic disease.

## Topical treatment
Not applicable.

## Intralesional treatment

Monthly steroid injections (triamcinolone acetonide 2.5 mg/ml) into the proximal nail fold and matrix area (even in the absence of associated chronic paronychia) may be useful.

## Systemic treatment

1. Oral vitamin E at dosages of 600 to 1200 IU daily for 6–18 months may induce a complete clearing of the nail changes (Fig. 11.4). Although the mechanism of action of vitamin E in yellow nail syndrome is still unknown, antioxidant properties of $\alpha$-tocopherol may account for its efficacy.[16]
2. Pulse therapy with itraconazole 400 mg daily for 1 week per month for 4 to 6 months.[17] Although the mode of action of itraconazole is still unknown, the drug may act by accelerating nail growth.

# Onychomycosis

For a review of the diagnosis and therapy of onychomycosis, see reference 18.

## Dermatophyte nail infections

These account for more than 90% of cases of onychomycosis. According to the modalities of the nail invasion, dermatophyte onychomycosis may be subdivided into four different types: superficial onychomycosis which is a superficial nail infection, and proximal

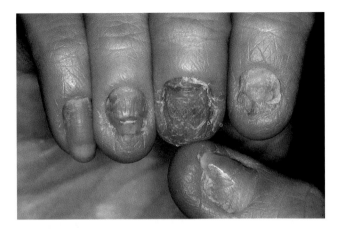

Figure 11.4

Yellow-nail-syndrome before (a) and after (b) treatment with vitamin E 1200 mg/day for 4 months.

a

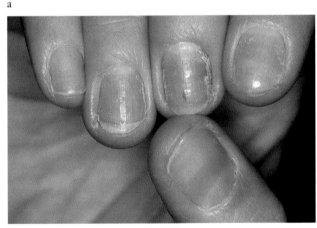

b

subungual onychomycosis (PSO), distal and lateral subungual onychomycosis (DLSO) and endonyx onychomycosis which are deep nail infections.[19]

**Topical treatment (applicable in superficial onychomycosis and in selected cases of DLSO)**

1. In superficial onychomycosis dermatophyte colonization is limited to the most superficial layers of the nail plate. Treatment of this condition is very easy, since it only requires scraping of the affected area followed by the application of a topical antifungal for 2 to 3 weeks.

2. Although distal subungual onychomycosis usually requires systemic antifungals, an exception to this rule may be represented by DLSO limited to the distal nail of a few

digits (fewer than three). This can be treated with one of the new transungual delivery systems containing topical antifungals. These include amorolfine 5% nail lacquer and ciclopirox 8% nail solution.[20-22] Amorolfine is applied once a week whereas ciclopirox requires daily application. Patients should be instructed to clean the surface of the affected nail with the lacquer remover before reapplying the medication. Treatment is continued for 6 to 12 months.

3. Despite the appearance of new potent antifungals and correct management of onychomycosis, all nails do not respond equally; some may remain unaffected by treatment especially those presenting with lateral nail plate invasion. Therefore, in some patients, particularly the elderly or those with only toenail involvement, simple grinding down of the mycotic nail plates may be the best therapy.

## Systemic treatment (applicable in DLSO and PSO)

In the last few years three new systemic antimycotics have been introduced onto the market: terbinafine, itraconazole and fluconazole. All these drugs have been shown to reach the distal nail soon after starting therapy and to persist in the nail plate for a long time (1 to 6 months) after interruption of treatment. The persistence of high post-treatment drug levels in the nail permits a short treatment period with fewer relapses and side effects. Partial nail avulsion and concomitant treatment with a topical antifungal agent further reduce duration of treatment.

Terbinafine is an allylamine derivative with primary fungicidal properties against dermatophytes. Recommended dosages are 250 mg/day for 6 weeks (fingernail infections) to 3 months (toenail infections). Terbinafine can also be administered as intermittent therapy at a dosage of 500 mg/day for 1 week every month for 2 to 4 months.[23] Terbinafine absorption is not affected by ingestion of food, but the drug delays gastric emptying.

Itraconazole is a triazole derivative with a broad spectrum fungistatic activity. Itraconazole is best administered as intermittent therapy at a dosage of 400 mg/day for 1 week every month. The duration of treatment ranges from 2 (fingernail infections) to 3–4 months (toenail infections). Accelerated nail growth has been reported during treatment with intermittent itraconazole. The drug should be administered with a high-fat meal to improve its absorption.[24]

Fluconazole is a triazole derivative with a broad action spectrum and a favourable adverse effects profile. Due to its long half-life, this drug can be administered on a once-weekly dosing regimen. The preferred dosage may be 150 or 300 mg weekly for 6 months up to 1 year.[25] Fluconazole may be a useful intermittent regimen in patients taking multiple medication and the once-weekly dosing may foster better patient compliance.

Patients treated with systemic antifungals should be followed for 4 to 12 months after discontinuation of therapy to evaluate efficacy. In fact, the nail will not be normal when therapy is discontinued but it will gradually improve as the new nail plate grows out. Clinical cure of onychomycosis can be established only when the new nail has completely regrown. This requires 6 months for fingernails and up to 1 year for toenails.

All the new systemic antifungals are very well tolerated. Most adverse reactions are of mild severity: gastrointestinal disturbances, pruritus, skin rashes, headache. Transitory loss of taste is not rare during terbinafine treatment. Symptomatic or asymptomatic hepatic damage is very rare and laboratory monitoring of patients during treatment is not mandatory.[26]

Since onychomycosis mostly affects elderly individuals who are usually taking several drugs, possible drug interactions of terbinafine, itraconazole and fluconazole should be considered before prescribing one of these drugs.[27]

Mycological cure rates of DLSO treated with terbinafine and itraconazole are >90% for fingernail infections and 60–90% for toenail infections according to different studies. Recurrences and/or reinfections are not uncommon (up to 20% of cured patients). They may be prevented by the application of topical antifungals on the previously affected nails, soles and toe webs.

## Onychomycosis due to non-dermatophytic moulds

For a more detailed description of the clinical features and treatment of onychomycosis due to non-dermatophytic moulds, see references 28 and 29.

### Topical treatment

Ciclopirox 8% nail lacquer is in our experience quite effective in PSO or DSO due to *Scopulariopsis brevicaulis*, *Fusarium* sp. and *Acremonium* sp. Chemical nail avulsion with 40% urea associated with 1% bifonazole in white petrolatum is also frequently successful. Infections due to *Scytalydium* sp. are usually unresponsive to treament.

### Systemic treatment

In our experience itraconazole and terbinafine are effective in nail infections due to *Aspergillus* sp. Systemic treatment is on the other hand scarcely useful for onychomycosis due to *Fusarium* sp, *S. brevicaulis* or *Scytalidium* sp.

## Candida onychomycosis

Onychomycosis due to *C. albicans* usually indicates an underlying immunological defect and is almost exclusively seen in chronic mucocutaneous candidiasis (CMCC) and HIV-infected patients. However, isolated *Candida* onychomycosis can be exceptionally observed in immunocompetent subjects.

## Topical treatment

Nail avulsion using urea-bifonazole ointment.

## Systemic treatment

Itraconazole 200 mg/day for 2 to 4 months is effective in treating *Candida* onychomycosis.

# Onychotillomania

This term includes nail biting, which is a very common habit in childhood, as well as all the other abnormalities produced by self-induced trauma to the nails and/or periungual tissues.

## Topical treatment

1. Frequent application of distasteful topical preparation such as 4% quinine in petrolatum to the nail and periungual skin can discourage patients from biting and chewing their fingernails. Possible alternatives include 1% clindamycin and quaternary ammonium derivatives.
2. Patients with severe onychotillomania can be helped to interrupt their habit by daily bandaging the injured fingers with micropore.

## Systemic treatment

Fluoxetine hydrochloride 20 mg/day orally can be useful.[30] In adults with onychotillomania, treatment of the underlying psychological disorder should be considered.

# Warts

Periungual and subungual warts are usually difficult to treat and frequently recur.

## Topical treatment

1. Topical anti-wart solutions containing salicylic and lactic acids are of moderate efficacy.
2. Topical immunotherapy with strong sensitizers (such as squaric acid dibutylester (SADBE) or diphencyprone is an effective and painless modality of treatment for multiple warts. SADBE or diphencyprone 2% in acetone are used for sensitization. After 21 days weekly applications are carried out with dilutions selected according to the patient's response. Complete cure usually requires 3 to 4 months (Fig. 11.5).

## Intralesional treatment

Bleomycin has been successfully used to treat viral warts for many years. The powder should be diluted to a concentration of 1 U/ml with saline. A bifurcate vaccination needle is utilized to introduce bleomycin into the. wart using the multiple puncture technique suggested by Shelley and Shelley.[31] After local anaesthesia, which may be obtained with a digital block, the bleomycin solution is dropped onto the wart, which is then punctured with the disposable bifurcated needle (Allergy Laboratory, Ohio Inc.) approximately

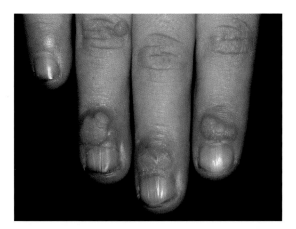

a

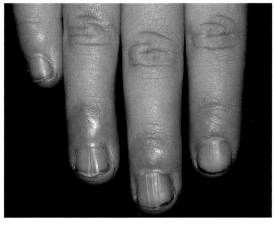

b

### Figure 11.5

Multiple periungual warts before (a) and after (b) topical immunotherapy with SADBE for 4 months.

40 times per 5 mm² area of the wart. No medications are required. Three weeks after treatment the eschar can be pared away and the area examined for residual warts, which can be re-injected if necessary. This technique minimizes the amount of bleomycin introduced into the skin and avoids introduction of the drug into the dermis.

## Surgical treatment

Subungual warts first require removal of the nail plate covering the wart under local anaesthesia. Curettage is then performed. This is followed by application of an antibiotic ointment and thick gauze padding. The $CO_2$ laser can successfully be used to treat subungual and periungual warts.

# Ingrowing nails

## Juvenile ingrowing nails

Ingrowing nails are a common complaint and usually affect the great toe of young adults.

### Topical treatment

1. Stage 1 ingrowing nails are treated with extraction of the embedded spicule and introduction of a package of non-absorbent cotton (soaked in a disinfectant) under the lateral corner of the nail. This medication should be replaced daily.
2. In stage 2 ingrowing nails the application of high potency steroids for a few days can promptly reduce the overgrowth of granulation tissue. Conservative treatment as for stage 1 can then be utilized.[32]

### Surgical treatment

Treatment of stage 3 ingrowing nails requires selective destruction of the lateral horn of the nail matrix. This may be achieved by phenol cauterization or by surgical lateral matrix excision.[33]

Phenol cauterization is applied after removal of the lateral strip of the offending nail. Haemostasis is achieved with a tourniquet and the blood is carefully cleared from the nail pocket. The surrounding skin is protected with petroleum jelly and a saturated solution of phenol is applied to the lateral matrix horn on a small cotton pack for

3 minutes, followed by neutralization with alcohol. The patient should be instructed to soak the foot twice daily in a quart of warm water containing three capsules of povidone-iodine (Betadine). This accelerates healing and prevents possible secondary infections.

Lateral matrix excision involves dissecting and excising the lateral matrix horn from the base of the phalanx (Haneke's technique).

## Distal nail embedding

This is a common complication of total nail plate avulsion or shedding.

### Topical treatment

Sculptured artificial nails can be used to override the distal nail wall.

### Surgical treatment

In severe cases, a crescent wedge tissue excision is carried out around the entire distal phalanx, and the defect is closed with 5-0 monofilament suture.

## Congenital malalignment of the great toenail

Management depends on accurate assessment of the degree of malalignment and associated changes. If the nail deviaton is mild, and in the absence of complications, the nail may overcome

the initial slight embedding produced
by the distal lip, as it hardens, and
sufficient normal nail may grow to the
tip of the digit to prevent further
secondary traumatic changes. Treatment should be conservative.

## Surgical treatment

If the deviation is marked and the nail
is buried in the soft tissues, the
patient may be disabled in later childhood and adult life. Although best
results are obtained when the congenital malalignment is corrected surgi-
cally before the age of 2 years, surgery
may be postponed provided photo-
graphic surveys are made at 6-month
intervals.

  Surgical rotation of the misdirected
matrix is essential to prevent permanent nail dystrophy, despite the possible favourable course of some cases. A
crescent, wedge-shaped resection
must be carried back proximal to and
below the nail bed and nail matrix
with special care in dissecting the
lateral horns of the latter. The
crescent has to be larger on the medial
than on the lateral aspect. A small
triangular area is also excised at the
start of the lateral incision line,
thereby enabling the whole nail
apparatus to be swung over the
resected area so that it may be
realigned and then sutured. When the
nail is medially deviated, the resected
crescent must be larger on the lateral
aspect than on the medial one, and a
small triangular area is also excised at
the start of the medial incision line.[34]

# References

1.   Colombo VE, Gerber F, Bronhofer M,
Floersheim GL, Treatment of brittle
fingernails and onychoschizia with biotin:
scanning electron microscopy. *J Am Acad
Dermatol* 1990: 23; 1127–32.

2.   Tosti A, Guerra L, Morelli R, Bardazzi
F, Role of foods in the pathogenesis of
chronic paronychia. *J Am Acad Dermatol*
1992: 27; 706–10.

3.   Tosti A, Piraccini BM, Paronychia. In:
Amin S, Lahti A, Maibach HI (eds) *Contact
urticaria syndrome*. Boca Raton: CRC Press,
1998; pp. 276–8.

4.   Baran R, Les onycholyses. *Ann Dermatol Venereol* 1986: 113; 159–70.

5.   de Berker D, Management of nail psoriasis. *Clin Exp Dermatol* 2000: 25; 357–62.

6.   Baran R, Dawber RPR, The nail in
dermatological diseases. In: Baran R,
Dawber RPR (eds) *Diseases of the nails and
their management, 2nd edn*. Oxford: Blackwell Scientific Publications, 1994, pp.
135–73.

7.   Tosti A, Morelli R, Bardazzi F, Piraccini BM, Psoriasis of the nails. In:
Dubertret L (ed) *Psoriasis*. Brescia: Ised,
1994, pp. 201–7.

8.   Baran R, Tosti A, Topical treatment of
nail psoriasis with a new corticoid-contain-
ing nail laquer formulation. *J Dermatol
Treatment* 1999: 10; 201–4.

9.   Tosti A, Piraccini BM, Cameli N et al,
Calcipotriol ointment in nail psoriasis: a
controlled double-blind comparison with
betamethasone dipropionate and salicylic
acid. *Br J Dermatol* 1998: 139; 655–9.

10.  de Berker DAR, Lawrence CM, A
simplified protocol of steroid infection for

psoriatic nail dystrophy. *Br J Dermatol* 1998: 138; 90–5.

11.   Piraccini BM, Tosti A, Jorizzo M, Misciali C, Pustular psoriasis of the nails: treatment and long term follow up of 46 patients. *Br J Dermatol* 2001: 144; 1000–5.

12.   Tosti A, Peluso AM, Zucchelli V, Clinical features and long-term follow-up of 20 cases of parakeratosis pustolosa. *Pediatr Dermatol* 1998: 15; 259–63.

13.   Tosti A, Peluso AM, Fanti PA, Piraccini BM, Nail lichen planus: clinical and pathological study of 24 patients. *J Am Acad Dermatol* 1993: 28; 724–30.

14.   Tosti A, Piraccini BM, Cambiaghi S, Jorizzo M, Nail lichen planus in children: clinical features, response to treatment and long term follow up. *Arch Dermatol* 2001: 137; 1027–32.

15.   Tosti A, Piraccini BM, Trachyonychia or twenty nail dystrophy. *Curr Opin Dermatol* 1996: 3; 83–6.

16.   Norton L, Further observation on the yellow nail syndrome with therapeutic effects of oral alpha-tocopherol. *Cutis* 1985: 36; 457–62.

17.   Luyten C, André J, Walraevens C et al, Yellow nail syndrome. Experience with itraconazole pulse therapy combined with vitamin E. *Dermatology* 1996: 192; 406–8.

18.   Baran R, Hay R, Haneke E, Tosti A (eds), Onychomycosis: the current approach to diagnosis and therapy. London: Martin Dunitz, 1999.

19.   Baran R, Hay RJ, Tosti A, Haneke E, A new classification of onychomycosis. *Br J Dermatol* 1998: 139; 567–71.

20.   Zaug M, Bergstraesser M, Amorolfine in the treatment of onychomycoses and dermatomycoses (an overview). *Clin Exp Dermatol* 1992: 17 (Suppl 1); 61–70.

21.   Ceschin-Roques CG, Hänel H, Pruja-Bougaret SM et al, Ciclopirox nail lacquer 8%: in vivo penetration into and through nails and in vitro effect on pig skin. *Skin Pharmacol* 1991: 4; 89–94.

22.   Baran R, Feuilhade M, Datry A et al, A randomized trial of amorolfine 5% solution nail lacquer combined with oral terbinafine compared with terbinafine alone in the treatment of dermatophytic toenail onychomycoses affecting the matrix region. *Br J Dermatol* 2000: 142: 1177–83.

23.   Tosti A, Piraccini BM, Stinchi C et al, Treatment of dermatophyte nail infections: an open randomized study comparing intermittent terbinafine therapy with continuous terbinafine treatment and intermittent itraconazole therapy. *J Am Acad Dermatol* 1996: 34; 595–600.

24.   De Doncker P, Decroix J, Pierard GE et al, Antifungal pulse therapy for onychomycosis. *Arch Dermatol* 1996: 132; 34–41.

25.   Gupta AK, Scher RK, Rich P, Fluconazole for the treatment of onychomycosis: an update. *Int J Dermatol* 1998: 37; 815–20.

26.   Hay RJ, Risk/benefit ratio of modern antifungal therapy: focus on hepatic reactions. *J Am Acad Dermatol* 1993: 29; 550–4.

27.   Brodell RT, Helewski BE, Clinical pearl: systemic antifungal drugs and drug interactions. *J Am Acad Dermatol* 1995: 33; 259–60.

28.   Tosti A, Piraccini BM, Lorenzi S, Onychomycosis due to non-dermatophytic moulds: clinical features and response to treatment. *J Am Acad Dermatol* 2000: 42; 217–24.

29. Hay RJ, Onychomycosis. Agents of choice. *Dermatol Clin* 1993: 11; 161–9.

30. Vittorio CC, Phillips KA, Treatment of habit-tic deformity with fluoxetine. *Arch Dermatol* 1997: 133; 1203–4.

31. Shelley WB, Shelley FD, Intralesional bleomycin sulfate therapy for warts. *Arch Dermatol* 1991: 12; 234–6.

32. Zaias N, Ingrown nails. In: Zaias N (ed) *The nail in health and disease*. New York: Appleton and Lange, 1988, pp. 83–5.

33. Haneke E, Baran R, Nail surgery and traumatic abnormalities. In: Baran R, Dawber RPR (eds) *Diseases of the nails and their management, 2nd edn*. Oxford: Blackwell Scientific Publications, 1994, pp. 345–415.

34. Baran R, Significance and management of congenital malalignment of the big toenail. *Cutis* 1996: 58; 181–4.

# 12

## Novel drugs for the treatment of skin cancer

*Christoph C Geilen,
Konstantin Krasagakis and
Constantinos E Orfanos*

## Introduction

There is a worldwide increasing incidence of all forms of skin cancer, both nonmelanoma skin cancer and also malignant melanoma. It has been reported, that 92,000 cases of melanoma and 2,750,000 cases of nonmelanoma skin cancer occur worldwide each year.[1] The increase in these disorders in the last decades can be considered, in part, as a result of the tremendous increase in the average individual dose of ultraviolet radiation since the 1950s. Sun damage of the skin may result from the fact that vacation times and time spent in sunnier parts of our world have increased considerably, and the fashion for being suntanned has prevailed in white Caucasian populations during the last decades.

Basal cell carcinomas and squamous cell carcinomas commonly arise on the head and neck of patients with fair skin and/or a history of long term sun exposure. In contrast, melanomas appear to be more related to episodes of acute sunburn, especially in childhood and in adolescence. Acute sun damage seems to induce the development of common and atypical nevi and leads to increased risk for developing cutaneous melanoma.[2] A further precipitating factor for the rising incidence of skin cancer may become the ongoing destruction of the ozone layer by nitrogen oxides, chlorofluorocarbons and other forms of environmental pollution.

In consequence, skin cancer is common today and may become an everyday finding in large population groups in the near future. Therefore, not only prevention and early diagnosis, but also adequate therapy appear necessary. In this chapter we outline possible new concepts for the treatment of skin cancer and melanoma, focusing on a selection of novel drugs which presently are under experimental investigation and/or in first clinical trials.

## Chemotherapeutic agents

Currently available anticancer drugs act mainly by interfering with mitotic activity or by preventing DNA synthesis in tumor tissue (Fig. 12.1). Anticancer agents can be divided into five

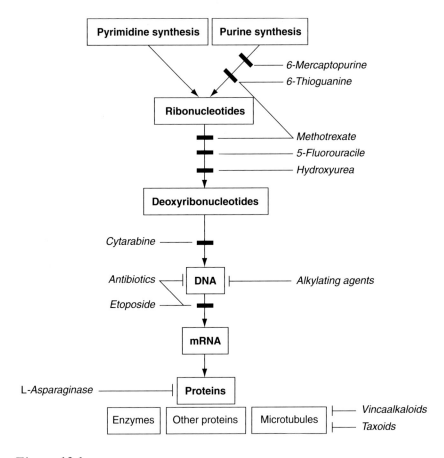

## Figure 12.1

Sites of action of anticancer drugs.

major classes (Table 12.1). Several new chemotherapeutic agents have been discovered in recent years. Taxoids are a new class of cytotoxic drugs with a novel mechanism of action: stabilization of tubulin polymers and promotion of microtubule assembly. In head and neck cancer, two compounds have been tested: docetaxel, extracted from the European yew (*Taxus baccata*), and paclitaxel, extracted from the Pacific yew (*Taxus brevifolia*). The chemical structure of paclitaxel is shown in Fig. 12.2. In a European multicentre phase II trial in 43 patients with advanced disease, docetaxel (100 mg/m² i.v.

## Table 12.1 Classification of anticancer drugs

| Alkylating agents | Antibiotics | Antimetabolites | Inhibitors of mitosis | Others |
|---|---|---|---|---|
| Carmustine | Bleomycin | Cytosine | Etoposide | L-Asparaginase |
| Chlorambucil | Daunorubicin | Arabinoside | Vinblastine | Hydroxyurea |
| Cisplatin | Doxorubicin | Fluorouracil | Vincristine | Procarbazine |
| Cyclophosphamide | Mitomycin C | Mercaptopurine | Vindesine | Miltefosine |
| Ifosfamide | | Methotrexate | Taxoids | |
| Melphalan | | | | |

every 3 weeks) showed a 32% response rate.[3] Paclitaxel (250 mg/m² as a 24-hour continuous infusion) was reported to induce a 40% response rate in 30 patients with head and neck cancer, but at this dose level serious hematological toxicity is observed.[4] Docetaxel has also been used for the treatment of advanced malignant melanoma in phase II studies. An overall response rate of 12–17% was reported for monotherapies.[5,6]

In a phase II study, the prodrug of methylimidazole carboxamide, temozolomide, was shown to be successful as an oral chemotherapeutic agent with an overall response rate of about 26%, as reported for malignant melanoma.[7,8]

The new pyrimidine antimetabolite gemcitabine (LY 188011) showed a 13% response rate in a multicentre phase II study in 54 patients.[9] In view of its low response rate but its favourable toxicity profile, gemcitabine has been proposed as a good candidate for combined chemotherapeutic schedules. Recently, the third-generation

platinum analogue, zeniplatin, in a monotherapy protocol showed modest activity in a first phase II trial in metastatic melanoma.[10]

Although tamoxifen, an antiestrogen used for the treatment of breast carcinoma, has little efficacy as a single agent in the treatment of melanoma, it probably acts synergistically with cisplatin through its calcium channel-blocking properties and may then overcome antitumour drug resistance. Indeed, removal of tamoxifen from a cisplatin-containing antimelanoma regimen (DBCT) resulted in a significant decrease in the response rate.[11]

Another recent advance is the development of cytoprotective substances that reduce the toxicity of chemotherapeutic agents in normal cells. Amifostine, developed as a radiation protector, may support cell survival by protecting nucleic acids from alkylation. Amifostine has been shown to reduce blood toxicity, neuropathy and nephrotoxicity in cyclophosphamide- and cisplatin-containing regimens.[12] Recently, the

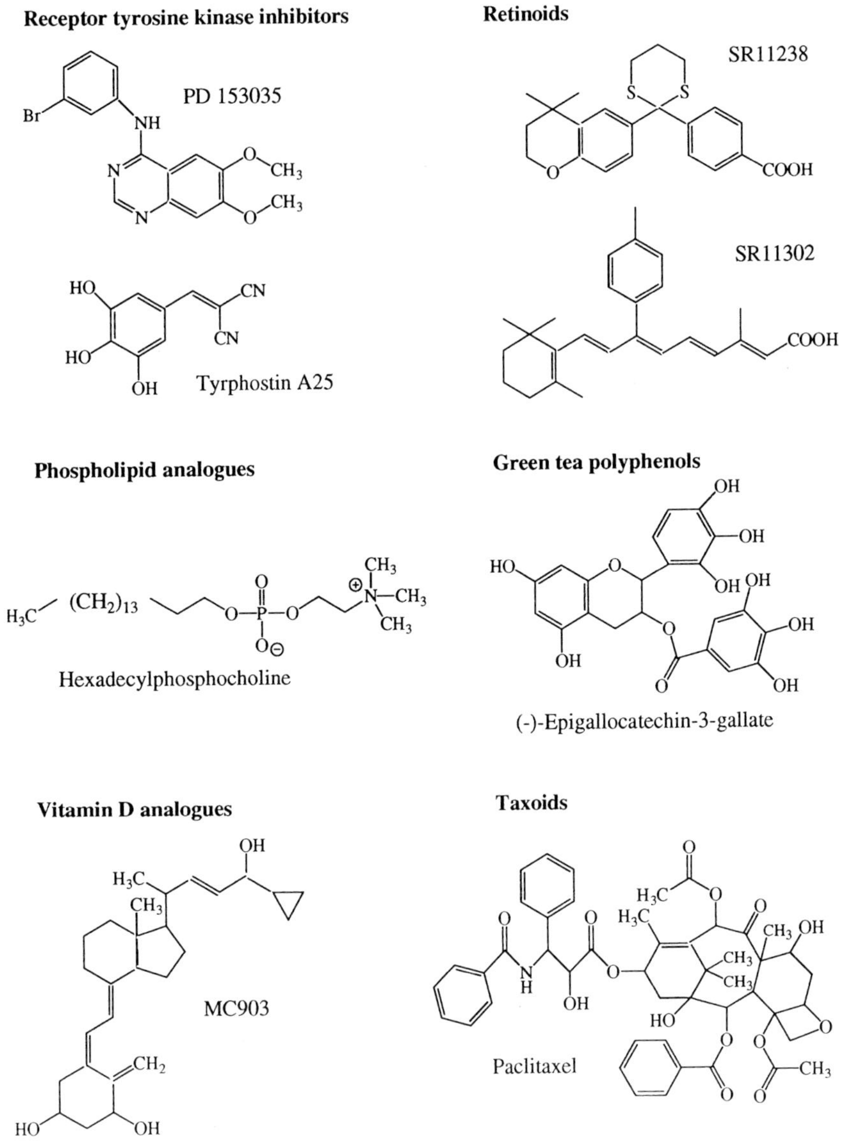

**Receptor tyrosine kinase inhibitors**

PD 153035

Tyrphostin A25

**Phospholipid analogues**

Hexadecylphosphocholine

**Vitamin D analogues**

MC903

**Retinoids**

SR11238

SR11302

**Green tea polyphenols**

(-)-Epigallocatechin-3-gallate

**Taxoids**

Paclitaxel

## Figure 12.2

Chemical structures of anticancer agents.

treatment of ten stage IV melanoma patients with amifostine and fotemustine in combination was reported.[13] Patients were treated with amifostine (740 mg/m²) prior to fotemustine chemotherapy (100 mg/m²). In this study, no patient developed severe myelosuppression, whereas with fotemustine monotherapy over 40% of patients have been reported to develop leukopenia and thrombocytopenia.

A novel approach in chemotherapy is the use of liposomal formulations. Such formulations of well known chemostatic drugs have been shown to be useful for treatment of skin cancer and skin metastases of other neoplasms. Promising results have been obtained using liposomal doxorubicin for the treatment of head and neck carcinomas.[14] Liposomal doxorubicin[15] and daunorubicin[16] have been reported to be effective in the treatment of Kaposi's sarcoma in HIV-infected patients.

# Cytokines, growth factors, antibodies and toxins

There is substantial evidence that the immune system plays an important role in maintaining prevention and control of cancer. The immune response alone is, however, often not sufficient to combat neoplasia if weak immunogenicity or the appearance of active immunosuppression induced by the malignant cells occur. A possible strategy for circumventing this problem is the amplification of the antitumour immune response by immunostimulatory cytokines, such as interleukin-2 (IL-2). In metastatic melanoma, IL-2 was found to be active with overall response rates of approximately 20% and an additive effect in combination with interferon α (IFN-α) has been demonstrated.[17] Recently, IFN alfa-2b given at high dose levels has been shown to prolong both relapse-free intervals and the overall survival of patients with high-risk resected cutaneous melanoma in an adjuvant setting.[18] A phase I trial exploring the effects of other cytokines has shown some activity of IL-12 against malignant melanoma[19] and further trials are planned to confirm these results.

Another strategy has been the use of tumour-specific antibodies which increase the immune response of the host against the tumour. In some initial clinical trials it was shown that this approach is able to reduce the tumour mass.[20] A phase I trial was performed in 11 patients with advanced cancer using a monoclonal antibody (FC-2.15) that recognized antigens present in breast cancer cells. The monoclonal antibody was administered by intravenous infusion with total doses between 2.5 and 5 mg/kg and one partial response was reported.[21]

Identification of several melanoma-associated antigens and molecular characterization of the sequences involved in immune recognition allowed the development of novel strategies for vaccination through the induction of specific cytotoxic T-lymphocytes.

Several phase I studies with synthetic melanoma-associated peptides have been initiated in recent years. Intradermal vaccination of ten advanced melanoma patients revealed disease stabilization in five patients and minor tumour regressions in two patients.[22] Optimization of vaccination protocols with cytokines or peptide-loaded antigen-presenting cells may improve response rates. Candidate genes for peptide vaccinations include Melan-A, tyrosinase, gp100 and MAGE 1–3. Also, induction of GM2 antibodies after vaccination of GM2 antibody-negative melanoma patients with GM2/BCG vaccine has been shown to be associated with prolonged disease-free intervals and overall survival rates.[23] Treatment with the murine monoclonal antibody R-24 which reacts with the ganglioside GD3 resulted in complete remission of meningeal melanoma in one of two patients after intrathecal administration, and in partial remission of advanced melanoma in two of nine patients after low-dose intravenous administration.[24]

Another new approach is to target therapeutic bacterial toxins to cancer cells by the use of chimeric proteins. In this approach, a toxin is linked to a cytokine which binds specifically to a subset of specific cells, e.g. cancer cells. Recently, a novel chimeric protein composed of *Pseudomonas* exotoxin and interleukin-13 has been shown to be highly toxic to human carcinoma cells. In different epithelial cancer cell lines, an $IC_{50}$ of 1 to 300 ng/ml was found in vitro.[25]

# Novel retinoids and retinoid combination therapies

Retinoids influence a wide range of biological processes including cell proliferation and the promotion of cell differentiation in various tissues.[26] They are of increasing importance as anticancer drugs as often suggested.[27,28] Synthetic retinoids have been shown to be beneficial in the treatment of basal cell and other epithelial tumours, but in contrast, no satisfactory therapeutic results have been reported for retinoid treatment of squamous cell carcinomas.[26] Recently, it was reported that a combination of 13-*cis*-retinoic acid (1 mg/kg per day) and IFN alfa-2a (3 or 6×10⁶ U/day) had a positive effect in 68% of patients with advanced squamous cell cancer.[29] Also, a similar combination of 60 mg 13-*cis*-retinoic acid daily and 6×10⁶ IFN-α five times per week with a 2-week IFN-free interval resulted in an overall response rate of 30% with 12% complete responses in patients with disseminated malignant melanoma.[30]

In another recent investigation, it was found that retinoid-mediated AP-1 inhibition leads to an antiproliferative effect in tumour cells which is independent of the receptor-transactivating potential of these compounds.[31] Using the mouse epidermal cell line JB6, it was shown that the new anti-AP-1 retinoids SR11238 and SR11302 (Fig. 12.2) block phorbol ester-induced cell transformation.[32] In the future, this new generation of retinoid compounds which selectively inhibit AP-1 may be used in the treatment of skin cancer.

## Vitamin D analogues

1α,25-Dihydroxyvitamin D$_3$ and other analogues (calcipotriol, tacalcitol) have been introduced for the treatment of benign hyperproliferative skin disease, such as psoriasis. The induction of a new signal transduction pathway, the sphingomyelin cycle, has been shown to be involved in mediating the antiproliferative effects of these interesting compounds.[33–36] In a new therapeutic approach, vitamin D analogues such as MC 903 (Fig. 12.2) and EB 1089, have been used to treat skin cancer.[37,38]

Very recently it has been demonstrated that the vitamin D analogue CB 1093 induces apoptosis in different malignant melanoma cell lines and may therefore be a promising new compound for the therapy of malignant melanoma in the future.[39]

## Phospholipid analogues

Phospholipid analogues are experimental agents with antineoplastic activities in vitro and in vivo.[40–43] In dermatology, alkylphosphocholines in particular have been investigated with respect to their antiproliferative properties.[44,45] Following these initial studies, different mechanisms of action have been shown including (1) inhibition of membrane phospholipid biosynthesis[46–48] and (2) modulation of cell–matrix interactions.[49]

In malignant cutaneous lymphomas, the benefit of topically applied hexadecylphosphocholine (miltefosine, Fig. 12.2) has been investigated. Among seven patients with cutaneous T-cell lymphoma, two with complete remission, two with partial remission, two with stable disease and one with progressive disease were observed. Among five patients with B-cell lymphoma, one with complete remission, three with partial remission and one with stable disease were seen. Furthermore, two patients with lymphomatoid papulosis treated with hexadecylphosphocholine showed complete remission.[45] The possible beneficial effect of hexadecylphosphocholine in patients with advanced basal cell carcinomas is now the subject of ongoing clinical investigation.

A new class of glucose-containing phospholipid analogues have been shown recently to inhibit cell proliferation of epidermal cells in vitro. Further studies are needed to investigate their possible therapeutic effect in skin cancer.[50–52]

## Antioxidants

The generation of free oxygen radicals is believed to play a major role in the pathogenesis of photoinduced skin cancer. This oxidative stress can be antagonized by antioxidants. The major naturally occurring antioxidant is vitamin E,[53] but also vitamin C has been found to be effective as an antioxidant in preventing the initiation of skin cancer, at least in experimental systems.[54]

# Green tea polyphenols

In recent years, green tea polyphenols isolated from green tea leaves have been shown in different animal tumour assay systems to protect against different chemical and UV light-induced skin cancers.

In BALB/C mice, topically applied green tea polyphenols protected significantly against 3-methylcholanthrene-induced skin cancer.[55] It has been demonstrated that (−)-epigallo-catechin-3-gallate (see Fig. 12.2) is the most potent compound among the different polyphenol derivatives.[56] Protection against UVB-induced photocarcinogenesis by green tea polyphenols has been shown by Wang et al.[57] In humans, epidemiological studies have indicated that individuals consuming green tea more frequently tended to have a lower risk for gastric cancer.[58,59] An increasing amount of experimental and epidemiological data suggest that green tea polyphenols possess anticancer activity and show potential as new agents for the prevention and treatment of skin neoplasia.[60]

# Modulators of cell signalling

Clinical as well as experimental evidence indicates that malignancy and cellular differentiation are inversely correlated. An increasing knowledge of mechanisms involved in the regulation of cell proliferation and differentiation would offer new therapeutic strategies for treating skin cancer. Among the regulators of growth and differentiation control are cytokines, hormones and growth factors which interact with specific receptors and communicate with the nucleus via a network of intracellular signalling pathways. Under pathological conditions, especially in cancer cells, these signalling pathways are frequently altered, leading to dysregulation of cell growth. Therefore, signalling pathways may provide potential targets for therapeutic interventions in treating neoplasia.[61-65]

In general, cell signalling events can be subdivided into different subcellular levels of signal transduction steps, as shown in Fig. 12.3, and any of these levels can become a particular target for anticancer drug therapy. For example, the agonist-receptor interaction can be blocked by neutralizing antibodies.[66] This approach has been tested using monoclonal antibodies raised against the extracellular domain of the EGF receptor. In these investigations, treatment of squamous cancer cells with antibodies inhibited their growth.[67-68] This approach is presently being investigated in phase I trials.

At the level of the receptor/effector interaction, tyrphostins have been used. These potently block cell proliferation mediated by receptor tyrosine kinases, e.g. the EGF receptor.[69] In dermatology, the first promising data have been published for the treatment of psoriatic keratinocytes with tyrphostins, e.g. tyrphostin A25 (Fig. 12.2).[70] New EGF receptor-specific tyrphostins, e.g. PD 153035 (Fig.

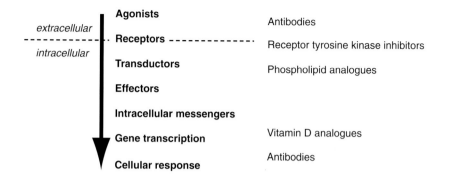

## Figure 12.3

Subcellular levels of signal transduction targets for anticancer compounds.

12.2), show clinical potential since they have been found to inhibit at picomolar concentrations.[71]

The plasma membrane NADH oxidase has been shown to be a possible therapeutic target in different malignant cell types, e.g. malignant melanoma cells. Synthetic retinoids and capsaicin inhibit this enzyme and this effect is paralleled by a strong antiproliferative effect.[72,73]

Bryostatin 1, a macrocyclic natural lactone isolated from a marine Bryozoan, has undergone phase I testing in humans. The mechanism of action of this compound depends in part on its ability to activate protein kinase C. Bryostatin 1 showed antitumoral activity after intravenous application in patients with advanced melanoma.[74] Bryostatin analogues 5 and 8 have shown similar antitumour activity but decreased side effects in vivo,[75] and are thus candidates for

clinical trials. Signal transduction-directed chemicals have entered first clinical trials in cancer patients in recent years. Early clinical experience gives cause for some optimism and indicates that inhibition of cell signalling pathways may be a new area for drug development worth further investigation.

## Conclusions

Over 40 approved anticancer agents are presently in clinical use. Nevertheless, chemotherapies are helpful in no more than 10 to 15% of patients with cancer. In dermatology, there is clearly an important need for new concepts to optimize melanoma treatment; conventional schedules are still not satisfactory. This requires new strategies and new types of anticancer agents. Most of the experimental approaches described in this chapter may still not have the power to completely inhibit malignant tumour growth, but combinations of such new concepts with established therapeutic regimens may provide a major check against skin cancer, particularly in patients with malignant melanoma.

# References

1.  Annstrong BK, Kricker A, Skin cancer. *Dermatol Clin* 1995: 13; 583–94.

2.  Garbe C, Büttner P, Weiss J et al, Risk factors for developing cutaneous melanoma and criteria for identifying persons at risk: multicenter case-control study on the central malignant melanoma registry of the German Dermatological Society. *J Invest Dermatol* 1994: 102; 695–9.

3.  Catimel G, Verweij J, Mattijssen V et al, Docetaxel (Taxotere): an active drug for the treatment of patients with advanced squamous cell carcinoma of the head and neck. *Ann Oncol* 1994: 5; 533–7.

4.  Forastiere A, Use of paclitaxel (Taxol) in squamous cell carcinoma of the head and neck. *Semin Oncol* 1993: 20 (Suppl 3); 56–60.

5.  Aamdal S, Wolff I, Kaplan S et al, Docetaxel (Taxotere) in advanced malignant melanoma: a phase II study of the EORTC early clinical trials group. *Eur J Cancer* 1994: 30A(8); 1061–4.

6.  Bedikian AY, Weiss GR, Legha SS et al, Phase II trial of docetaxel in patients with advanced cutaneous malignant melanoma previously untreated with chemotherapy. *J Clin Oncol* 1995: 13; 2895–9.

7.  Bleehen NM, Newlands ES, Lee SM et al, Cancer research campaign phase II trial of temozolomide in metastatic melanoma. *J Clin Oncol* 1995: 13; 910–3.

8.  Marzolini C, Decosterd LA, Shen F et al, Pharmacokinetics of temozolomide in association with fotemustine in malignant melanoma and malignant glioma patients: comparison of oral, intravenous, and hepatic intra-arterial administration. *Cancer Chemother Pharmacol* 1998: 42; 433–40.

9.  Catimel G, Vermorken JB, Clavel M et al, A phase II study of gemcitabine (LY 188011) in patients with advanced squamous cell carcinoma of the head and neck. EORTC Early Clinical Trials Group. *Ann Oncol* 1994: 5; 543–7.

10.  Olver I, Green M, Peters W et al, A phase II trial of zeniplatin in metastatic melanoma. *Am J Clin Oncol* 1995: 18; 56–8.

11.  McClay EF, Mastrangelo MJ, Sprandio JD et al, The importance of tamoxifen to a cisplatin-containing regimen in the treatment of metastatic melanoma. *Cancer* 1989: 63; 1292–5.

12.  Capizzi RL, Protection of normal tissues from the cytotoxic effects of chemotherapy by amifostine (Ethyol): clinical experiences. *Semin Oncol* 1994: 21; 8–15.

13.  Mohr P, Makki A, Breitbart E, Schadendorf D, Combined treatment of stage IV melanoma patients with amifostine and fotemustine – a pilot study. *Melanoma Res* 1998: 8; 166–6.

14.  Uziely B, Jeffers S, Isacson R et al, Liposomal doxorubicin: antitumor activity and unique toxicities during two complementary phase I studies. *J Clin Oncol* 1995: 13; 1777–85.

15.  Bergin C, O'Leary A, McCreary C et al, Treatment of Kaposi's sarcoma with liposomal doxorubicin. *Am J Health Syst Pharm* 1995: 52; 2001–4.

16.  Tulpule A, Yung RC, Wernz J et al, Phase II trial of liposomal daunorubicin in the treatment of AIDS-related pulmonary Kaposi's sarcoma. *J Clin Oncol* 1998: 16; 3369–74.

17.  Garbe C, Perspectives of cytokine treatment in malignant skin tumors. *Recent Results Cancer Res* 1995: 139; 349–69.

18.  Kirkwood JM, Strawderman MH, Ernstoff MS et al, Interferon alfa-2b adjuvant therapy of high-risk resected cutaneous melanoma: the Eastern Cooperative Oncology Group Trial EST 1684. *J Clin Oncol* 1996: 14; 7–17.

19.  Atkins MB, Robertson IMJ, Gordon MS et al, Phase I evaluation of intravenous recombinant human interleukin 12 (RHIL-12) in patients with advanced malignancies. *Proc Am Soc Clin Oncol* 1996: 15: 270.

20.  Bystryn JC, Clinical activity of a polyvalent melanoma antigen vaccine. *Recent Results Cancer Res* 1995: 139; 337–48.

21.  Mordoh J, Siva C, Albarellos M et al, Phase I clinical trial in cancer patients of a new monoclonal antibody FC-2.15 reacting with tumor proliferating cells. *J Immunother Emphasis Tumor Immunol* 1995: 17: 151–60.

22.  Jäger E, Ilsemann C, Hagedorn M et al, Spezifische Immuntherapie des malignen Melanoms mit synthetischen Melanom-assoziierten Peptiden. *Z Hautkr* 1996: 71; 875 (abstract).

23.  Livingston PO, Wong GY, Adluri S et al, Improved survival in stage III melanoma patients with GM2 antibodies: a randomized trial of adjuvant vaccination with GM2 ganglioside. *J Clin Oncol* 1994: 12; 1036–44.

24.  Dippold W, Bernhard H, Meyer zum Buschenfelde KH, Immunological response to intrathecal and systemic treatment with ganglioside antibody R-24 in patients with malignant melanoma. *Eur J Cancer* 1994: 30A; 137–44.

25.  Debinski W, Obiri NI, Pastan I, Puri PK, A novel chimeric protein of interleukin 13 and Pseudomonas exotoxin is highly cytotoxic to human carcinoma cells expressing receptors for interleukin 13 and interleukin 4. *J Biol Chem* 1995: 270; 16775–80.

26.  Orfanos CE, Zouboulis ChC, Almond-Roesler B, Geilen CC, Current use and future potential of retinoids in dermatology. *Drugs* 1997: 53; 358–88.

27.  Bollag W, Holdener EE, Retinoids in cancer prevention and therapy. *Ann Oncol* 1992: 3; 513–26.

28.  Kurie JM, Lippman SM, Hong WK, Potential of retinoids in cancer prevention. *Cancer Treat Rev* 1994: 20; 1–10.

29.  Eisenhauer FA, Lippman SM, Kavanagh JJ et al, Combination 13-cis-retinoic acid and interferon alpha 2a in the therapy of solid tumors. *Leukemia* 1994: 8; 1622–5.

30.  Fierlbeck G, Schreiner T, Rassner G, Combination of highly purified human leukocyte interferon alpha and 13-cis-retinoic acid for the treatment of metastatic melanoma. *Cancer Immunol Immunother* 1995: 40; 157–64.

31.  Fanjul A, Dawson MI, Hobbs PD et al, A new class of retinoids with selective inhibition of AP-1 inhibits proliferation. *Nature* 1994: 372; 107–11.

32. Li JJ, Dong Z, Dawson M, Colburn NH, Inhibition of tumor promotor-induced transformation by retinoids that transrepress AP-1 without transactivating retinoic acid response element. *Cancer Res* 1996: 56; 483–9.

33. Geilen CC, Bektas M, Wieder T, Orfanos CE, The vitamin D3 analogue, calcipotriol, induces sphingomyelin hydrolysis in human keratinocytes. *FEBS Lett* 1996: 378; 88–92.

34. Geilen CC, Bektas M, Wieder T et al, $1\alpha,25$ Dihydroxyvitamin $D_3$ induces sphingomyelin hydrolysis in HaCaT cells via tumor necrosis factor $\alpha$. *J Biol Chem* 1997: 272: 8997–9001.

35. Geilen CC, Wieder T, Orfanos CE, Ceramide signalling: regulatory role for cell proliferation and apoptosis in human epidermis. *Arch Dermatol Res* 1997: 289; 559–66.

36. Wu S, Geilen CC, Tebbe B, Orfanos CE, $1\alpha,25$-Dihydroxyvitamin $D_3$: its role for the homeostasis of keratinocytes. *J Nutr Biochem* 1996: 7; 642–9.

37. Hansen CM, Maenpaa EB 1089, a novel vitamin D analog with strong antiproliferative and differentiation-inducing effects on target cells. *Biochem Pharmacol* 1997: 54; 1173–9.

38. Yu J, Papavasiliou V, Rhim J et al, Vitamin D analogs: new therapeutic agents for the treatment of squamous cancer and its associated hypercalcemia. *Anticancer Drugs* 1995: 6; 101–8.

39. Danielson C, Fehsel K, Polly P, Carlberg C, Differential apoptotic response of human melanoma cells to $1\alpha,25$-dihydroxyvitamin $D_3$ and its analogues. *Cell Death Differ* 1998: 5; 946–52.

40. Berdel WE, Membrane-interactive lipids as experimental anticancer drugs. *Br J Cancer* 1991: 64; 208–11.

41. Berdel WE, Munder PG, Antineoplastic actions of ether lipids related to platelet-activating factor. In: Snyder F (ed) *Platelet-activating factor and related lipid mediators.* New York: Plenum Press, 1987, p. 449–67.

42. Berdel WE, Andreesen R, Munder PG, Synthetic alkyl-phospholipid analogs; a new class of antitumor agents. In: Kuo JF (ed) *Phospholipids and cellular regulation, vol II.* Boca Raton: CRC Press, 1985, p. 41–73.

43. Wieder T, Reutter W, Orfanos CE, Geilen CC, The effect of hexadecylphosphocholine on the proliferation of human keratinocytes in vitro and in vivo. *Drugs Today* 1998: 34; 97–105.

44. Detmar M, Geilen CC, Wieder T et al, Phospholipid analogue hexadecylphosphocholine inhibits proliferation and phosphatidylcholine biosynthesis of human epidermal keratinocytes in vitro. *J Invest Dermatol* 1994: 102; 490–4.

45. Dummer R, Röger J, Vogt T et al, Topical application of hexadecylphosphocholine in patients with cutaneous lymphomas. *Prog Exp Tumor Res* 1992: 34; 160–9.

46. Geilen CC, Haase A, Wieder T et al, Phospholipid analogues: side chain- and polar head group-dependent effects on phosphatidylcholine biosynthesis. *J Lipid Res* 1994: 35; 625–32.

47. Geilen CC, Wieder T, Orfanos CE, Antiproliferative phospholipid analogues act via inhibition of phosphatidylcholine biosynthesis. In: Vanderhoek JY (ed) *Frontiers of bioactive lipids.* New York: Plenum Press, 1996, p. 245–50.

48. Wieder T, Haase A, Geilen CC, Orfanos CE, The effect of two synthetic phospholipids on cell proliferation and

phosphatidylcholine biosynthesis in Madin-Darby canine kidney cells. *Lipids* 1995: 30; 389–93.

49.   Schön M, Schön MP, Geilen CC et al, Cell-matrix interactions of normal and transformed human keratinocytes in vitro are modulated by the synthetic phospholipid analogue hexadecylphosphocholine. *Br J Dermatol* 1996: 135; 696–703.

50.   Mickeleit M, Wieder T, Buchner K et al, Glyceroglycophospholipid (Glc-PC), a new type of glucosidic phospholipid. *Angew Chem Int Ed Engl* 1995: 34; 2667–9.

51.   Mickeleit M, Wieder T, Arnold M et al, A glucose-containing ether lipid (Glc-PAF) which acts as an antiproliferative analog of platelet-activating factor. *Angew Chem Int Ed Engl* 1998: 37; 351–3.

52.   Wieder T, Reutter W, Orfanos CE, Geilen CC, Mechanisms of action of phospholipid analogs as anticancer compounds. *Prog Lipid Res* 1999: 38; 249–59.

53.   Nachbar F, Korting HC, The role of vitamin E in normal and damaged skin. *J Mol Med* 1995: 7–17.

54.   Slaga TJ, Inhibition of skin tumor initiation, promotion, and progression by antioxidants and related compounds. *Crit Rev Food Sci Nutr* 1995: 35; 51–7.

55.   Wang ZY, Khan WA, Bickers DR, Mukhtar H, Protection against polycyclic aromatic hydrocarbon-induced skin tumor initiation in mice by green tea polyphenols. *Carcinogenesis* 1989: 10; 411–5.

56.   Katiyar SK, Agarwal R, Wang ZY et al, (–)-Epigallocatechin-3-gallate in *Camelia siensis* leaves from Himalayan region of Sikkim: inhibitory effects against biochemical events and tumor initiation in

SENCAR mouse skin. *Nutr Cancer* 1992: 18; 73–83.

57.   Wang ZY, Agarwal R, Bickers DR, Mukhtar H, Protection against ultraviolet B radiation-induced photocarcinogenesis in hairless mice by green tea polyphenols. *Carcinogenesis* 1991: 12; 152–30.

58.   Kono S, Ikeda M, Tokudome S, Kuratsune M, A case-control study of gastric cancer and diet in Northern Kyushu. *Jpn J Cancer Res* 1988: 79; 1067–74.

59.   Ogani I, Nasu K, Yamamoto S, Nomura T, On the antitumor activity of fresh green tea leaf. *Agric Biol Chem* 1988: 52; 1879–80.

60.   Mukhtar H, Katiyar SK, Agarwal R, Green tea and skin – anticarcinogenic effects. *J Invest Dermatol* 1994: 102; 3–7.

61.   Brunton VG, Workman P, Cell-signaling targets for antitumor drug development. *Cancer Chemother Pharmacol* 1993: 32; 1–19.

62.   Geilen CC, New therapeutic strategies in dermatology by modulating signal transduction pathways. *Z Hautkr* 1996: 71; 427–32.

63.   Langdon SP, Smyth JE, Inhibition of cell signalling pathways. *Cancer Treat Rev* 1995: 21; 65–89.

64.   Levitzki A, Signal-transduction therapy. A novel approach to disease management. *Eur J Biochem* 1994: 226; 1–13.

65.   Powis G, Signalling pathways as target for anticancer drug development. *Pharmacol Ther* 1994: 62; 57–95.

66.   Baselga J, Mendelsohn J, Receptor blockade with monoclonal antibodies as anticancer therapy. *Pharmacol Ther* 1994: 64; 127–54.

67.  Aboud-Pirak E, Hurwitz E, Pirak ME et al, Efficacy of antibodies to epidermal growth factor receptor against KB carcinoma in vitro and nude mice. *J Natl Cancer Inst* 1988: 80; 1605–11.

68.  Masui H, Kawamoto T, Sato JD et al, Growth inhibition of human tumor cells in athymic mice by anti-epidermal growth factor receptor monoclonal antibodies. *Cancer Res* 1984: 44; 1002–7.

69.  Yoneda T, Lyall R, Alsine MM et al, The antiproliferative effects of tyrosine kinase inhibitor tyrphostin on a human squamous cell carcinoma in vitro and in nude mice. *Cancer Res* 1991: 51; 4430–5.

70.  Ben-Bassat H, Vardi DV, Gazit A et al, Tyrphostins suppress the growth of psoriatic keratinocytes. *Exp Dermatol* 1995: 4; 82–8.

71.  Fry DW, Kraker AJ, McMichael A et al, A specific inhibitor of the epidermal growth factor receptor tyrosine kinase. *Science* 1994: 265; 1093–5.

72.  Dai S, Morré DJ, Geilen CC et al, Inhibition of plasma membrane NADH oxidase activity and growth of HeLa cells by natural and synthetic retinoids. *Mol Cell Biochem* 1997: 166; 101–9.

73.  Morré DJ, Sun E, Geilen CC et al, Capsaicin inhibits plasma membrane NADH oxidase and growth of human and mouse melanoma lines. *Eur J Cancer* 1996: 32A; 1995–2003.

74.  Philip PA, Rea D, Thavasu P et al, Phase I study of bryostatin 1: assessment of interleukin 6 and tumor necrosis factor alpha induction in vivo. The Cancer Research Campaign Phase I Committee. *J Natl Cancer Inst* 1993: 85; 1812–8.

75.  Kraft AS, Woodley S, Pettit GR et al, Comparison of the antitumor activity of bryostatins 1, 5, and 8. *Cancer Chemother Pharmacol* 1996: 37; 271–8.

# 13

## The status of antiviral drugs for skin disorders

*Leslie S Baumann,*
*Christiane Machado,*
*Melissa Lazarus and*
*Francisco A Kerdel*

## Introduction

Recent advances in antiviral therapy have facilitated treatment of viral conditions. This chapter concentrates on the treatment and prevention of viral conditions that have dermatologic manifestations (Table 13.1).

## DNA viruses

### Herpes virus family

The herpes virus family consists of DNA viruses that are morphologically indistinguishable and share a number of properties, including a remarkable propensity for establishing latent infections that persist for the life of the host.

The members of the herpes virus family that are pathogenic for humans include herpes simplex virus types 1 and 2 (HSV-1 and -2), varicella zoster virus (VZV), cytomegalovirus (CMV), Epstein-Barr virus (EBV), human herpes virus types 6 (HHV-6), and the recently recognized human herpes virus type 8 (HHV-8). Each of these viruses, with the exception of CMV, encodes for the enzyme thymidine kinase (TK) which is important in viral replication. Many of the new antiviral therapies are directed against this enzyme and selectively inhibit viral replication. Unfortunately, TK-negative strains of HSV and VZV are emerging, particularly in immunocompromised hosts, and these strains are resistant to the more commonly used antivirals such as acyclovir. For this reason, new antiviral agents are being developed which target different sites in the replication cycle.

### Table 13.1 Antiviral drugs used in herpes virus infections

|  | HSV | VZV | CMV | EBV |
|---|---|---|---|---|
| Aciclovir | + | + | + | + |
| Valaciclovir | + | + | – | – |
| Famciclovir | + | + | – | – |
| Idoxuridine | + | – | – | – |
| Trifluridine | + | + | – | – |
| Foscarnet | + | + | + | – |
| Vidarabine | + | – | – | – |
| Ganciclovir | – | – | + | – |

+ indicated, – not indicated

## Herpes simplex viruses 1 and 2

HSV-1 and -2 are DNA viruses that cause vesicular and erosive lesions in the skin and mucosa. HSV-1 usually causes recurrent lesions in the facial–oral area, whereas HSV-2 usually causes recurrent lesions in the genital area. HSV-1 may also cause lesions in the genital area but is associated with milder symptoms and fewer recurrences than is HSV-2. HSV-1 and -2 are closely related viruses and share many of the same surface glycoproteins having about 50% of nucleotide sequences in common. The HSV genome encodes a number of viral enzymes that can be selectively inhibited without causing an effect on the human cellular enzymes. Examples of these viral enzymes include viral TK, DNA polymerase, ribonucleotide reductase, and alkaline DNAse. In the last decade several antiviral drugs have been developed that safely and selectively inhibit these viral enzymes. Currently ten antiviral agents have been approved by the US Federal Drug Administration (FDA) for the therapy of herpes virus infections.[1]

Aciclovir (Zovirax, Fig. 13.1) is currently the most widely used antiviral drug in the world.[2] It is a synthetic acyclic purine nucleoside analogue that selectively inhibits viral DNA replication in infected cells and inactivates viral DNA polymerase resulting in the termination of DNA synthesis. Aciclovir must be converted to the monophosphate form by viral TK found in the herpes virus-infected cells and not in

uninfected cells. Aciclovir exhibits specific activity against HSV-1 and -2 and VZV which express TK.[3] Aciclovir can be administered intravenously, orally, or topically. Although intravenous aciclovir has increased bioavailability and is therefore more effective, its use is limited to those patients with severe or systemic infections that require hospitalization. Patients with severe HSV infection are frequently immunocompromised. Patients with severe HSV infection are treated with a dose of 5 mg/kg over 1 hour every 8 hours for 7 days (Table 13.2).

The most common side-effects seen with intravenous aciclovir include inflammation at the i.v. site, nausea, and uncommonly reversible elevation in the serum creatinine level and renal dysfunction.[4] The effects on the kidney can be minimized by ensuring proper hydration of the patient during aciclovir therapy. Oral aciclovir is indicated in initial and recurrent HSV infection episodes. The bioavailability of the oral form is dose dependent and

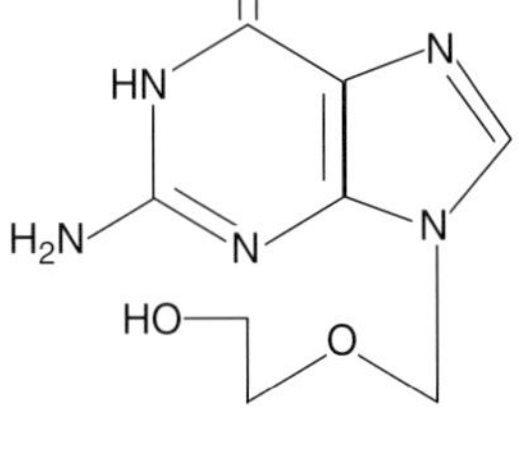

## Figure 13.1

Chemical structure of aciclovir.

## Table 13.2 Common dosing schedules to treat herpes virus infections

| Drug | HSV | | VZV | CMV[a] | EBV |
| --- | --- | --- | --- | --- | --- |
| | Initial | Prophylaxis | | | |
| Aciclovir | 200 mg orally every 4 h × 10 days | 400 mg orally twice daily | 800 mg orally every 4 h × 7 days | NSD | NSD |
| Valaciclovir | 500 mg orally twice daily | 500 mg orally daily | 1 g orally three times daily × 7 days | NI | NI |
| Famciclovir | NI | 125 mg orally three times daily | 500 mg orally three times daily × 7 days | NI | NI |
| Idoxuridine | Topical application | NI | NI | NI | NI |
| Trifluridine | Topical application | NI | Topical application | NI | NI |
| Foscarnet | 40 mg/kg i.v. every 8 h × 10 days | NI | 40 mg/kg i.v. every 8 h × 10 days | 60 mg/kg i.v. every 8 h × 2 weeks | NI |
| Vidarabine | Topical application | NI | NI | NI | NI |
| Ganciclovir | NI | NI | NI | 5 mg/kg i.v. every 12 h × 14–21 days | NI |

[a]Does not include required maintenance dosing
NSD, no standard dose; NI, not indicated

decreases with increasing dosages. For this reason, immunocompromised patients who require higher plasma levels of aciclovir for suppression of HSV infection may not be adequately treated with the oral preparation. The oral form has been found to have very few side-effects and is the most commonly used form of aciclovir. Initial and recurrent active infections are treated with 200 mg five times a day for 10 days for an initial episode and for 5 days for recurrent outbreaks. For chronic suppressive therapy a dose of 400 mg twice daily has been shown to decrease the number of HSV recurrences by 80–90%[5] and reduce viral shedding by 95%.[6] Topical aciclovir is available as a 5% ointment. It is generally not as effective because the drug is not able to reach the infected nerve. It is currently indicated only in initial HSV-2 infections since it may decrease viral shedding; however, its application has been associated with a burning sensation.

Valaciclovir (Valtrex, Fig. 13.2) received FDA approval in 1995 for treatment of herpes zoster infections and later it was approved for the episodic treatment of recurrent genital herpes at a dose of 500 mg twice a day for 5 days and for the first episode of genital herpes at a dose of 1000 mg twice a day for 10 days. Recently, valaciclovir 500 mg once a day was approved for suppression of recurrent genital HSV infection. Valaciclovir is a valine ester of aciclovir. After oral administration, it is rapidly converted to aciclovir in the gut wall and liver by the enzyme valacyclovirase. The mode of action and action spectrum are identical to those of aciclovir but higher plasma levels are achieved and less-frequent dosing schedules can be used. Studies comparing valaciclovir to aciclovir in the episodic treatment of HSV infections demonstrated valaciclovir 1 g twice daily to be as effective as aciclovir 200 mg five times daily without added toxicity.[7] Valaciclovir has been associated with thrombotic thrombocytopenic purpura in immunocompromised patients, so caution should be taken in this population.[8]

Famciclovir (Famvir, Fig. 13.3) is the diacetyl 6-deoxy derivative of the active antiviral compound penciclovir

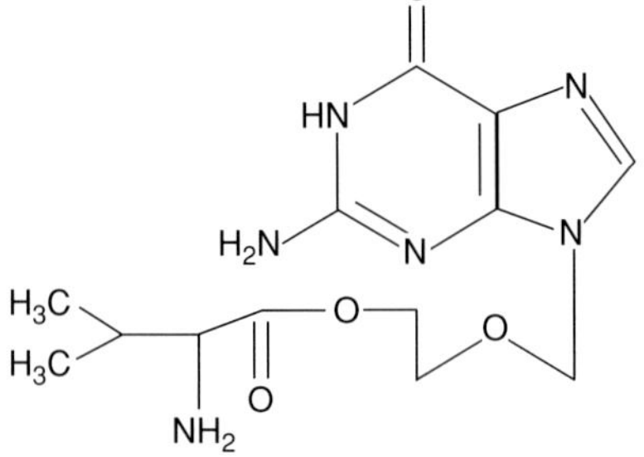

Figure 13.2

Chemical structure of valaciclovir.

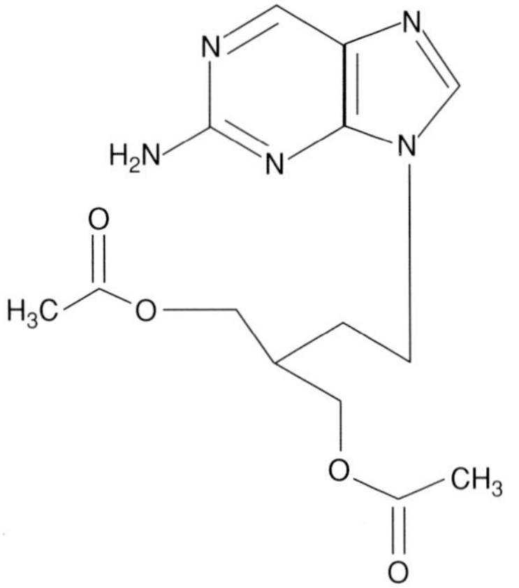

Figure 13.3

Chemical structure of famciclovir.

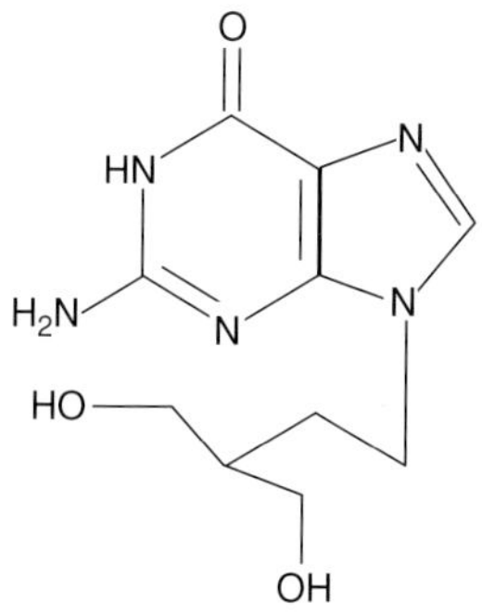

**Figure 13.4**

Chemical structure of penciclovir.

(Fig. 13.4). It has been approved by the FDA for treatment of herpes zoster and also for the treatment of genital HSV infection at a dose of 125 mg twice a day for 5 days and 250 mg twice a day for suppression of recurrent genital herpes. Famciclovir, like aciclovir, must be phosphorylated by viral encoded TK before it can competitively inhibit the incorporation of the natural substrate deoxyguanosine triphosphate into the DNA chain. Penciclovir is phosphorylated much more efficiently and more rapidly than aciclovir in herpes virus-infected cells in which viral TKs are present due to penciclovir's higher affinity for the enzyme.[9] Famciclovir also has a longer intracellular half-life than aciclovir (7–20 hours versus 0.7–1 hour). Therefore a less-frequent dosing schedule is possible.[10] Furthermore, the bioavailability of penciclovir after oral administration is 77%. In culture,

inhibition of HSV–2 replication takes place with low doses of famciclovir and new viral replication does not occur for many hours after exposure to the drug even when the drug has been removed from the culture medium. This seems to be a unique property of penciclovir that may enhance its efficacy.[11] Famciclovir is well tolerated with few side-effects and a safety profile comparable to placebo in clinical trials.[12] Penciclovir has a similar spectrum of antiviral activity as aciclovir for HSV and VZV infections and the majority of resistance to aciclovir will also occur to penciclovir, although this is not the rule.[13] A topical form of penciclovir is also available and is FDA approved for episodic treatment of herpes labialis in healthy patients.[14]

Idoxuridine (Idu, Herplex, Stoxil), also known as 5-iodo-2'-deoxyuridine, has shown inhibitory effects on nearly all DNA viruses. Idoxuridine resembles thymidine, and is phosphorylated to the triphosphate form within cells. Triphosphate-idoxuridine is incorporated into newly synthesized DNA and disrupts normal functioning by making the DNA molecule structurally unstable and fragile. Unfortunately, it is toxic when administered systemically and it is currently only FDA approved for topical use in the treatment of herpes keratitis. It is distributed in a 0.5% ophthalmic ointment and a 0.1% ophthalmic solution. Topical formulations with DMSO are available in many countries.

Trifluridine (Viroptic), 2'-deoxy-5-(trifluoromethyl)uridine, is a fluorinated pyrimidine deoxynucleoside. It is phosphorylated to a triphosphate form and is incorporated into newly synthesized viral DNA where it disrupts viral replication. Because this drug must be phosphorylated to become active, it is dependent on the presence of viral TK in the infected cells to be effective. It is currently used for HSV-1 and HSV-2 primary keratoconjunctivitis and recurrent epithelial keratitis. Trifluridine has also been reported as a successful treatment for HSV mucocutaneous infections refractory to aciclovir and foscarnet (see below) in AIDS patients.[15] It is currently available as a 1% ophthalmic solution.

Foscarnet sodium (Foscavir, phosphonoformic acid) has currently been approved for the treatment of CMV infections and aciclovir-resistant strains of HSV. Unlike the previously described antiviral drugs, foscarnet is not dependent on the presence of TK to be effective. Foscarnet is an organic analogue of inorganic pyrophosphate that exerts its antiviral activity through selective inhibition at the pyrophosphate binding site on virus-specific DNA polymerases and reverse transcriptases at concentrations that do not affect cellular DNA polymerases. This reversibly inhibits viral DNA polymerase and viral reverse transcriptase thus preventing viral replication. This drug may become more important as TK-resistant herpes virus strains become more prevalent. In 1991 a controlled trial comparing the efficacy of foscarnet with that of vidarabine (see below) in AIDS patients with aciclovir-

resistant HSV showed tht foscarnet had a superior efficacy and less serious toxicity when compared to vidarabine.[16] Once the foscarnet was stopped, however, a high frequency of relapse was seen. The dose of foscarnet used in this study was 40 mg/kg i.v. every 8 hours for 10 days (Table 13.3). The side-effects of foscarnet include fever, gastrointestinal symptoms, anemia, nephrotoxicity, genital ulcerations and alterations in serum concentration of calcium and phosphate ions.[17]

Foscarnet can also be effective in the topical form. Swetter et al[18] reported a case of aciclovir-resistant TK-deficient HSV infection in an immunocompetent patient presenting as a vulvar ulceration which healed completely with the application of 1% foscarnet cream with no recurrence during 24 months follow up.

Vidarabine (Vira A, Ara-A), also known as 9-D-arabinofuranosyladenine, is an organic analogue of the purine nucleoside adenosine. Vidarabine was one of the first systemic agents against HSV to be licensed.[19] Vidarabine, like foscarnet, does not require activation by TK to be effective and therefore is not a selective inhibitor of virus replication as it also effects cellular DNA polymerase.[20] It has been used in aciclovir-resistant HSV infections in the immunocompromised patient but its use is limited by neurotoxic side-effects. It is also used topically as a 3% ophthalmic ointment.

Cidofovir (HPMPC) is a new nucleoside analogue of deoxycytidine monophosphate with activity against a wide spectrum of DNA viruses including HSV. Cidofovir diphosphate, the active metabolite, has similarities with nucleotides and acts as a competitive inhibitor and an alternative substrate for viral DNA polymerase. It is incorporated into the viral DNA strand, blocking DNA synthesis. Its action does not depend on HSV TK allowing it to be used in aciclovir- and foscarnet-resistant HSV infections in immuno-compromised patients. Lo Presti et al[21] recently reported a case of an immuno-suppressed patient who developed HSV-1 mucositis resistant to aciclovir and foscarnet. The patient received i.v. cidofovir (5 mg/kg once weekly) and after three doses the mucositis cleared. Unfortunately, cidofovir can be neph-rotoxic when administered intravenously but this can be minimized with saline hydration and oral probenecid.

A cidofovir gel is also being evaluated by the FDA for the treatment of refractory HSV infection. Lateef et al[22] reported a case of a child with AIDS with aciclovir-resistant and foscarnet-unresponsive mucocutaneous HSV infection who responded to topical cidofovir 1%. Several studies are in progress to further evaluate the efficacy of and indications for this drug.

Interferon is a naturally produced glycoprotein with both antiviral and antineoplastic activity. The interferons ($\alpha$, $\beta$ and $\gamma$) upregulate proteins that inhibit transcription and protein translation, leading to antiviral activity.[23] The interferons also upregulate the expression of major histocompatibility antigens, possibly by facilitating recog-

nition of virally infected cells by the host's immune system. The mechanism of action can be directly antiviral or due to the activation of macrophages and natural killer cells.[24] Synergistic action of interferon and nucleoside analogues against HSV has been reported both in vivo and in vitro[25] and is presumed to be due to the effect of interferon-$\alpha$ on nucleoside metabolism in the infected cell.

More than 50 different HSV vaccines have been developed but their precise role in HSV diseases has yet to be defined, although partial protection can be achieved in those treated. A recombinant glycoprotein vaccine for HSV-2 containing glycoproteins gD2 and gB2 combined with the novel MF59 adjuvant emulsion was created and it has been shown to induce both humoral and cellular responses to HSV-2 that are greater or equal to those seen in naturally acquired infection.[26] The vaccine was well tolerated with few side-effects.

Another strategy is the use of genetically disabled HSV with deletion in the glycoprotein gH gene which is able to complete only one cycle of replication in normal cells, stimulating humoral and cell-mediated antiviral immune responses. Studies using an animal model showed a high degree of protection against recurrent disease.[27] Adenovirus containing HSV gB and gD have also shown promising responses in clinical and in animal studies.

Sorivudine is a synthetic deoxy-thymidine nucleoside analogue which is very potent against VZV and also effective against HSV-1 but with little activity against HSV-2. It acts as an inhibitor of virus-encoded DNA polymerase and it is also dependent on viral TK. The oral bioavailability is around 60% and the half-life is 5–6 hours. It has been used in clinical trials mostly for the treatment of varicella and herpes zoster, but due to significant adverse drug interactions, further studies and development have been terminated.

## Varicella virus

VZV is a DNA virus that is a member of the herpes virus family. Varicella infection (chickenpox) is an acute highly contagious eruption consisting of macules and papules that progress to vesicles, pustules and crusted lesions. This infection is spread by close contact and by respiratory droplet infection to individuals who have no prior history of varicella infection. Varicella zoster (herpes zoster or shingles) is caused by the same DNA virus, but herpes zoster infection occurs when the latent form of the varicella virus is reactivated in the sensory ganglia. Herpes zoster is seen in individuals with a prior history of chickenpox and results in a unilateral vesicular eruption in a dermatomal distribution with ipsilateral radicular pain. The radicular pain persists in 10–15% of patients after the skin lesions have healed and is known as postherpetic neuralgia. Elderly patients frequently develop postherpetic neuralgia but it usually spontaneously remits in 1 to 6 months. Many of the new antiviral agents, if used during acute herpes zoster, may shorten the duration of postherpetic neuralgia.[28]

Aciclovir is commonly used in herpes zoster infections. Severe infections in immunocompromised patients are treated with i.v. aciclovir at a dose of 10–12 mg/kg every 8 hours for 7 to 10 days (Table 13.4). In a placebo-controlled, double-blind study in immunocompromised zoster patients, i.v. aciclovir halted the progression of lesions after a 1-week course and hastened the clearance of viral particles from the vesicle fluid.[29] For immunocompetent patients the standard oral dose is 800 mg five times daily for 7 days. This treatment has been shown by multiple studies to reduce healing time for the lesions, the duration of viral shedding, and the duration of pain.[30] Although aciclovir has been shown to be effective in herpes zoster infections, several reports have demonstrated, as in HSV infections, altered or deficient TK activity of VZV isolates in patients with HIV disease on long-term suppressive doses of aciclovir.[31,32]

Aciclovir has also been shown to shorten the course of chickenpox in otherwise healthy children by 25–33% in three placebo-controlled trials in the US.[33,34] The treatment should be started within 24 hours of development of the lesions. The recommended dosage for children is 20 mg/kg and for adults the average dose is 800 mg five times daily for 7 days. Studies evaluating the cost-benefit ratio of this treatment are ongoing. There also is concern that treatment of chickenpox with aciclovir will blunt the immune response, leaving the patient susceptible to future reinfection, but recent studies have shown durability of immunity in these patients.[35] Prophylactic doses of 40 mg/kg daily in four divided doses for 5 days given 9 days after exposure to varicella has been shown to decrease the incidence of acquisition of chickenpox.[36] Low titres of VZV IgG were seen in these patients but it is unknown if these low titres would provide immunity to future VZV infections. Further studies are warranted.

Valaciclovir, the valine ester of aciclovir, has received initial approval from the FDA for use in herpes zoster infections. In a large trial, the efficacy and safety of oral valaciclovir was compared to aciclovir for the treatment of zoster in patients over 50 years of age. The data showed valaciclovir and aciclovir to be essentially comparable in regard to time to new lesions, cessation of new lesions, time to 50% crusting, and cessation of viral shedding. The increased bioavailability of valaciclovir allows a more convenient dosing schedule and may be effective in reducing the length of postherpetic neuralgia. The patients treated with valciclovir had a median of 40 days of pain after healing of the skin lesions compared to those treated with aciclovir that had a median of nearly 60 days.[37] The recommended dose of valciclovir is 1 g by mouth three times daily for 7 days.

Famciclovir was approved by the FDA in June 1994 for the treatment of herpes zoster at a dosing schedule of 500 mg by mouth three times daily for 7 days. In a similar manner to the drugs mentioned above, famciclovir accelerates the time to healing, decreases the duration of viral shedding and significantly reduces the occurrence of postherpetic neuralgia.[38]

Trifluridine is available in an ophthalmologic solution. Severe side-effects, however, prevent systemic usage. A case report described the treatment with a combination of trifluridine and interferon-α in an AIDS patient with aciclovir-resistant VZV infection who could not tolerate foscarnet.[39] Although trifluridine is dependent on the presence of TK, it is thought to have synergistic effects with interferon due to the effects of interferon on nucleoside metabolism. The trifluridine solution was placed topically on the lesions and interferon-α was given intralesionally. The lesions cleared after 3 months of therapy and did not recur in the 6 months following cessation of the therapy.

Foscarnet is indicated for use against aciclovir-resistant strains of VZV which occasionally occur in AIDS patients. Lokke Jensen reported successful treatment of VZV with foscarnet in an AIDS patient that was refractory to aciclovir treatment.[40] Vidarabine is infrequently used in VZV infections due to its serious neurotoxic side-effects.

Varicella vaccine was licensed by the FDA in 1995 and is available for use in individuals aged 12 months and older who have not had varicella. It has been found to be safe and effective in preventing serious cases of varicella.[41] The vaccine should not be given to immunocompromised patients, to household contacts of immunocompro-mised patients, pregnant patients, and individuals with an allergy to neomycin because trace amounts are included in the vaccine.

## Cytomegalovirus

CMV is also a member of the herpes virus family. The CMV genome is the most complex of the DNA viruses and is 50% larger than that of HSV. Unlike the other viruses in the herpes virus family, CMV does not express TK, therefore many of the commonly used antiviral agents are not effective in this disease. The majority of the population has been infected with CMV and carry it in a latent form. Sexual intercourse is the primary mode of transmission of CMV in adults but CMV infections rarely affect the skin. Perianal ulcers and less frequently, verrucous plaques, nodular lesions, palpable purpuric papules, vesicles, bullae, morbiliform and maculopapular eruptions and hyperpigmented indurated plaques have been described in immunocom-promised patients as manifestations of CMV infection.[42]

Although aciclovir is not very effec-tive in the treatment of active CMV infection, it does appear to suppress CMV replication and therefore is useful as prophylaxis against CMV. It is currently being used in AIDS patients and transplant patients to prevent CMV infection.

Ganciclovir (Cytovene, 9-(1,3-dihydroxy-2-propoxymethyl)guanine) is a nucleoside analogue that differs from aciclovir structurally only by the addition of a hydroxymethyl group on the 3' position of the acyclic side chain. Ganciclovir does not require activation by TK and the mechanism of action in CMV-infected cells is not completely understood. Ganciclovir is phosphory-lated and made active by CMV-specific protein kinase. The active form inhibits CMV DNA polymerase by inducing premature chain termination into newly synthesized DNA. It has in vitro activ-ity against all herpes viruses but, due to its side effects, is currently indicated only for treatment of CMV retinitis in immunocompromised patients. The oral bioavailability is less than 5% necessitating i.v. administration. The dose for CMV retinitis is 5 mg/kg i.v. every 12 hours for 14–21 days with a maintenance dose of 5 mg/kg daily for 5 days each week. The common side-effects include granulocytopenia, neutropenia and thrombocytopenia due to bone marrow suppression. The incidence of the hematological side-effects increases when ganciclovir and zidovudine are used concurrently which is often the case in AIDS patients. Ganciclovir is virostatic and not viroci-dal, so patients may relapse when the therapy is discontinued.

Foscarnet has been used successfully to treat CMV infections. It is currently indicated for the treatment of CMV retinitis. A study comparing the efficacy of foscarnet and ganciclovir in CMV retinitis showed a more prolonged survival in those patients treated with foscarnet.[43] Side-effects included nephrotoxicity and anaemia.

Interferon-α has been successfully used to prevent seropositive transplant patients from developing active CMV infection. CMV hyperimmune globulin has also been used to prevent CMV infection in transplant patients. The entire CMV viral genome has been sequenced and several types of vaccines for this virus are being developed and studied.[44]

Cidofovir is also approved for the treatment of CMV retinitis and other CMV infections and is used mainly in the setting of ganciclovir- and foscarnet-resistant strains of CMV in patients with AIDS.

Fomivirsen is the first antisense drug approved for the treatment of CMV retinitis. Although presently only available for ophthalmological use, a dermatological antisense drug for the treatment of other CMV infections may be available in the future.

Epstein-Barr virus

EBV is a DNA virus and a member of the herpes virus family. EBV is the causal agent of infectious mononucleosis and is associated with African Burkitt's lymphoma, nasopharyngeal carcinoma, lymphoproliferative syndromes, and chronic fatigue syndrome; additionally, oral hairy leucoplakia is associated with an EBV infection in HIV-positive individuals, and it is a prognostic marker for progression to AIDS. The skin findings that occur in EBV infec-

tion are seen primarily in infectious mononucleosis. It occurs in 3–16% of patients and consists of a maculopapular rash in the majority of the cases. The trunk and upper arms are most commonly affected but the whole skin can become involved. Erythematous, vesicular, morbilliform, petechial and purpuric exanthems have also been described. The treatment of these patients is largely supportive and symptomatic. In most EBV infections the use of antiviral therapy is not warranted.

Aciclovir acts on the lytic phase of EBV infection and has only shown benefit in decreasing viral replication in oropharyngeal infections.[45] Aciclovir has shown minimal effect on the symptoms of infectious mononucleosis and treatment has little effect in diminishing the number of EBV-infected B cells in the peripheral circulation. Aciclovir is, however, effective in patients with oral hairy leucoplakia.[42] A subunit vaccine consisting of the EBV gp350 envelope glycoprotein has been effective in animal studies and is awaiting clinical trials.

Human herpesvirus-6

HHV-6 is the cause of exanthem subitum, also known as roseola infantum. HHV-6 differs from the other members of the herpes virus family because the genome is linear and composed of double-stranded DNA. Roseola is seen in children 6 months to 2 years of age and consists of a maculopapular rash that is preceded by 3 to 5 days of high fever. The disease is mild and self limited and usually requires symptomatic treatment only. In vitro testing has shown foscarnet and ganciclovir to be more effective against HHV-6 than aciclovir.[46]

## Human herpesvirus-8

HHV-8 is a newly described member of the herpes virus family. Herpes virus-like DNA sequences have been found in lesions of Kaposi's sarcoma patients. These sequences have homology to other members of the herpes virus family; therefore, the agent has been given the name HHV-8. Further studies are ongoing. Interferon-$\alpha$ is licensed for use in treating Kaposi's sarcoma in HIV patients. It has been used alone and in combination with vinblastine[47] and also with zidovudine[48] with response rates up to 40%. Patients with higher CD4 counts have demonstrated higher response rates. A study is currently being designed to evaluate the potential use of cidofovir for the treatment of Kaposi's sarcoma.[49] There are also reports suggesting a possible role of foscarnet in the treatment of the epidemic variant of this disease.[50]

In an in vitro study comparing the potency of cidofovir, aciclovir, foscarnet and ganciclovir against HHV-8, cidofovir was the most potent inhibitor.[51]

## Papillomaviruses

The papillomaviruses are doubled-stranded DNA viruses that do not encode a DNA polymerase or TK and therefore are not susceptible to aciclovir and related antiviral agents. More than 70 different genotypes of the human papilloma virus (HPV) are recognized. The genotypes can be divided into three large categories: HPV trophic for nongenital regions include HPV 1, 2, 3, 4, 10, 28, 29 and 57; HPV trophic for genital-mucosal regions include HPV 6, 11, 16, 18, 31, 33 and 35; and epidermodysplasia verruciformis-related types include HPV 5 and 8. Many treatment modalities have been employed, most of which involve physical destruction, including surgery, cryosurgery, laser surgery, cantharidin, dinitrochlorobenzene, podophyllin, salicylic acid, trichloroacetic acid, lactic acid, and topical retinoids. Topical 5-fluorouracil has been shown to be effective in some cases of flat warts and condyloma accuminata[52] and intralesional bleomycin has been shown to be useful in eradicating common warts.[53]

Recombinant interferon-$\alpha$ is indicated as an intralesional injection for refractory genital warts. Double-blind trials have shown that intralesional interferon-$\alpha$, at doses in the range 1–5 MU per treatment, is much more effective than placebo at eradicating condyloma accuminata.[54] The major side-effects noted include fever, myalgia, lethargy, and headaches. These side-effects can be diminished by pretreatment with acetaminophen. Controlled trials with recombinant HPV protein vaccines are also in development.

Imiquimod (Aldara), a recently approved drug, is a heterocyclic amine which stimulates human peripheral blood mononuclear cells, macrophages and keratinocytes to release several subtypes of interferon-α and other cytokines such as interleukins 1, 6, 8, 10 and 12. It therefore acts as a topical immune modulator. It can cause 90% reduction in wart area when used in patients with condyloma accuminata. Aldara cream is applied three times a week and left on the skin for 6–10 hours. The treatment should be continued until total clearance of the warts or for a maximum of 16 weeks. Local skin reactions are common, particularly erythema.

## Parvovirus

Parvovirus B19, a single-stranded DNA virus, belongs to the family Parvoviridae. It is the cause of a common disease known as Fifth disease or erythema infectiosum which is characterized by a low-grade fever, pink 'slapped cheek' appearance, erythematous eruption on trunk and extremities, and arthralgia. It has been associated with aplastic crisis, chronic anaemia, and fetal hydrops. Immunocompromised patients may develop chronic anaemia and have been shown to benefit from intravenous gammaglobulin.[55] Erythema infectiosum is a mild, benign condition that usually requires only symptomatic treatment.

### Poxviruses

Poxviruses are the aetiological agents in molluscum contagiosum, orf, and

Milker's nodules. The poxvirus is a large DNA virus that replicates in the cytoplasm of infected cells. The molluscum contagiosum virus is the most commonly seen poxvirus infection. Molluscum contagiosum presents as dome-shaped papules with a central umbilication on mucocutaneous surfaces. In immunocompetent patients, the condition is self limited and treatment is often not necessary; however, the disease can be recalcitrant in immunocompromised patients. Multiple destructive modalities have been employed in the treatment of molluscum contagiosum. Intralesional interferon-α has been shown to be effective in eliminating lesions in immunocompetent patients, but appears to be less effective in immunocompromised patients.[56]

Orf, caused by the parapoxvirus member of the poxvirus family, is a zoonotic infection that consists of cutaneous nodules that heal in 35 days without treatment. Milker's nodules, caused by the paravaccinia virus member of the poxvirus family, is a zoonotic infection that is seen when there is human contact with cattle. The disease presents as red papules on the hands and forearms that heal without treatment.

## RNA viruses

### Enterovirus

Enteroviruses a subgroup of the picornaviruses, are a common cause of viral exanthems. Polioviruses, coxsackie viruses, echoviruses and reoviruses are grouped under the classification of enteroviruses because of their similarities and their common habitat in the human enteric tract. Hand-foot-and-mouth disease (HFMD) is an epidemic disease usually associated with coxsackie virus A16 or enterovirus 71. Characteristics of HFMD include low-grade fever, malaise, abdominal pain, respiratory symptoms and ulcerative oral lesions. Red papules and vesicles appear on the hands and feet. The lesions usually disappear after a 10-day course and resolve without scarring. As this disease is benign and self limited, no treatment is necessary.

Herpangina is an exanthem consisting of grey–white papulovesicular lesions on the anterior pillars of the tonsillar fauces, the soft palate, the uvula, and the tonsils and is caused by six types of coxsackie group A viruses (A2, A4, A5, A6, A8, A10). Herpangina resolves spontaneously in 7 days and does not require treatment.

## Rubeola

Rubeola, also known as measles, is caused by a paramyxovirus. The illness consists of fever, cough, coryza, conjunctivitis and, pathognomonic for the disease, Koplik's spots in the buccal mucosa. The rash consists of red macules and papules that begin on the forehead and behind the ears and progress to the trunk and extremities. Patients with rubeola may develop serious complications such as encephalitis, purpura due to thrombocytopenia, or rarely subacute sclerosing panencephalitis. Fortunately, the disease is usually self limited and therapy consists only of supportive care. The incidence of measles has greatly decreased since the licensing of the measles vaccine in 1963. In unvaccinated individuals who have been exposed to measles, immune serum globulin may be used to modify or prevent disease but must be given within 6 days of exposure.

Vitamin A supplements are believed to reduce the morbidity and mortality in children in underdeveloped areas with severe measles at a dose of 400,000 IU.[57]

## Rubella

Rubella, or German measles, is caused by a member of the togaviridae family. It is a common infection of children characterized by a short prodromal period, lymphadenopathy and a rash. The lymphadenopathy usually involves the cervical, suboccipital, and postauricular glands. The rash, consisting of pink-red macules and papules, begins on the face before spreading to the trunk and extremities and usually resolves in 3 days. Fine desquamation may occur following resolution of the rash. Rubella is generally a benign disease and does not require treatment; however, development of the disease during pregnancy can have devastating consequences on the fetus. Complications include microcephaly, cataracts, deafness, and congenital heart disease. Prevention is key in this disease and can be accomplished by routine vaccination with the rubella vaccine which is usually given in combination with the measles and mumps vaccine (MMR). The person given the vaccine does not shed sufficient virus to infect susceptible individuals; therefore, it is safe to administer the vaccine to close contacts of a pregnant individual. Women who are given the vaccine should avoid pregnancy for at least 3 months after receiving the vaccine.

# Retroviruses

## Human immunodeficiency virus

HIV is a virus that contains an RNA genome, an RNA-dependent DNA polymerase, and is a member of the family Retroviridae. It causes an immunosuppressed state that leads to multiple complications that are beyond the scope of this chapter. Many different treatments have been used to treat the complications and to increase longevity in these patients.[58] Currently there are a multitude of approved antiretroviral drugs to treat HIV patients belonging to three categories: nucleoside analogues (zidovudine, lamivudine, didanosine, zalcitabine and stavudine), non-nucleoside analogues (nevirapine, delavirdine) and protease inhibitors (saquinavir, indinavir, ritonavir and nelfinavir). A new category of nucleotide reverse transcriptase

inhibitors is expected to be available in the near future. Highly active antiretroviral therapy is a regimen, introduced in 1997, consisting of a combination of one or more nucleoside reverse transcriptase inhibitors and a protease inhibitor or a non-nucleoside reverse transcriptase inhibitor. This approach causes significant suppression of viral replication and prolonged elevations of CD4 cells thereby reducing morbidity and mortality in HIV patients. This is currently the regimen of choice at the time of initial diagnosis of HIV infection.

The risk of acquiring HIV after accidental exposure depends on several factors such as: volume of blood involved in the exposure, stage of disease, plasma HIV RNA level in the patient, location and also mechanism of exposure. The revised Collaborative Zidovudine Chemoprophylaxis Study Group protocol is: zidovudine 200 mg three times a day, lamivudine 150 mg twice a day and indinavir 800 mg every 8 hours for 28 days, starting immediately following exposure.

The most common opportunistic viral infections in HIV patients causing cutaneous involvement are the result of infection with herpes viruses, poxviruses and papillomaviruses. These diseases usually present in a more aggressive and disseminated form and may be extremely resistant to treatment.

Due to the growing rate of aciclovir-resistant HSV in the HIV population, it is extremely important to give these patients the full dose of aciclovir until complete healing of the lesions and then continue a suppressive regimen for life at a dose of 200 mg orally twice a day.[59] Resistance to aciclovir must be suspected in patients who develop progressive HSV disease despite 10–14 days of aciclovir and this should be confirmed by culture. Alternative drugs are foscarnet, vidarabine or cidofovir. Lalezari et al reported a double-blind placebo-controlled study using cidofovir 1% gel in 30 patients with AIDS and aciclovir-resistant HSV infection.[60] Complete healing occurred in 30% in the cidofovir group compared to none in the placebo group and 50% of the patients in the cidofovir group had at least a 50% improvement. Negative viral cultures were obtained in 87% of the cidofovir-treated patients within 2 days.

Foscarnet resistance can also occur, and in such cases high oral doses or i.v. aciclovir with or without concurrent foscarnet may result in healing.[61] Cidofovir is another option in such cases, as is topical trifluridine. Herpes zoster should be treated with i.v. aciclovir in HIV patients, particularly if the disease is disseminated or there is ophthalmological involvement or visceral involvement, at a dose of 10 mg/kg three times a day until lesions are healed. Famciclovir can also be effectively used. Foscarnet is the drug of choice and should be administered for ten or more days in cases of VZV resistant to aciclovir at a dose of 40–60 mg/kg three times a day for ten or more days.

Molluscum contagiosum can become very disfiguring in AIDS patients, and its prevalence increases as the immune system deteriorates. Patients can present with more than 100 lesions which can grow to as much as 1 cm in diameter. Destructive methods are usually employed, such as cryotherapy, caustic agents, carbon dioxide laser and others. Interferon-α (1 MU) intralesionally for 4 weeks has been shown to produce good results within 6 weeks.[62]

Meadows et al reported three HIV patients with disfiguring molluscum contagiosum who responded to cidofovir. Two of them were receiving cidofovir for CMV retinitis and cleared their concurrent molluscum lesions. The third patient was treated with cidofovir 3% cream three times a week with excellent results.[63]

In the HIV population the spectrum of HPV disease is extensive and can be particularly difficult to treat. Several destructive methods are used such as surgery, laser, electrosurgery, cryosurgery, acids as well as local chemotherapeutics (5-fluorouracil, podophyllin), retinoids and cimetidine. The results are variable but the recurrence rates are high in this specific population.

Interferon-α is the only FDA-approved genital wart therapy with truly antiviral activity. It is administered intralesionally, requiring 9 to 16 injections over a period of 3–8 weeks and it takes a few weeks for the clinical results to be seen. Imiquimod (Aldara) may also be useful in this setting.

Cidofovir was evaluated by Douglas et al in the topical form for the treatment of condyloma acuminata in patients with AIDS and resulted in complete or partial responses in 65% of the patients.[64] More clinical trials are ongoing to further evaluate the role of this promising drug.

## Human T-cell lymphotropic virus type 1

Human T-cell lymphotropic virus type 1 (HTLV-1) is associated with a variety of human diseases such as adult T-cell leukaemia (ATL), myelopathy/tropical spastic paraparesis, uveitis and other not so well defined conditions. HTLV-1 is endemic in Japan and in the Caribbean, occurs sporadically in Africa, Latin America, Middle East and in the United States. ATL is characterized by the presence of HTLV-1 antibodies in the patients' serum, monoclonal integration of the virus in the malignant cells, lymphadenopathy, epatosplenomegaly, cutaneous lesions and hypercalcaemia. Malignant lymphocytes contain a characteristic indented or convoluted nucleus (flower cells) and are found in the peripheral blood.

ATL can present in four different clinical subtypes with different prognosis: smouldering and chronic forms have a median survival of 2 years or more, whereas the acute and lymphomatous form have a survival rate ranging from 3 to 6 months. The last two forms are very aggressive, respond poorly to chemotherapy and when they do respond it usually is not long-lasting.

In order to evaluate alternative therapy for this subset of patients, Gill et al conducted a study using the combination of interferon-α (5–10 MU subcutaneously daily) and zidovudine (200 mg orally five times a day) in 19 patients.[65] Partial responses were observed in 58% of the patients and five patients had a complete response. The median survival among the responders was 13 months. Even those patients who did not respond, experienced a significant reduction in the number of circulating leukaemic cells. In another study, all of five previously untreated patients with ATL treated with the same regimen achieved complete or partial remissions.[66] The exact mechanism of action of this regimen is not completely clear. Zidovudine and interferon may block the production of the HTLV-1 viruses but also act as cytotoxic agents. Relapses after this therapy was discontinued suggest the need for a maintenance treatment. Further studies are needed to define the optimal doses and duration of this therapy.

## References

1.  Evans TY, Tyring SK, Advances in antiviral therapy in dermatology. *Dermatol Clin* 1998: 16: 409–20.

2.  Memar O, Antiviral agents in dermatology: current status and future prospects. *Int J Dermatol* 1995: 34(9); 597–606.

3. O'Brien JJ, Acyclovir: an update review of its antiviral activity, pharmacokinetic properties and therapeutic efficacy. *Drugs* 1989: 37; 233–309.

4. Laskin O, Acyclovir, pharmacology and clinical experience. *Arch Intern Med* 1984; 144; 1241–6.

5. Goldberg L, Long-term suppression of recurrent genital herpes with acyclovir. A five-year benchmark. *Arch Dermatol* 1993: 129; 582–7.

6. Wald A, Asymptomatic viral shedding of genital herpes simplex is significantly reduced by acyclovir suppression. American Society for Microbiology, 34th Interscience Conference on Antimicrobial Agent and Chemotherapy, Orlando, October 1994 (Poster).

7. McCrary M, Memar O, Drugs with antiviral activity used in clinical dermatology. *Fitzpatricks J Clin Dermatol* 1995; 3(6); 44–51.

8. Pereira FA, Herpes simplex: evolving concepts. *J Am Acad Dermatol* 1996: 35; 503–20.

9. Vere Hodge RA, Cheng YC, The mode of action of penciclovir. *Antivir Chem Chemother* 1992: 36(9); 2037–8.

10. Earnshaw DL, Mode of antiviral action of penciclovir in MRC-5 cells infected with HSV-1, HSV-2, and varicella-zoster virus. *Antimicrob Agents Chemother* 1992: 36; 2747–57.

11. Weinberg A, Bate JB, Masters HB et al, In vitro activities of penciclovir and acyclovir against herpes simplex virus types 1 and 2. *Antimicrob Agents Chemother* 1992; 36(9); 2037–8.

12. Tyring S, Efficacy and safety of fanciclovir in the treatment of patients with herpes zoster: results of the first placebo-controlled study. 33rd Interscience Conference on Antimicrobial Agents Chemother, New Orleans, October 1993; p. 1540 (poster).

13. Alrabiah FA, Sacks SL, New antiherpesvirus agents. *Drugs* 1996: 52(1); 17–32.

14. Spruance SL, Rea TL, Thoming C et al, Penciclovir cream for the treatment of herpes simplex labialis. *JAMA* 1997: 277; 1374–9.

15. Murphy M, Morley A, Eglin RP, Monteiro E, Topical trifluridine for mucocutaneous acyclovir-resistant herpes simplex 2 in AIDS patients. *Lancet* 1992: 340; 1040.

16. Safrin S, A controlled trial comparing foscarnet with vidarabine for acyclovir-resistant mucocutaneous herpes simplex in the acquired immunodeficiency syndrome. *N Engl J Med* 1991: 325; 551–5.

17. Seidel EA, A dose escalation study to determine the toxicity and maximally tolerated dose of foscarnet. *AIDS* 1993: 7; 941–5.

18. Swetter SM, Hill EL, Kern ER et al, Chronic vulvar ulceration in a immunocompetent woman due to acyclovir-resistant, thymidine-kinase-deficient herpes simplex virus. *J Invest Dermatol* 1998: 177; 543–50.

19. Meamar O, Antiviral agents in dermatology: current status and future prospects. *Int J Dermatol* 1995: 34(9); 597–606.

20. Dolin R, Antiviral chemotherapy and chemoprophylaxis. *Science* 1985: 227; 1296–303.

21. LoPresti AE, Levine JF, Munk GB et al, Successful treatment of an acyclovir and foscarnet-resistant herpes simplex virus type 1 lesion with intravenous cidofovir. *Clin Infect Dis* 1998: 28; 513–14.

22.   Lateef F, Don PC, Kaufmann M et al, Treatment of acyclovir-resistant, foscarnet-unresponsive HSV infection with topical cidofovir in a child with AIDS. *Arch Dermatol* 1998: 134; 1169–70.

23.   Gresser I, Biological effects of interferons. *J Invest Dermatol* 1990: 95; 66S–71S.

24.   Kunder SC, Biological response modifier-mediated resistance to herpesvirus infections requires induction of interferon. *Antiviral Res* 1993: 21; 129–39.

25.   Birch CJ, Clinical effects and in vitro studies of trifluirithymidine combined with interferon alpha for treatment of drug resistant and sensitive herpes simplex virus infections. *J Infect Dis* 1992: 166; 108–12.

26.   Langenberg A, A recombinant glyco-protein vaccine for herpes simplex type 2: safety and efficacy. *Ann Intern Med* 1995: 122; 889–98.

27.   McLean CS, Ertwk M, Jennings R et al, Protective vaccination against primary and recurrent disease caused by herpes virus type 2 using a genetically disabled HSV 1. *J Infect Dis* 1994: 170; 1100–9.

28.   Gilden D, Herpes zoster with postherpetic neuralgia – persisting pain and frustration. *N Engl J Med* 1994: 330(13); 932–3.

29.   Balfour H, Acyclovir halts progression of herpes zoster in immunocompromised patients. *N Engl J Med* 1983: 308; 1448–53.

30.   Beutner K, Antivirals in the treatment of pain. *J Geriatr Dermatol* 1994: 6(Suppl A); 23A–28A.

31.   Pahwa S, Biron K, Lim W et al, Continuous varicella-zoster infection associated with acyclovir resistance in a child with AIDS. *JAMA* 1988: 260; 2879–82.

32.   Linnemann CC, Biron KK, Hoppenjans WG, Solinger AM, Emergence of acyclovir-resistant varicella zoster virus in an AIDS patient on prolonged acyclovir therapy. *AIDS* 1990: 4; 577–9.

33.   Dunkle LM, A controlled trial of acyclovir for chickenpox in normal children. *N Engl J Med* 1991: 325; 1539–44.

34.   Balfour HH, Acyclovir treatment of varicella in otherwise healthy adolescents. *J Pediatr* 1992: 120; 627–33.

35.   Englund JA, Acyclovir treatment for varicella does not lower gpI and IE-62 antibody responses to VZV in normal children. *J Clin Microb* 1990: 28; 2327–30.

36.   Huang Y, Acyclovir prophylaxis of varicella after household exposure. *Pediatr Infect Dis J* 1995: 14(2); 152–4.

37.   Beutner K, Valaciclovir compared with acyclovir for improved therapy for herpes zoster in immunocompromised adults. *Antimicrob Agents Chemother* 1995: 39; 1546–53.

38.   Tyring S, Famciclovir for the treatment of acute herpes zoster. Effects on acute disease and postherpetic neuralgia. *Ann Intern Med* 1995: 123; 89–96.

39.   Rossi S, The treatment of acyclovir-resistant herpes zoster with trifluorothymidine and interferon alpha. *Arch Dermatol* 1995: 131; 24–6.

40.   Lokke Jensen B, Atypical varicella-zoster infection in AIDS. *Acta Derm Venereol* 1993: 73; 123–4.

41.   Committee of Infectious Diseases, Recommendations for the use of live attenuated varicella vaccine. *Pediatrics* 1995: 95(5); 791–6.

42. Castano-Molina C, Cockerell C, Diagnosis and treatment of infectious diseases in HIV infected hosts. *Dermatol Clin* 1997: 15; 267–83.

43. [No authors listed], Mortality in patients with the acquired immunodeficiency syndrome treated with either foscarnet or ganciclovir for cytomegalovirus retinitis. Studies of Ocular Complications of AIDS Research Group, in collaboration with the AIDS Clinical Trials Group. *N Engl J Med* 1992: 326; 213–20.

44. Plotkin S, Vaccines for VZV and CMV – recent progress. *Science* 1994: 265; 1383–5.

45. Ernberg I, Andersson J, Acyclovir efficiently inhibits oropharyngeal excretion of EBV in patients with acute infectious mononucleosis. *J Gen Virol* 1986: 67; 2267–72.

46. Burns WH, Sandford GR, Susceptibility of human herpes-6 to antivirals in vitro. *J Infect Dis* 1990: 162; 634–7.

47. Krown SE, AIDS-associated Kaposi's sarcoma: pathogenesis, clinical course and treatment. *AIDS* 1988: 2; 71–80.

48. Fischl MA, Antiretroviral therapy in combination with interferon for AIDS-related Kaposi's sarcoma. *Am J Med* 1991: 90 (Suppl 4A); 2S–7S.

49. Zabawski EJ, Cockerell CJ, Topical and intralesional cidofovir: a review of pharmacology and therapeutic effects. *J Am Acad Dermatol* 1998: 39; 741–5.

50. Morfeldt L, Torssander J, Long term remission of Kaposi's sarcoma following foscarnet treatment in HIV-infected patients. *Scand J Infect Dis* 1994: 26(6); 749–52.

51. Kedes DH, Ganem D, Sensitivity of Kaposi's sarcoma-associated herpesvirus replication to antiviral drugs. Implications for potential therapy. *J Clin Invest* 1997: 99; 2082–6.

52. Goette DK, Topical chemotherapy with 5-fluorouracil. *J Am Acad Dermatol* 1981: 4; 633–49.

53. Shumer SM, O'Keefe EJ, Bleomycin in the treatment of recalcitrant warts. *J Am Acad Dermatol* 1983: 9; 91–6.

54. Friedman-Kien AE, Natural interferon alfa for treatment of condylomata acuminata. *JAMA* 1988: 259; 533–8.

55. Koch WC, Massey G, Russell CE, Adler SP, Manifestations and treatment of human parvovirus B19 infection in immunocompromised patients. *J Pediatr* 1990: 116; 355–9.

56. Memar O, Cutaneous viral infections. *J Am Acad Dermatol* 1995: 33; 2.

57. Hussey GO, Klein M, A randomized, controlled trial of vitamin A in children with severe measles. *N Engl J Med* 1990: 323; 160–4.

58. Collier A, Coombs R, Treatment of human immunodeficiency virus infection with saquinavir, zidovudine and zalcitabine. *N Engl J Med* 1996: 334; 1011–7.

59. Berger TG, Greene I, Bacterial, viral, fungal and parasitic infections in HIV disease and AIDS. *Dermatol Clin* 1991: 9; 465–92.

60. Lalezari J, Jaffe HS, Schaker T et al, A randomized, double-blind, placebo controlled trial of cidofovir for the treatment of acyclovir-unresponsive mucocutaneous herpes simplex virus infection in patients with AIDS. *J Infect Dis* 1997: 76; 892–8.

61. Safrin S, Kenmerly S, Plotkin B et al, Foscarnet-resistant HSV infection in

patients with AIDS. *J Infect Dis* 1994: 169; 193–6.

62.   Nelson MR, Chard S, Barton SE, Intralesional interferon for the treatment of recalcitrant molluscum contagiosum in HIV antibody positive individuals. A preliminary report. *Int J STD AIDS* 1995: 6; 351–2.

63.   Meadows KP, Tyring SK, Pavia AT et al, Resolution of recalcitrant molluscum contagiosum virus lesions in human immunodeficiency virus-infected patients treated with cidofovir. *Arch Dermatol* 1997: 133; 987–90.

64.   Douglas J, Tyring S et al, A phase 1/2 study of cidofovir topical gel for refractory condyloma acuminatum in patients with HIV infection. Poster Presented at the Fourth Conference on Retrovirus and Opportunistic Infections, Washington DC, 1997 Jan 2–26, poster 334.

65.   Gill PS, Harrington W Jr, Kaplan MH, Ribeiro RC et al, Treatment of adult-T-cell leukemia-lymphoma with a combination of interferon alfa and zidovudine. *N Engl J Med* 1995: 29; 1744–8.

66.   Hermine O, Bouscary D, Gessain A, et al, Brief report: treatment of adult T-cell leukemia-lymphoma with zidovudine and interferon alfa. *N Engl J Med* 1995: 29; 1749–51.

# 14

## Update on topical corticosteroids

*Ronald Marks*

## Introduction

Hydrocortisone was made generally available as a topical medication in the early 1950s and it is a tribute to its efficacy and safety that it is still being used in routine dermatological practice. This short chapter does not attempt to review all the developments that have taken place in topical or corticosteroid research, and should any reader wish to read a more comprehensive and systematic treatment of the subject they are recommended to Chaffman (1999)[1] and Maibach and Surber (1992).[2] Here, I have selected some important developments that have taken place in the past two decades to emphasize the continuing importance of this group of agents in a time of expanding novel pharmaceutical approaches.

One issue that continually recurs in the vast literature concerning topical corticosteroids is their propensity to cause significant adverse side-effects (see Table 14.1 for a list of the common adverse side-effects). This has dominated thinking about these agents and has been one of the major motivating factors in corticosteroid research. Other directions taken in recent research on topical corticosteroids have been the search for higher potency preparations as well as the investigation of specific therapeutic properties possessed by different corticosteroid molecules.

## Novel molecules and their actions

The search for topical corticosteroids with greater potency has led to the development and eventual licensing of clobetasol-17-propionate, halcinonide and difluocortolone pivalate. These agents seem equally extremely potent clinically, but also equally hazardous when used without due regard to their potential for causing adverse side-effects. They should only be used in special situations and should not be used merely as alternative treatments if other topical corticosteroids do not appear to be working sufficiently quickly.

The indications for corticosteroids in general are reviewed later, but it is worth mentioning here the main reasons for using one of the very potent agents. The obvious and most important indication for their use is disease processes that seem to only respond to these very potent agents and these

Table 14.1 Main adverse reactions from the use of topical corticosteroids

| Adverse reaction | Mechanism | Comment |
|---|---|---|
| Pituitary–adrenal axis suppression with potential adrenal failure | Percutaneous penetration of corticosteroid | Predictable with many potent and very potent agents |
| Cushingoid state | Percutaneous penetration of corticosteroid | Uncommon. Occurs with excessive use of potent agents over long periods |
| Skin thinning, telangiectasia, fragility, impaired healing. When used on face causes intense redness and telangiectasia | Suppression of dermal synthetic activities | Predictable after few weeks with potent and very potent preparations. Mostly slowly reversible |
| Striae distensae | Rupture of elastic fibres due to weakening of surrounding collagen in areas of maximal skin tension | Particularly frequent around joints and on trunk when potent agents used in adolescents and pregnant women |
| Tinea incognito | Suppression of usual eczematous response to dermatophyte infection by inappropriate application of topical corticosteroids | Results from misdiagnosis of ringworm |
| Dermatitis medicamentosa | Allergic contact dermatitis to the corticosteroid molecule | Suspect when patient worsens after treatment. Becoming more frequent |

include lichen sclerosus et atrophicus and cutaneous mastocytosis. There are other very recalcitrant localized inflammatory dermatoses such as chronic discoid lupus erythematosus and localized cutaneous sarcoidosis that sometimes respond to one of the potent agents, but may only respond to the very potent topical corticosteroid preparations. They are also useful as a treatment for exuberant and prominent scar formation, although my personal experience with the treatment of hypertrophic and keloid scars has been disappointing. It has also been suggested that regular intermittent treatment of stubborn plaque-type psoriasis with halcinonide or clobetasol propionate – a kind of 'pulse therapy' – is safe and effective.[3] In view of the possibility of severe rebound and even pustular psoriasis because of this, as well as the ever present danger of hypercortisonism and pituitary adrenal axis suppression and skin thinning, this treatment should be regarded with the same hesitations and concerns as systemic methotrexate or cyclosporin.

Apart from potency, safety has been a major aim of the pharmaceutical chemists involved with steroid molecules and some very interesting corticosteroids have evolved from their efforts in this area. Essentially they have been able to manipulate percutaneous penetration and the speed and direction of metabolism of the molecule after penetration into the skin.[4,5] Two such agents are methyl prednisolone aceponate (MPA) and prednicarbate. The first is a non-halogenated diester of 6-α-methyl-prednisolone and is available as a 0.1% cream, an ointment and as a fatty ointment. It has enhanced lipophilicity and penetrates the skin readily.[6] It is rapidly metabolized in the skin to 17-methyl-prednisolone propionate which is the active and potent anti-inflammatory agent, although it has relatively little skin-thinning activity.[7] When the molecule reaches the systemic circulation, it is rapidly glucuronidated and thus effectively inactivated. Studies of plasma cortisol levels have shown that there appears to be relatively little pituitary adrenal axis suppression compared to the effects of other corticosteroids of comparable clinical potency.[7] It has been promoted specifically for use in eczematous disorders and all the published studies do indeed appear to be in eczematous disorders though there is no a priori reason for believing that it would not be active in psoriasis or other usually corticosteroid-responsive dermatoses.

Prednicarbate (used as a 0.25% ointment) is also moderately potent 'combining the potent anti-inflammatory action of topical corticosteroids with a greatly reduced potential for antiproliferative activity and systemic effects'.[8] It has also been used successfully in the treatment of atopic dermatitis.[9] There have been few other attempts at channelling plain topical corticosteroid preparations towards specific diseases save as mentioned above in the broadest general terms. One that may be mentioned, however, is the use of once-daily 0.1% mometasone furoate for seborrhoeic dermatitis. In a trial of this agent compared with twice-daily 1% hydrocortisone in patients with seborrhoeic dermatitis, the symptoms/sign score of 93% of the mometasone furoate-treated patients and 85% of the hydrocortisone-treated patients improved, i.e. there were no major differences.[10]

There is no special theoretical reason for believing that one or another corticosteroid should be especially active in a particular inflammatory skin disorder but eczema, psoriasis, lichen planus and discoid lupus erythematosus are sufficiently different from the pathodynamic stand-point to hope that some characteristic of a new steroid molecule will particularly suit one or another disease.

# New formats and combinations

The pharmaceutical industry has striven to keep pace with patients preferences driven in large part by the cosmetics industry. Ever more creamier creams and lighter, non-tacky ointments have been the results of this trend. The exception to this has been the development of 'fatty ointments'. These have been popular in particular in North West Europe and mainly for the treatment of psoriasis.

Special attention has been given to scalp applications. There has been some popularity of alcohol-based lotions containing various corticosteroids including betamethasone-17-valerate, clobetasol-17-propionate and fluocinolone acetonide. Their use certainly avoids messing up the hair with creams and ointments, but they do cause stinging in some patients. Another approach has been the development of a betamethasone-17-valerate-containing mousse (Bettamousse) for the treatment of scalp psoriasis and seborrhoeic dermatitis which appears to work effectively and is certainly quite popular with patients. Fluocinolone acetonide has also been formulated in a shampoo.[11]

It is surprising that no new corticosteroid-impregnated adhesive tape preparations have appeared on the market. The one impregnated tape that is available (flurandrenolone is the impregnating steroid) is quite useful for the treatment of localized recalcitrant inflammatory disorders and is a popular first-line treatment for keloid scars.

Corticosteroids have been formulated with antimicrobial compounds for many years, and such combinations continue to appear despite their relative unpopularity amongst some dermatologists who complain that if an anti-infective agent is required it is best to either prescribe an appropriate systemic agent or a topical antimicrobial independently of the corticosteroid after taking a swab to identify the infecting agent. This certainly gives greater flexibility and decreases the likelihood of the antimicrobial compound being used unnecessarily. Topical corticosteroid/antimicrobial combinations are most often prescribed by general practitioners when they are confronted with a red, scaling and/or oozing rash which defies their diagnosis clinically.

Although in my view such combination products are overused, I believe that there is a place for them, especially in seborrhoeic dermatitis and infectious eczematoid dermatitis where invasion of the skin by pathogenic bacteria or yeasts may well be playing an aetiological role. It is also true that patients with atopic dermatitis are prone to infection with *Staphylococcus aureus* and some effort to combat the infection with a staphylococcocidal agent incorporated into the topical product is worthwhile. To avoid producing resistance and selecting antibiotic resistant strains of staphylococci it is best to choose a steroid combination with a non-antibiotic antimicrobial such as Vioform or one of the imidazoles. Furthermore, a bacterial swab should be taken before treatment begins to determine sensitivities if possible. The use of a combination product for suspected patches of ringworm or because there is difficulty in making a clinical diagnosis is strongly deprecated.

Topical corticosteroids are also formulated together with urea (Calmurid HC and Alphaderm) and these do appear to have slightly greater clinical potency than the hydrocortisone alone. It is my impression that these are especially useful for patients with mild atopic dermatitis. Other combination products that are currently available include combinations with salicylic acid (e.g. betamethasone-21-propionate with 2% salicylic acid as Diprosalic) and with tar (e.g. hydrocortisone with a tar extract as Alphosyl HC). The salicylic acid appears to enhance the penetration of the betamethasone[12] and the formulation may be useful for inflammatory dermatoses complicated by hyperkeratotic scaling. The combinations with tar are used for both chronic eczema and in some patients for flexural and/or scalp psoriasis.

Eurax-Hydrocortisone (crotamiton 10% and hydrocortisone 1%) is one other combination product worth mentioning not because of its recent introduction (it must be at least 30 years old!), but because it is one of the very few topical products especially for itching dermatoses. Doxepin hydrochloride 5% (Xepin) is also promoted as an antipruritic topical antihistamine. Would there be any gain by combining it with a mild or moderately potent corticosteroid?

In the recent past two other corticosteroid combination treatments have been described which enhance the therapeutic activities of both agents. The first is the vitamin D analogue calcipotriol. When used once daily in the mornings alongside halobetasol 0.05% ointment once daily at night, the clinical response rate was better than for either component alone and there was less skin irritation.[13] The results after 6 months treatment showed that the combined regimen had a 76% remission rate compared to 40% for the steroid/placebo regimen.[14]

There is also enhanced efficacy and decreased adverse side-effects when the topical retinoid tazarotene is combined with topical corticosteroids.[14] It seems that the best results therapeutically are from a combination of tazarotene with a mid-potency corticosteroid such as mometasone furoate both used once daily. Response rates of nearly 90% at 12 weeks can be expected from this use of the two active agents. It should be noted that there is good evidence that the concomitant use of a topical retinoid does prevent skin thinning from the topical corticosteroid.

Until relatively recently the frequency of application of topical corticosteroids had never been seriously questioned – they were always recommended for twice daily use. Many of the newer agents, e.g. fluticasone and mometasone furoate, have been used once daily in clinical trials and found as effective as when used twice daily. Even the older agents can be used just once daily without detriment.

# Indications for topical corticosteroids

There has been little change in the way that topical corticosteroids are used in the treatment of eczema in recent years. There has been some reluctance on the part of dermatologists to recommend highly potent corticosteroid materials for two main reasons. Firstly, potent agents have a greater tendency to cause serious adverse side-effects

both local and systemic and secondly there is a greater likelihood of sudden and severe relapse after using really powerful topical corticosteroids. It has been claimed that some of the new potent compounds cause fewer problems than the older ones. Fluticasone, for example, has been claimed to cause less skin thinning than might be expected of a similarly clinically potent agent. The 'soft steroids' such as methyl prednisolone aceponate[7] or prednicarbate[8] are much less likely to cause pituitary-adrenal axis suppression than older corticosteroids of similar potency and also cause less skin thinning. It is also true that given the chance most cases of eczema – from whatever cause – respond well to moderately potent corticosteroids so that it would be unusual to need a very potent topical corticosteroid. The major exception to this is the distressingly itchy condition known as lichen simplex chronicus. This rarely seems to respond to any topical application, although if it does it fares best with potent topical corticosteroids.

Psoriatic lesions in the flexures, on the genitalia or the face often do respond to weak or moderately potent corticosteroids, but psoriatic plaques are altogether a different problem – they require the heavy artillery of potent and very potent agents. Pulse therapy with potent or very potent corticosteroids, in which these agents are used three times weekly at 12-hour intervals, has been proposed as a way of avoiding serious adverse side-effects.[3] Pulse therapy is instituted after an initial 3–4-week induction phase in which the steroid is initially used twice daily. A major problem with this scheme is that a substantial proportion of patients do not achieve satisfactory remission.

One of the issues concerning the treatment of psoriasis with topical corticosteroids is the phenomenon of tachyphylaxis in which a psoriatic patch will no longer respond to one topical corticosteroid, but will respond to another. It was claimed that this was also observed experimentally both in depression of DNA synthesis and the human vasoconstrictor test.[15,16] More recently, doubt has been expressed as to whether this fascinating pharmacological problem actually occurs in the clinical treatment of psoriasis. It has been suggested that what has been taken to be tachyphylaxis is actually a mixture of poor therapeutic efficacy and lack of patient compliance.[17]

# References

1. Chaffman MO, Topical corticosteroids: a review of properties and principles in therapeutic use. *Nurse Practitioner Forum* 1999: 10(2); 95–105.

2. Maibach HI, Surber Ch, *Topical corticosteroids.* Basel: Karger, 1992.

3. Katz HI, Hien NT, Prawer SE et al, Betamethasone dipropionate in an optimised vehicle: intermittent pulse dosing for extended maintenance in treatment of psoriasis. *Arch Dermatol* 1987: 123; 1308–11.

4. Bodor N, The application of soft drug approaches to the design of safer corticosteroids. In: Christophers E, Kligman AM,

Schopf E, Staughton RB (eds) *Topical corticosteroid therapy. A novel approach to safer drugs.* New York: Raven Press, 1988, pp. 13–26.

5. Flower RJ, A molecular biology approach to the design of solar steroid like drugs. In: Christophers E, Kligman AM, Schopf E, Staughton RB (eds) *Topical corticosteroid therapy. A novel approach to safer drugs.* New York: Raven Press, 1988, pp. 27–34.

6. Zaumzeil RP, Kecskes A, Täuber U, Töpert M, Methylprednisolone aceponate (MPA) – a new therapeutic for eczema: A pharmacological overview. *J Dermatol Treat* 1992: 3(Suppl 2); 3–8.

7. Ortonne JP, Safety aspects of methylprednisolone aceponate (MPA) treatment. *J Dermatol Treat* 1992; 3(Suppl 2); 21–6.

8. Dehavay J, Pierard GE, Lapiére ChM, Evaluation of the potential atrophogenicity of 0.25% prednicarbate cream. In: Christophers E, Kligman AM, Schopf E, Staughton RB (eds) *Topical corticosteroid therapy. A novel approach to safer drugs.* New York: Raven Press, 1988, pp. 119–26.

9. Lawlor F, Black AK, Greaves M, Prednicarbate 0.25% ointment in the treatment of atopic dermatitis: a vehicle controlled double-blind study. *J Dermatol Treat* 1995: 6; 233–5.

10. Medansky RS, Lepaw MI, Shavin JS et al, Mometasone furoate cream 0.1% vs hydrocortisone cream 1% in the treatment of seborrhoeic dermatitis. *J Dermatol Treat* (1992): 3; 125–8.

11. Ramirez RG, Dorton D, Double-blind, placebo controlled multicentre study of fluocinolone acetonide shampoo (FS shampoo) in scalp seborrhoeic dermatitis. *J Dermatol Treat* 1993: 4; 135–7.

12. Marks R, What do you do with a topical corticosteroid. In: Marks R (ed) *Topics in topicals*. Lancaster: MTP Press, 1985, pp. 47–60.

13. Lebwohl M, Topical application of topical calcipotriene and corticosteroid combination regimens. *J Am Acad Dermatol* 1997: 37; S55–8.

14. Lebwohl M, Tazarotene in combination with topical corticosteroids. *J Am Acad Dermatol* 1998: 39; S139–43.

15. Du Vivier A, Stoughton RB, Tachyphylaxis to the action of topically applied corticosteroids. *Arch Dermatol* 1975: 111; 581–3.

16. Du Vivier A, Tachyphylaxis to topically applied steroids. *Arch Dermatol* 1976: 112; 1245–8.

17. Miller JJ, Roling D, Margolis D, Guzzo C, Failure to demonstrate therapeutic tachyphylaxis to topically applied steroids in patients with psoriasis. *J Am Acad Dermatol* 1999: 41; 546–9.

# 15

# Laser hair removal

*Nicholas J Lowe, Donna Lee and Gary Lask*

## Introduction

Initial interest in laser hair removal began when the Q switched ruby laser used for tattoo removal was also noted to have a sustained effect on the hair follicles. Further research has shown that this mechanism of follicular injury is based on the theory of selective photothermolysis. Many laser systems and light sources have been since introduced and the technology of laser hair removal has expanded rapidly and significantly.

## Principles of laser hair removal

Laser hair removal is based on the principle of selective photothermolysis. This theory, proposed by Anderson and Parrish, holds that the thermal injury will be confined to a specific target if there is preferential absorption of the light at an appropriate wavelength and the pulse duration or width is shorter than the thermal relaxation time of the target.[1] Thermal relaxation time is defined as the time it takes for the target to cool to 50% of its peak temperature.

The primary targets for laser hair removal are the hair follicle and the hair bulb. The endogenous target is melanin, which is located mainly in the hair shaft as well as in smaller amounts in the inner and outer root sheaths. A variety of chromophores have been used, e.g. carbon rich lotion, or proposed, e.g. photoactive dyes used as a modified use of photodynamic therapy. Theoretically, laser or light energy directed primarily at the pigment of the hair shaft, melanin or the lotion, is absorbed and transferred to the surrounding follicle and perifollicular tissue, causing conductive thermal damage to the follicle. Adequate damage is required to cause long-term hair removal. A better understanding of hair biology in the future should also produce other targets that may more efficiently cause hair removal.

## Hair removal laser systems

With most of the current hair removal laser systems, histological assessments have shown that the thermal damage is confined to the follicular epithelium and that the coagulative follicular epithelial destruction appears to correlate with clinical efficacy. Permanent or long-term hair reduction is defined as a lasting reduction in terminal hairs for a period of time greater than the complete hair cycle of the hairs in a given body site.

It is important, then, to understand the hair cycle in order to plan an efficient strategy of hair removal with laser systems. Hair follicles undergo asynchronous repeated sequences of growth (anagen) and rest (telogen) phases, called the hair cycle.[2] In the active phase, anagen, melanocytes transfer melanin to the matrix cells in the lower portion of the hair bulb. The matrix cells then give rise to the hair shaft as well as the inner and outer root sheaths as they move into the upper part of the hair bulb. At the end of anagen, the follicular bulb moves up to the superficial portion of the dermis as melanization is completed. Telogen, the rest phase, then follows, which appears to be a relatively consistent period given a specific body site. Because of the high concentration of melanin in the anagen hair, laser energy is better absorbed during this phase.

The duration of anagen also varies according to multiple factors including body location, patient age, gender and genetics, hormonal effects and seasons.[3-7] This may be significant in that the anagen hairs are especially sensitive to environmental challenges and physical, chemical or inflammatory insults. This has been proven by mouse model studies by Lin et al, where only the actively growing anagen hairs were significantly sensitive to hair removal by a ruby laser.[8]

Multiple experiments have also shown that the location of the damage to the follicle may be important in determining the effectiveness of hair removal. Initially it was thought that the matrix cells and the dermal papilla were the only important sites involved in preserving hair follicle regeneration, but more recent transection experiments have shown that the isthmus of the follicle is also needed for hair follicle regeneration.[9] These results and future research may lead to more efficient hair removal by targeting different sites of the follicle for destruction from those utilized today.

# Key elements in achieving good results

There are three key elements in achieving effective laser-assisted hair removal: wavelength, pulse duration and fluence.

## Wavelength

Wavelengths between 700 and 1064 nm are selectively absorbed by melanin. Oxyhaemoglobin, a competing chromophore, absorbs less energy at these wavelengths. The currently available lasers for hair removal utilize these wavelengths.

## Pulse duration

The optimal pulse width for hair removal is in the order of tens of milliseconds. This pulse duration is shorter than the thermal relaxation time of the hair follicle (40–100 ms for terminal hair follicles of 200–300 μm diameter) but longer than that of the epidermis (3–10 ms), allowing some preservation of the epidermis from thermal damage.[10,11]

*Fluence*

The fluence also determines the ability of the laser system to cause follicular damage. Significant energy must be delivered at the appropriate wavelength and pulse duration in order to induce adequate follicular destruction. Insufficient energy may merely heat the hair shaft causing temporary epilation without causing long-term hair loss.

# Hair removal laser systems

There are four main wavelength-type lasers available for hair removal. They include the ruby (694 nm), alexandrite (755 nm), diode (800 nm) and neodymium:yttrium-aluminium-garnet (Nd:YAG, 1064 nm) lasers. These lasers are described below and are summarized in Table 15.1

## Table 15.1 Some lasers used for hair removal

| Laser type and wavelength | Pulse duration | Spot sizes (mm) | Maximum fluence ($J/cm^2$) | Chromophore target |
|---|---|---|---|---|
| Alexandrite lasers (755 nm) | | | | |
| Apogee | 5, 10, 20 ms | 7, 10, 12.5 | 50 | Melanin |
| Epitouch | 2 ms | 5, 10 | 25 | Melanin |
| Gentlelase | 3 ms | 8, 10, 12, 15 | 100 | Melanin |
| Photogenica | 5, 10, 20 ms | 7, 10 | 40 | Melanin |
| Diode lasers (800 nm) | | | | |
| Lightsheer | 5–30 ms | 9 × 9 | 40 | Melanin |
| Nd:YAG (1064 nm) | 10–30 ms | Varied | Varied | Melanin |
| Nd:YAG + Softlight | 10 ns | 7 | 3 | Topical carbon dye |
| Ruby lasers (694 nm) | | | | |
| Chromos | 1.2 ms | 7, 10 | 20 | Melanin |
| Epilaser | 3 ms | 7, 10 | 40 | Melanin |
| Epitouch Silk Laser | 1.2 ms | 5, 6 | 40 | Melanin |
| Epilight Light Source | Variable | 10 × 45, 8 × 35 | 65 | Melanin |

## Long-pulsed ruby lasers

There are several ruby lasers with varying parameters of pulse width, fluence and spot size. These units emit light of wavelength 694 nm which is strongly absorbed by melanin and only slightly by haemoglobin. The efficacy of these lasers for hair removal has been demonstrated in several studies.[11-14]

The first pilot study carried out with a long-pulsed ruby laser was by Grossman et al.[11] In this study, 13 patients received a single treatment on the thigh or the back at fluences ranging from 30 to 60 J/cm². They were followed at 1, 3 and 6 months with manual terminal hair counts. At 6 months, four patients showed <50% regrowth, and of these patients, two showed no regrowth. Follow-up observations of seven of these patients at 2 years showed four patients with significant sustained hair growth arrest. Long-term fluence-dependent hair loss was also noted. Histologically, heterogeneous injury to the follicular epithelium was noted initially after treatment followed by the subsequent development of vellus-like hairs.

An additional study by Dierckx also found that 72 of 100 patients achieved long-term hair loss when fluences of 30 J/cm² or more were used (personal communication, 1998). They were also followed for long-term effects at 6, 9 and 12 months, and were found to have sustained hair loss. Adverse effects included immediate erythema and oedema which lasted less than 24 hours, and transient dyspigmentation which was inversely related to skin type. No scarring was noted.

### Epilaser

The Epilaser offers a 3 ms pulse width, 5 Hz repetition rate and fluences ranging between 10 and 40 J/cm².[10] A 7 or 10 mm spot size can be used. The epidermis, including its melanin, is cooled, allowing preservation from thermal injury, by a sapphire cooling handpiece which is directly applied to the skin.[11,15] This crystal has a high thermal conductivity which provides cooling of the epidermis before, during and after the laser energy is delivered. This reduces patient discomfort during the procedure, which allows higher fluences to be delivered. The concomitant direct pressure applied with the cool tip also flattens the epidermis which decreases the distance that the laser light energy has to traverse in the dermis to target the lower portion of the hair follicle. It also temporarily constricts the blood vessels underlying the tip which displaces the oxyhaemoglobin, the competing chromophore. The tip must be routinely cleansed during the treatment to minimize collection of debris on the lens which can cause epidermal injury. The area to be treated also must be closely shaven to lessen the singeing and accumulation of the hairs on the lens surface.

### Epitouch

Epitouch is another ruby laser that is effective for hair removal.[13] The highest fluence is 40 J/cm² with spot size options in the range 4–6 mm. The pulse duration is 1.2 ms. A pretreatment of a water-based gel is applied to cool the skin. Using fluences of 18–25 J/cm² on the arms, Lask et al noted 40–80% hair regrowth at 12 weeks.[14] The results of this study are summarized in Table 15.2. Nestor treated arms, legs and the bikini area once at 25 J/cm² and reported 60% regrowth at 3 months, and with two treatments found 25% regrowth.[13] After a third session, less than 10% regrowth was noted at 1-year follow-up. The same fluences in the moustache and beard areas at 1 month yielded regrowths of 55%, 40% and 25% after one, two and three treatments, respectively. However, there was no longer term follow-up in these patients.

## Chromos 694

Another ruby laser is the Chromos 694, for which at the present time no adequate efficacy data are available.[13,16]

## *Long-pulsed alexandrite lasers*

Two long-pulsed alexandrite laser systems currently available are the Epitouch and Gentlelase lasers. They emit light of wavelength 755 nm with varying spot sizes and fluences. Theoretically, the epidermal melanin absorbs this wavelength less than the ruby laser wavelength (694 nm ) which may allow a safer therapy in dark-skinned patients.[17] These lasers utilize a cooling mechanism to minimize the risk of thermal damage to the superficial melanin-containing epidermis.

## Table 15.2 Ruby hair removal laser (Epitouch) study: results summary[14]

Multicentre study groups of more than 100 patients

One year follow-up, multiple treatment sessions

First treatment results
   Average 60% growth, 3 months after treatment: arms, bikini, legs
   Average 55% growth, 1 month after treatment: upper lip, chin

Second treatment (performed on hair growth) results
   Average 24% growth, 3 months after second treatment: arms, bikini, legs
   Average 40% growth, 1 month after treatment: upper lip, chin

Third treatment results
   Less than 10% growth, 3 months after third treatment: arms, bikini, legs
   Average 25% growth, 1 month after third treatment: upper lip, chin

Pretreatment shaving further protects the epidermis from undesirable thermal injury.

Promotional data for these Alexandrite lasers indicate that 80–100% hair reduction can be achieved by three or four treatments 4–6 weeks apart using fluences up to 40 J/cm².[16] The Epitouch has a cool tip handpiece and offers 1–40 J/cm² fluence, 5, 10 or 20 ms pulse durations, and 7 or 10 mm spot sizes.

The Gentlelase offers fluences of 10–100 J/cm² at 3 ms pulse duration and optional 8, 10, 12 and 15 mm spot sizes.[18] It has a novel dynamic cooling device which consists of a burst of cryogen spray that protects the epidermis (Figure 15.1). The Epitouch 5100

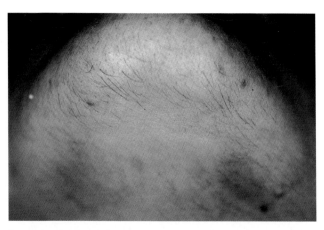

a

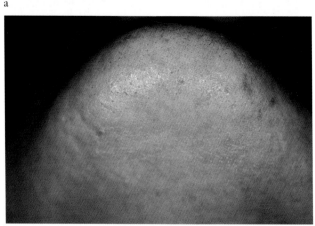

b

Figure 15.1

(a) Chin hirsutes pretreatment. (b) Following treatment with long-pulsed alexandrite laser with dynamic cooling.

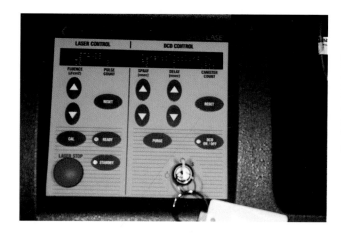

**Figure 15.2**

Long-pulsed
alexandrite laser.
Typical settings for
hair removal for dark
hair with a light skin
colour: 30 J/cm² 
dynamic cooling,
70 ms, 15 mm
diameter spot size.

performs at a 2 ms pulse duration at
5 Hz with a 5 or 10 mm spot size. It also
offers a scanner with high repetition
rates for rapid treatments. It uses a
water-based gel as a 'heat sink' to cool
the epidermis to decrease its risk of
injury. Finkel et al reported 5–15%
regrowth of hair at 3 months after three
treatments using 20–40 J/cm² at intervals of 1 to 2½ months (Figure 15.2).[18]

Comparable clinical efficacy as well
as adverse effects have been found
between these laser systems and the
ruby lasers. The adverse effects of
these lasers are few. They include post-
treatment erythema and oedema lasting
less than 4 hours, transient discomfort
during the procedure and epidermal
changes in 10–15% of patients (dark-
skinned or tanned individuals).[17,18]

## Diode lasers

The Lightsheer diode laser emits light
of wavelength of 800 nm and also
causes hair removal by effectively
targeting melanin while deeply
penetrating the dermis.[16] It offers a
pulse duration of 5–30 ms, which is
comparable to the thermal relaxation
time of the follicle. Fluences range
from 10 to 40 J/cm² and the spot size is
9 cm². A contact cooling sapphire tip,
as described for the Epilaser, is also
employed to effectively cool the epidermis. This has many advantages
discussed previously. Clinical studies
have shown that higher fluences can be
better delivered with fewer adverse
effects using this cooling system. This
may allow a safer treatment in dark-
skinned individuals.

Dierickx (personal communication,
1998) reported a study of 100 subjects
using a combination of fluences and
pulse widths in eight test sites, mostly
on the back and thighs. Patients were
followed at 1, 3, 6, 9 and 12 months.
All patients had temporary epilation
which lasted up to 1–3 months at all
fluences used. Of the 100 patients, 89

had long-term hair loss at 1 year follow-up, fulfilling the criteria for long-term hair reduction described above. The efficacy was also fluence-dependent. Those who did not respond adequately were patients with blonde hair which contains less melanin and therefore less chromophore. These subjects had in addition to decreased absolute number of hairs, lighter and thinner regrowing hairs which added to the apparent clinical hair reduction. Histological evaluation confirmed the clinical findings by showing a reduction in size of hair follicles and granulomatous degeneration of the follicle epithelium with consequent fibrosis. In the study, a fixed fluence–pulse duration combination was employed regardless of the patient's skin type. This parameter was therefore not matched to the characteristics of each patient probably leading to a higher incidence of adverse effects. A 6% epidermal change and 3% textural change (mostly at higher fluences), both of which had resolved by 3 months, were noted. Transient dyspigmentation was noted in 10% of patients, mostly in dark-skinned and tanned individuals.

The clinical efficacy of the diode laser has also been confirmed by Adrian who treated 125 patients with the laser. Most had <60% long-term (6 months) hair reduction after two or three treatments (personal communication, 1998). The treated areas included the lip, face, neck, axilla and back. Subsequent treatments were given when significant clinical regrowth of hair was noted at 1–3 months

## Nd: YAG lasers

The Q-switched Nd:YAG laser produces light at 1064 nm in the near-infrared spectrum. Water, haemoglobin and melanin are poorly absorbed at this wavelength,[19] and because of this, the laser was initially employed in combination with a topical pigmented carbon-based suspension as an exogenous chromophore.[10,17,20,21] This method provides a selective target that is independent of the colour of the hair shaft. This potentially permits effective treatment of even light-haired individuals who lack significant hair melanin, the main chromophore for other laser systems.

Softlight was the first FDA-approved laser-assisted hair removal system. It provided fluences of 2–4 J/cm$^2$ at 10 ns pulse duration and a rapid 10 Hz repetition rate with a 7 mm spot size.[16] The original treatment technique required the skin to be first waxed, theoretically allowing the carbon-rich lotion to be placed into the 'empty' follicles.[17,20] The carbon then targeted with the laser beam caused a photomechanical and photothermal injury to the follicle as the carbon particles were vaporized. This produced a 40–70% hair loss at 3 months in 35 patients after a single session, but the patients had full regrowth of hair at 6 months.[17] This process is also time consuming and is now little used in the USA.

More recently, Nanni and Alster have reviewed the efficacy of the treatment parameters.[22] While they observed adequate delay in hair regrowth in all patients, they noted that neither the pretherapy waxing nor the carbon-based lotion significantly affected the efficacy of the laser treatment at 3 months after a single session. At this time, further studies that better predict the parameters and the efficacy of this laser are needed.[23] Nd:YAG laser with longer pulsed width are also being used.[24,25]

## Non-laser light sources

A variety of intense pulse light sources with variable spectrum between 550 and 1100 nm have recently been claimed to be successful for hair removal. The treatment frequency and permanence of hair removal remains to be determined. Various presentations have shown between 50–60% hair reduction, with treatment frequency up to every 2 weeks.

## Eflornithine hydrochloride

A new cream has been approved in the USA which delays hair follicle regrowth. This cream, eflornithine hydrochloride, will delay hair regrowth and may be used following laser or light hair removal.[26]

# References

1.  Anderson RR, Parrish JA, Selective photothermolysis: precise microsurgery by selective absorption of pulsed radiation. *Science* 1983: 220; 524–7.

2.  Olsen EA, *Disorders of hair growth: diagnosis and treatment.* New York: McGraw-Hill, 1994; pp. 1–19.

3.  Seago SV, Ebling FJG, The hair cycle on the human thigh and upper arm. *Br J Dermatol* 1985: 113; 9–16.

4.  Randall VA, Ebling FJG, Seasonal changes in human hair growth. *Br J Dermatol* 1991: 24; 146–51.

5.  Eaton P, Eaton MW, Temperature and the growth of hair. *Science* 1937: 86; 354.

6.  Saitoh M, Uzuka M, Sakamoto M, Human hair cycle. *J Invest Dermatol* 1970; 54; 65–81.

7.  Trotter M, The cycle of hair in selected regions of the body. *Am J Phys Anthropol* 1924: 7; 427–37.

8.  Lin TY, Manuskiatti W, Dierickx CC et al, Hair growth cycle affects hair follicle destruction by ruby laser pulses. *J Invest Dermatol* 1998: 111(1); 107–13.

9.  Kim J-C, Choi Y-C, Hair follicle regeneration after horizontal resectioning: implications for hair transplantation. In: Stough DB, Haber RS (eds) *Hair replacement: surgical and medical.* St Louis: Mosby-Year Book, 1995, pp. 358–63.

10. Wheeland RG, Laser-assisted hair removal. *Dermatol Clin* 1997: 15; 459–77.

11. Grossman MC, Dierickx C, Farinelli W et al, Damage to hair follicles by normal-mode ruby laser pulses. *J Am Acad Dermatol* 1996: 35; 889–94.

12. Dierickx CC, Grossman MC, Farinelli WA, Anderson RR, Permanent hair removal by normal pulsed ruby laser. *Arch Dermatol* 1998: 134; 837–42.

13. Nestor MS, Laser hair removal: clinical results and practical applications of

selective photothermolysis. *Skin Aging* 1998: 1; 34–40.

14.   Lask G, Elman M, Slatkine M et al, Laser-assisted hair removal by selective photothermolysis. *Dermatol Surg* 1997: 23; 737–9.

15.   Alster TS, Nanni CA, Laser-assisted hair removal with long-pulsed ruby and alexandrite lasers. In: Keller TS (ed) *Lasers in facial plastic surgery*. New York: Thieme, 1998.

16.   Olsen EA, Methods of hair removal. *J Am Acad Dermatol* 1999: 40; 143–58.

17.   Nanni CA, Alster TS, A practical review of laser-assisted hair removal using the Q-switched Nd:Yag, long-pulsed ruby, and long-pulsed alexandrite lasers. *Dermatol Surg* 1998: 24; 1–7.

18.   Finkel B, Eliezri YD, Waldman A, Slatkine M, Pulsed alexandrite laser technology for noninvasive hair removal. *J Clin Laser Med Surg* 1997: 15; 225–9.

19.   Dover JS, Arndt KS, *Illustrated cutaneous laser surgery: a practitioner's guide*. Norwalk: Appleton & Lange, 1990.

20.   Goldberg DJ, Topical suspension-assisted Q-switched Nd:Yag laser hair removal. *Dermatol Surg* 1997: 23; 741–5.

21.   Goldberg DJ, Topical solution assisted laser hair removal. *Lasers Surg Med* 1995: 7; 47.

22.   Nanni CA, Alster TS, Optimizing treatment parameters for hair removal using a carbon-based solution and a 1064 nm Q-switched neodymium:Yag laser energy. *Arch Dermatol* 1997: 133; 1546–9.

23.   Sumian CC, Pitre FB, Gauthier BE et al, A new method to improve penetration depth of dyes into the follicular duct: potential application for laser hair removal. *J Am Acad Dermatol* 1999: 41; 172–5.

24.   Kilmer SL, Laser hair removal with the long pulse 1064 nm Coolglide* laser system. *J Cut Laser Therapy* 2000: 2; 99.

25.   Liew SH, Gault DT, Laser-assisted hair removal at 1064 nm without added chromophore. *Br J Dermatol Surg* 1999: 52; 322–30.

26.   Shapiro J, Lui H, Vaniqa-eflornithine 13.9% cream. *Skin Therapy Lett* 2001: 6; 1–5.

# 16

# Review of surgical advances

*Barry I Resnik and*
*Sorrel S Resnik*

The trend in cutaneous surgical techniques in the last 10 years has become tightly focused on cosmetic surgery. Aging baby-boomers are providing an ever-increasing population intent upon maintaining youthful appearances. Our ability to remove imperfections with less disturbance of the overlying epidermis has grown in step with demand for these procedures. Some of the newest and most exciting techniques for rejuvenation and augmentation of the skin are discussed, with special attention paid to laser technology.

## Laser resurfacing

Laser resurfacing using the pulsed $CO_2$ laser has been in clinical use for approximately 5 years and is one of the most requested cosmetic procedures today. Great strides have been made in the areas of wound healing and optimization of technique. Pretreat-

ment has long been thought to contribute to postoperative healing and a better result. Recent reports in the literature suggest pretreatment using tretinoin or glycolic acid combined with hydroquinone is not as effective as originally thought. Further, any inhibition of postinflammatory hyperpigmentation gained by pretreatment is removed along with the epidermis on the first pass of the laser.[1,2] The concept of pretreatment was carried over from chemical peels, where the use of exfoliating agents combined with hydroquinone was found to enhance healing and the final result in clinical studies.[3-6] It appears that the irritation seen as a result of pretreatment tretinoin may actually enhance and accentuate the postoperative erythema.[7]

A new wound care technique developed by Ruiz-Esparza et al has demonstrated that postoperative erythema can be significantly reduced by leaving intact the last layer of carbonless char. This last layer of desiccated tissue is used as a biologic dressing, and is covered by bland emollients and an interpositional dressing, forming a mask.[7-9] The mask would automatically separate in approximately 48 hours, revealing almost complete reepithelialization. The results are impressive, reducing duration of erythema to several weeks, rather than several months. They suggest that vigorous removal of the last layer of carbonless char produces more erythema than leaving the layer in place. Antioxidants such as vitamins C and E have been used anecdotally as topical treatments to diminish postoperative erythema. Recent work has indeed shown vitamin C to be beneficial in erythema resolution.[10]

The erbium:YAG laser was developed to answer several of the pulsed $CO_2$ laser's shortcomings: uncomfortable postoperative healing phase and prolonged erythema. It produces excellent results in minimally damaged skin, and can be used safely to treat darker-skinned patients. It has also been shown to be safe and effective in the rejuvenation of non-facial areas such as the neck, areas where the $CO_2$ laser can and does cause scarring.[11] Erbium:YAG resurfacing also has some benefits not available with $CO_2$ laser. With a wavelength of 2960 nm, it has a much greater affinity for water, providing true ablation. It does not, however, have the depth of penetration and collagen remodeling force available with the $CO_2$ laser because it lacks a thermal component. Additionally, without that thermal component, there is no hemostasis. This obscures the operative field and can compromise the ability to work more deeply in severely damaged skin.

It has been exciting to watch the gap between $CO_2$ and erbium:YAG resurfacing systems narrow in the last years. In a recent study by Goldman et al, it was shown that patients treated with two passes of the $CO_2$ laser, followed by two more passes with the erbium:YAG laser had significantly shorter healing times, as well as shorter times for erythema resolution.[12] The clinical results were thought to be comparable to complete $CO_2$ resurfacing. It was postulated that the two final passes with the erbium:YAG laser removed the non-specific thermal damage produced by the $CO_2$ laser, substantially reducing postoperative erythema while retaining thermal collagen shrinkage.

Two new lasers appear to provide the best of both lasers in one package. The Derma-K laser (ESC Medical Systems, Needham, MA) combines an erbium:YAG with a continuous wave superpulsed $CO_2$ laser. The $CO_2$ laser is pulsed in between the erbium:YAG pulse, allowing true ablation with thermal collagen shrinkage. The Contour laser (Sciton, Palo Alto, CA) is a dual beam erbium:YAG laser. One beam provides ablation, while the other provides adjustable levels of coagulation. These combination lasers marry the shorter recovery times and ablative powers of the erbium:YAG laser with the hemostatic, tissue-tightening and deeper penetration of the $CO_2$ laser.[13] These are exciting developments and will undoubtedly receive further clinical evaluation.

# Thermescent skin treatment

Until now, attention has been focused primarily on water as the chromophore of choice in laser resurfacing. A new technique called Thermescent skin treatment may change that focus. This technique targets collagen as the chromophore in an attempt to cause remodelling with little or no epidermal disruption. An Nd:YAG laser (Cooltouch, Byron Medical, Tucson, AZ) emitting light at a wavelength of 1320 nm, combined with a thermocouple-controlled liquid nitrogen spray, cools the epidermis while heating the dermis. Collagen contraction is initiated while epidermal slough is prevented. The process requires several treatments and takes several months to see results, but may be the next step in the evolution of skin resurfacing. Epidermal solar dyschromia and fine lines will still require additional treatment.

mild to severe photodamage in Fitzpatrick classes 1–3 were treated in periorbital and perioral sites. Significant improvement was seen in wrinkles for both the periorbital and perioral sites, with greater change for patients with more severe wrinkles at the start of the study. Of note was a slightly increased incidence of hypertrophic scarring as compared to laser resurfacing procedures. The authors attributed this to the novelty of the treatment for most of those performing the procedures. They expect that this rate would probably go down with experience.[15]

## Electrosurgical facial resurfacing

In the quest for resurfacing modalities that have less down-time and fewer side-effects, coblation may be the answer. Coblation, or cold ablation, is also called electrosurgical facial resurfacing. Low-power radio frequency energy generated by a RF unit first utilized in arthroscopic procedures reacts with the skin to cause dermal remodeling. Saline is used as the conductive medium. This lower energy resurfacing technique produces less collateral damage and appears to induce collagen remodeling similar to that found with the resurfacing lasers. In initial trials, it produced modest tissue remodeling with minimal complications, usually in the form of temporary dyspigmentation.[14]

In a multicenter, prospective, noncomparative study, 95 patients with

## Light-assisted hair removal

This technique continues to grow at a startling pace, driven by high patient demand. In light of its somewhat temporary nature, it seems more correct to refer to the procedure as reduction rather than removal because the duration of clearance is still not well established. Endogenous melanin in the hair bulb is the chromophore. The light treatments appear to force the hairs into a prolonged telogen phase. The technique works only on dark hairs in anagen, so several treatments are required to catch the greatest number of hairs during the growth phase. Side-effects can include postinflammatory hypo- and hyperpigmentation, as well as foot-printing and superficial burns. Permanent changes are rare.

The FDA has approved several systems including the long-pulsed ruby and alexandrite lasers for this treatment. The diode laser at 810 nm has also proven effective.[16] The Epilight high-intensity pulsed light source uses a flashlamp and filters under computer control to achieve selective photothermolysis. Advantages of this system include a large rectangular footprint and wavelengths in a range from 650 to 1200 nm. The light output can be fine-tuned according to several parameters, possibly enhancing treatment in darker-skinned individuals.

All the available systems have advantages particular to each model, but results appear to be similar: reduction of growth and diminution of hair shaft caliber after several treatments. All require maintenance treatments as well. While permanence and hair removal remain elusive, recent work with the ruby and the alexandrite lasers has shown hair loss to be persistent in treated areas at two-year follow up.[17–19]

The long-pulsed Nd:YAG laser appears to be more effective than previous hair removal lasers in that its wavelength is effective in all skin types. The longer pulse, in the range of 40–100 ms, allows deeper penetration to the dermal papilla, with preservation of epidermis. Patients with types 4 through 6 skin in particular will benefit from this new technology.

# Light-assisted hair transplantation

The $CO_2$ and erbium:YAG lasers have been evaluated as time-saving devices in the formation of the recipient sites. This work arose from their use as bloodless scalpels in standard plastic surgical techniques such as blepharoplasty and brow- and face-lifts.[20,21] Unger and David laid the groundwork for laser-assisted hair transplantation, a more apt descriptor, in 1992.[22,23] Suggested advantages include ablation of alopecic scalp in creating the 1–2 mm sites, alleviation of slit graft 'compression', less graft handling and resultant trauma, less bleeding and injury to the blood supply because of the thermal cautery effect, and sealed nerve endings with resultant decreased pain. It has been shown to be effective in transplantation of cicatricial alopecia. It has been shown to cause minimal disruption of the surrounding tissues, crucial to the successful transplantation of scarred skin.[24]

Disadvantages include the production of a noxious plume requiring the use of a suction device, delay of hair growth, increased postoperative crusting, and reduced hair growth which has been reported to have occurred in several patients after their laser sessions. The reason for the last is unclear, but might be attributed to less than optimal laser settings or other peri- and postoperative variables.

Clinical evaluation has shown the value of laser-generated recipient sites in high-count transplantation sessions, and the results appear to be comparable to those of scalpel-driven transplantation.[25-27] Due to its size and price, however, it is unclear whether this technique will become widely used.

# Microdermabrasion

Microdermabrasion has attracted a great deal of attention in the last year. This procedure is analogous to a mild sandblasting of the skin. Silica or aluminum oxide crystals running through a closed loop system abrade the skin as a handpiece is held against and moved across the skin. There is very little erythema if done superficially and the patient can return to work after the treatment. A series of six to ten sessions is recommended. This technique is usually performed by allied health personnel, and can be a useful adjunct in the treatment of acne and melasma, among other conditions. Although clinical studies are lacking, the technology appears to hold some value, and may find a niche between superficial and medium-depth chemical peels.[28] Combining this therapy with Thermescent skin treatment might be a way to offer non-ablative skin resurfacing where laser treatment may be undesirable.

# Botox®

*Clostridium botulinum*-A exotoxin, Botox® (Allergan, Irvine, CA), is a neurotoxin that causes reversible paralysis in striated muscle. It has been well documented as an effective therapy in the treatment of lines of facial expression.[29-32] It is extremely effective for the relaxation of glabellar and periocular rhytids. It is also useful in the relaxation of platysmal bands, allowing unopposed upward movement of the neck and lower facial skin, providing a non-surgical neck lift.

In an exciting development, it has now been found to be effective in the treatment of axially, plantar and palmar hyperhidrosis.[33,34] Small amounts (2–4 U/0.1 ml) were injected superficially into the affected areas. Relief is usually seen within 5 days, and can persist for as long as 7 months. Although costly and temporary, this treatment can be effective where other therapies such as topical aluminum chloride and iontophoresis have failed, and surgical intervention is not desired.

# Chelated trichloroacetic acid

The TCA Accupeel (ICN Pharmaceuticals, Costa Mesa, CA) is a new formulation of TCA available in 11% and 16% strengths. This easily managed form of TCA provides increased control over acid penetration with a superior safety profile. Advantages over conventional aqueous TCA include ease of application without fear of dripping and evenness of blanche, which eliminates hot spots and skip-areas. It has proven highly effective both alone and in combination with pretreatment regimens such as Jessner's solution in the treatment of actinic degeneration, dyschromia and superficial wrinkles in over 85 patients studied.[35] When combined with laser resurfacing, it can produce results equivalent to full-face laser resurfacing, with local anesthesia and a shorter, less involved, healing period.[36]

# Soft tissue augmentation

Bovine collagen (Zyderm and Zyplast, Collagen Corporation, Palo Alto, CA) has been a popular filler substance for over 10 years. Patients are pleased with its 'instant' correction, but it is temporary and its allergic potential requires a skin test. Dermalogen (Collagenesis Corporation, Beverly, MA) appears to have overcome these drawbacks. It is a new autologous injectable collagen product derived from human cadaver skin. It is composed of intact collagen and elastin fibers in a matrix form and appears to have little to no allergic potential. The tissue is obtained from federally certified tissue banks and exhaustively screened for viral contamination including HIV and hepatitis. It also undergoes two stages of antiviral treatment before the collagen matrix is extracted. Although clinical data are limited, it appears to be comparable to bovine collagen and may have more longevity.[37] It is placed mid-dermally in a series of three sessions 2 weeks apart. While most people tolerate the injections well, it is not mixed with lidocaine and local anesthesia may be necessary.

Isolagen (Isolagen Technologies, Paramus, NJ) and Restylane (Q-Med, Uppsala, Sweden) are different approaches in tissue augmentation. Isolagen is a substance developed from culturing dermal fibroblasts from the patient's skin. Initial studies show only mild improvement of facial lines as compared to bovine collagen.[38] It is also more expensive and time-consuming as compared to collagen, due to its culturing requirements and limited shelf life. Restylane is a hyaluronic acid-containing gel used extensively in Europe. Anecdotal reports have been favorable, with side-effects including postoperative erythema and burning. No clinical studies are available.

SoftForm (Collagen Corporation, Palo Alto, CA) is a hollow tubular implant made from expanded polytetrafluoroethylene (ePTFE) designed to provide a stable and permanent augmentation for the mesolabial folds and the vermilion border. It is available in several diameters and is provided ready-mounted on a tissue trocar for subdermal placement. Fibrous tissue grows on and around the tube, helping to anchor it in place and provide more augmentation. Success with SoftForm is dependent on operator skill, and scattered reports of extrusion have been noted.

# Hair transplantation

Hair transplantation has undergone tremendous refinement since Norman Orentreich first transplanted 4-mm grafts of hair-bearing skin from occiput to bald frontal scalp.[39,40] Refinements over the years have allowed denser and more natural-appearing transplantation of hair. Today's transplant techniques use smaller grafts, slits and receptor holes for the recipient sites. In an effort to duplicate the look of natural growth, transplantation of tissue containing single follicular units has become increasingly popular. Some transplant surgeons consider mega-sessions of up to 3000 single-hair grafts as the only viable method for full head restoration.

Orentreich's original technique involved 4–4.5-mm circular hair-bearing grafts placed into slightly smaller punched-out recipient sites. Graft sizes have decreased in size from 4.5 mm to 1 mm as the technique has evolved. Graft sizes of 2, 1.75 and 1.5 mm are now commonly used. Healing with all sizes has been excellent, with nearly 100% graft take and virtually no infection. The classic punch donor technique utilizes different-sized punches to prepare hair-bearing skin plugs rapidly and uniformly, with minimal bleeding or trauma to the plugs. While decidedly low-tech, it is reliable and requires no mechanization. The resultant grid pattern is visible only if the hair is lifted. If care is used to contain the donor area with the 'safety zone' where alopecia is not expected to progress, they will remain invisible.

Many hair transplant surgeons now favor the strip donor, or total excision, technique exclusively.[41–44] Thousands of grafts can be harvested utilizing algorithms developed to calculate how many hair-bearing grafts can be obtained per unit area of scalp. A specially designed multi-bladed knife, with spacers of varying dimensions, allows multiple strips of a desired width to be harvested simultaneously, and variations on this theme have been developed to maximize yield.[45] The preparation of grafts from strips is more involved and time-consuming, and may be delegated to trained nurses and technicians using dissecting microscopes or small light tables with disposable transparent plastic cutting surfaces. The scar is invisible after healing, and subsequent strip donor harvesting always incorporates the previous scar. The strip donor technique can also allow additional sessions in patients whose donor sites have been depleted by previous punch-graft transplantation sessions.

Improvements in technique have stimulated the development of new time-saving instruments. The Lightning Knife (Swann Morton Company, Sheffield, UK, and A to Z Surgical, Santa Clara, CA) is an alternative to the conventional scalpel. It combines the razor-sharp edge of the scalpel with depth-of-incision control, allowing the surgeon to create sites more rapidly and uniformly. The Rapid Fire Hair Implanter Carousel can atraumatically place large numbers of follicular grafts much more rapidly than by hand and has eased the repetition of mega-sessions.[46]

# Tumescent liposuction

Liposuction is one of the most common office-based procedures performed today. The most commonly treated areas in women are the abdomen, inner and outer thighs, buttocks and chin. Men usually request treatment for abdominal and pectoral fat. Complications are rare, and include infection, hematoma, seroma, and the as-yet-unreported possibility of viscus perforation.[47,48] The tumescent technique for local anesthesia revolutionized liposuction in the late eighties and early nineties.[48,49] This technique has now given us the ability to provide adequate local anesthesia for larger reconstructive and cosmetic procedures and to perform them in the office.[50]

Ultrasonic liposculpture is a technique that has been performed in Europe for several years, and was brought to the United States some years ago.[51–53] It utilizes a titanium probe attached to an ultrasonic generator to liquefy adipose deposits. Anesthesia is achieved using the tumescent technique, which also increases lipolysis. A titanium probe is inserted through conventional stab wounds and passed into the areas to be treated. The tip has a small indented cutting edge to sever fibrous attachments to the overlying dermis, to facilitate a true skin lifting effect. This may also help reduce the appearance of cellulite by obliterating the fibrous bands that form the peau d'orange appearance. The adipose tissue, when in contact with the probe and ultrasonic energy, undergoes violent and irreversible damage, congealing into an oily emulsion.[54] This emulsion is manually forced out of the incision sites during the remodeling phase of the procedure. This controlled removal is felt to be less traumatic, and would appear to facilitate the sparing of vascular and nervous structures to allow a nearly bloodless procedure.

Although ultrasonic liposculpture appears to have less blood loss than standard liposuction techniques, there are concerns of heat injury generated from the ultrasonic waves. Ischemic necrosis and burns have been reported.[55] Studies have shown that while the temperatures in the subcutaneous adipose sites do rise during ultrasonic liposuction, they remain well below the core body temperature.[56] It has been postulated that ischemic skin complications are more likely the result of injury to the subdermal plexus rather than a temperature-induced thermal injury.

It has been used externally and combined with standard tumescent liposuction in an effort to avoid these concerns.[53,57] This technique is still being evaluated, and more studies are needed. While ultrasonic liposuction is a successful procedure, its advantages over standard tumescent liposuction have not yet been fully appreciated.[58–60]

# Conclusion

Dermatologic surgery has expanded dramatically over the last 10 years. It now embraces a widening spectrum of cosmetic procedures as well as classic neoplasm excision and closure techniques. This growth is not, however, without cost. There are currently no Federal or State regulations in place regarding who may use or purchase the latest technology, who is qualified to use it, or even what constitutes proper training. Cursory training does not prepare the dermatologic surgeon for the side-effects and risks encountered with even the most basic of cosmetic surgical procedures. Monitored and rigorous training, proper and complete preoperative counseling, and meticulous attention to postoperative care all combine to produce the best possible outcome for patient and surgeon. We must keep foremost in our minds the maxim 'first, do no harm'.

# References

1. West TB, Alster TS, Effect of pretreatment on the incidence of hyperpigmentation following cutaneous $CO_2$ laser resurfacing. *Lasers Surg Med* 1999: 10(Suppl); 55.

2. Weinstein C, Ramirez O, Pozner J, Postoperative care following $CO_2$ laser resurfacing. *Dermatol Surg* 1998: 24; 51–6.

3. Mandy SH, Tretinoin in the preoperative and postoperative management of dermabrasion. *J Am Acad Dermatol* 1986: 15; 878–9.

4. Hung VC, Lee JY, Zitelli JA, Hebda PA, Topical tretinoin and epithelial wound healing. *Arch Dermatol* 1989: 125; 65–9.

5. Hevia O, Nemeth AJ, Taylor JR, Tretinoin accelerates healing after trichloroacetic acid chemical peels. *Arch Dermatol* 1991: 127; 678–82.

6. Popp C, Kligman AL, Stoudemayer TJ, Pretreatment of photoaged forearm skin with topical tretinoin accelerates healing of full thickness wounds. *Br J Dermatol* 1995: 132; 46–9.

7. Ruiz-Esparza J, A safe and easy pre- and post-laser resurfacing routine. *Cosmet Dermatol* 1999: 12; 47–53.

8. David L, Ruiz-Esparza JL, Fast healing after laser skin resurfacing. The minimal mechanical trauma technique. *Dermatol Surg* 1997: 23; 359–61.

9. Ruiz-Esparza J, Gomez JM, Gomez de la Torre OL et al, Erythema after laser skin resurfacing. *Dermatol Surg* 1998: 24; 31–4.

10. Alster TA, West TB, Effect of topical vitamin C on postoperative laser resurfacing erythema. *Dermatol Surg* 1998: 24; 331–4.

11. Goldman MP, Fitzpatrick RE, Manuskiatti W, Laser resurfacing of the neck with the erbium:YAG laser. *Dermatol Surg* 1999: 25; 164–8.

12. Goldman MP, Manuskiatti W, Combined laser resurfacing with the 950-msec pulsed $CO_2$ + Er:YAG lasers. *Dermatol Surg* 1999: 25; 160–3.

13. Dover JS, Hruze GJ, Arndt KA, Lasers in skin resurfacing. *Semin Cutan Med Surg* 2000: 19(4); 207–20.

14. Burns RL, Carruthers A, Langtry JA, Trotter MJ, Electrosurgical skin resurfacing: a new bipolar instrument. *Dermatol Surg* 1999: 25; 582–6.

15. Grekin RC, Tope WD, Yarborough JM Jr et al, Electrosurgical facial resurfacing: a prospective multicenter study of efficacy and safety. *Arch Dermatol* 2000: 136; 1309–16.

16. Campos VB, Dierickx CC, Farinelli WA et al, Hair removal with an 800-nm pulse diode laser. *J Am Acad Dermatol* 2000: 43(3); 442–7.

17. Dierickx CC, Grossman MC, Farinelli WA, Anderson RR, Permanent hair removal with the ruby laser. *Arch Dermatol* 1998: 143; 837–42.

18. Polderman MC, Pavel S, le Cessie S et al, Efficacy, tolerability, and safety of a long-pulsed ruby laser system in the removal of unwanted hair. *Dermatol Surg* 2000: 26(3); 240–3.

19. Lloyd JR, Mirkov M, Long-term evaluation of the long-pulsed alexandrite laser for the removal of bikini hair at shortened treatment intervals. *Dermatol Surg* 2000: 26(7); 633–7.

20. Glassberg E, Babapour R, Lask G, Current trends in laser blepharoplasty: results of a survey. *Dermatol Surg* 1995: 21; 1060–4.

21. Baker SS, Pham RTH, Lateral canthal tendon suspension using the carbon dioxide laser: a modified technique. *Dermatol Surg* 1995: 21; 1071–3.

22. Unger W, David L, Laser hair transplantation. *J Dermatol Surg Oncol* 1994: 20; 515–21.

23. Unger W, Laser hair transplantation II. *Dermatol Surg* 1995: 21; 759–65.

24. Podda M, Spieph K, Kaufmann R, Er:YAG laser-assisted transplantation in cicatricial alopecia. *Dermatol Surg* 2000: 26; 1010–14.

25. Bernstein RM, Rassman WR, Laser hair transplantation: is it really state of the art? (letter). *Lasers Surg Med* 1996: 19; 233–5.

26. Smithdeal CD, Carbon dioxide laser-assisted hair transplantation. The effect of laser parameters on scalp tissue – a histologic study. *Dermatol Surg* 1997: 23; 835–40.

27. Villnow MM, Feriduni B, Update on laser-assisted hair transplantation. *Dermatol Surg* 1998: 24; 749–54.

28. Tsai RY, Wang CN, Chan HL, Aluminum oxide crystal microdermabrasion. A new technique for treating facial scarring. *Dermatol Surg* 1995: 21; 539–42.

29. Carruthers J, Stubbs HA, *Botulinum* toxin for benign essential blepharospasm. *Can J Neurol Sci* 1987: 14; 42–5.

30. Carruthers J, Carruthers A, Treatment of glabellar frown lines with *C. botulinum*-A exotoxin. *J Dermatol Surg Oncol* 1992: 18; 17–21.

31. Klein AW, Glogau PG, Botulinum: beyond cosmesis. *Arch Dermatol* 2000: 136; 487–90.

32. Trindade de Almeida AR, Kadunc BV, Martins de Oliveira EM, Improving botulinum toxin therapy for palmar hyperhidrosis: wrist block and technical considerations. *Dermatol Surg* 2001: 27; 34–6.

33. Glogau RG, Botulinum A neurotoxin for axillary hyperhidrosis. *Dermatol Surg* 1998: 24; 817–19.

34. Shelley WB, Talanin NY, Shelley ED, Botulinum toxin therapy for palmar hyperhidrosis. *Arch Dermatol* 1998: 38; 227–9.

35. Chiarello S, Resnik BI, Resnik SS, The TCA Creme Masque and Jessner's solution: a new medium-depth chemical peel. *Dermatol Surg* 1996: 22; 687–90.

36. Resnik BI, Resnik SS, TCA cream peel and segmental $CO_2$ laser resurfacing: effective combination treatment of rhytids and solar dyschromia. *Cosmet Dermatol* 1999: 12; 31–4.

37. Elson ML, Soft tissue augmentation with allogeneic human tissue matrix. *Cosmet Dermatol* 1998: 11; 24–8.

38. Alkek D, Isolagen, a new autologous collagen. *Cosmet Dermatol* 1998: 11; 30–2.

39. Orentreich N, Hair transplants. Long-term results and new advances. *Arch Otolaryngol* 1970: 92; 576–7.

40. Orentreich N, Hair transplantation: the punch graft technique. *Surg Clin North Am* 1971: 51; 511–18.

41. Bisaccia E, Scarborough D, Hair transplantation by incisional strip harvesting. *J Dermatol Surg Oncol* 1994: 20; 443–9.

42. Unger WP, Total excision techniques in donor area harvesting for hair transplantation. *Am J Cosmet Surg* 1994: 11; 15–22.

43. Rassman WR, Carson S, Micrografting in extensive quantities. The ideal hair restoration procedure. *Dermatol Surg* 1995: 21; 306–11.

44. Villnow M, 2300 grafts/laser sessions. *Hair Transplant Forum* 1994: 4; 6–7.

45. Alkek DS, Combining vertical strips and the ellipse in saving time and follicles. *Dermatol Surg* 1998: 24; 1061–3.

46. Rassman WR, Bernstein RM, Rapid Fire Hair Implanter Carousel. A new surgical instrument for the automation of hair transplantation. *Dermatol Surg* 1998: 24; 623–7.

47. Hanke CW, Bernstein G, Bullock S, Safety of tumescent liposuction in 15,336 patients. National survey results. *Dermatol Surg* 1995: 21; 459–62.

48. Klein JA, Tumescent technique chronicles. Local anesthesia, liposuction, and beyond. *Dermatol Surg* 1995: 21; 449–57.

49. Klein JA, Tumescent technique for regional anesthesia permits lidocaine doses of 35 mg/kg for liposuction. *J Dermatol Surg Oncol* 1990: 16; 248–63.

50. Namias A, Kaplan B, Tumescent anesthesia for dermatologic surgery. Cosmetic and noncosmetic procedures. *Dermatol Surg* 1998: 24; 755–8.

51. Zocchi M, Ultrasonic liposculpturing. *Aesthetic Plast Surg* 1992: 16; 287–98.

52. Zocchi ML, Ultrasonic assisted lipoplasty. Technical refinements and clinical evaluations. *Clin Plast Surg* 1996: 23; 575–98.

53. Havoonjia H, Luftman D, Menaker G, Moy R, External ultrasonic tumescent liposuction. A preliminary study. *Dermatol Surg* 1997: 23; 1201–6.

54. Lawrence N, Coleman W 3rd, The biologic basis of ultrasonic liposuction. *Dermatol Surg* 1997: 23; 1197–200.

55. Grolleau JL, Rouge D, Chavoin JP, Costagliola M, Severe cutaneous necrosis after ultrasound lipolysis. Medicolegal aspects and review. *Ann Chir Plast Esthet* 1997: 42; 31–6.

56. Ablaza VJ, Gingrass MK, Perry LC et al, Tissue temperatures during ultrasound-assisted lipoplasty. *Plast Reconstr Surg* 1998: 102; 534–42.

57. Igra H, Satur NM, Tumescent liposuction versus internal ultrasonic-assisted tumescent liposuction. A side-to-side comparison. *Dermatol Surg* 1997: 23; 1213–18.

58. Lack E, Safety of ultrasonic-assisted liposuction (UAL) using a non-water-cooled ultrasonic cannula. A report of six cases of disproportionate fat deposits treated with UAL. *Dermatol Surg* 1998: 24; 871–4.

59. Rohrich RJ, Beran SJ, Kenkel JM et al, Extending the role of liposuction in body contouring with ultrasound-assisted liposuction. *Plast Reconstr Surg* 1998: 101; 1090–102.

60. [No authors listed], Statement on ultrasonic liposuction. Task Force on Ultrasonic Liposuction of the American Society for Dermatologic Surgery. *Dermatol Surg* 1998: 24; 1035.

# 17

## Cosmetic dermatology

*Leslie S Baumann, Irina Daza, Annia C Lourenço and Melissa Lazarus*

## Introduction

Over the past several years, many advances have been made in methods to improve the appearance of the face and skin. Many dermatologists are now converting large parts of their practice to these procedures and academic institutions are beginning to research and teach these methods. This chapter reviews the available methods used for rejuvenation of the face and skin except for laser surgery which is discussed in a separate chapter.

## When to use which method

It is very important to interview the patient and listen carefully to his or her concerns and expectations. To be happy with the results of any cosmetic procedure, the physician must fix the problem the patient complains of and the patient needs to know what results to expect. If a patient presents with tiny wrinkles, sun damage, and small areas with hyperpigmented macules, a chemical peel would be the treatment of choice. For a younger patient with 'wrinkles in motion' in the upper part of the face, botulinum toxin is indicated. For those patients with 'wrinkles at rest' soft tissue augmentation should be considered. Of course, all of these methods can be used in combination according to the individual patient's needs and desires.

## Chemical peels

Chemical peels can be used to improve the texture of the skin and to decrease hyperpigmentation. They may improve mild wrinkling of the skin as well. Chemical peels can be subdivided into superficial, medium and deep peels. Superficial peels create necrosis of part or all of the epidermis, anywhere from the stratum granulosum to the basal cell layer. Medium peels create necrosis of the epidermis and part or all of the papillary dermis. In deep peels, the necrosis extends into the reticular dermis.[1] Superficial and medium peels are the ones performed most commonly today as the deeper peels have been largely replaced by laser resurfacing and dermabrasion. Superficial and medium peels do not improve deep wrinkles or sagging skin, but can improve the color and texture of the skin imparting a more youthful appearance to the skin. In this chapter the most commonly used types of superficial and medium peels are discussed.

## Superficial peels

Although a number of agents have been demonstrated to be useful for superficial peeling, alpha hydroxy acids (AHAs), beta hydroxy acid (BHA), Jessner's solution, and trichloroacetic acid (TCA) are currently the most commonly used in-office peels. AHAs and BHA are also popular additives in home-use products.

### Hydroxy acids

The AHAs are naturally occurring organic acids. Glycolic (hydroxyacetic) acid, the most commonly used, is derived from sugar cane. Lactic acid is derived from sour milk, malic acid from apples, citric acid from acid fruits and tartaric acid from grapes.[2] The only BHA is salicylic acid, which is derived from willow bark, wintergreen leaves and sweet birch,[3] but is also available as a synthetic product.

The common structure of all AHAs is a terminal carboxyl group with one or two hydroxyl groups on the second or alpha carbon and a variable-length carbon chain. A single hydroxyl group is found in glycolic and lactic acids, whereas two carboxyl groups are found in malic and tartaric acids.[4] Salicylic acid is an aromatic carboxylic acid with a hydroxy group in the beta position; and it is therefore known as a beta hydroxy acid.[3]

The strength of these acids derives from their ability to donate protons and is measured in terms of the pKa which is the pH at which the amount of free acid equals the amount of salt of the acid (Fig. 17.1). The acid form predominates when the pH is less than the pKa, while the salt form predominates when the pH is greater than the pKa. The lower the pKa, the stronger the acid. It is the free acid form that causes the exfoliation of the skin. A difference in one unit represents a 10-fold difference of strength. The pKa for salicylic acid is 2.97 and for the AHAs is 3.83.[4,5] Because of the different pKas of these two acid families, it is difficult to formulate a combination product containing both with an optimal pH. In other words, if a combination product with a pH of 3.5 contained AHA and BHA, the AHA acid form would predominate but the BHA salt form would predominate. Therefore the effects of BHA would be suboptimal. Understanding how the pH and pKa affect the functioning of superficial chemical peels is crucial in order to perform safe and efficacious peels.

Topical preparations containing AHAs have been shown to exert pro-

$$PH = pKa + \log[\text{salt concentration} / \text{acid concentration}]$$

## Figure 17.1
Relationship between pH and pKa.

found effects on epidermal keratinization.[6] AHAs and BHA exert their influence on corneocyte cohesiveness at the lower levels of the stratum corneum.[7] These acids act on the skin by changing the pH of the stratum corneum.[8] When applied to the skin in high concentrations, AHAs and BHA cause detachment of keratinocytes and epidermolysis, while application at lower concentrations reduces intercorneocyte cohesion immediately above the granular layer, promoting desquamation and thinning of the stratum corneum. Ditre et al[9] have shown that application of AHAs causes a significant increase in thickness of the epidermis, reversal of basal cell atypia, and dispersal of melanin pigmentation. AHAs also increase glycosaminoglycans and collagen synthesis, improve the quality of elastic fibers and promote fibroblast proliferation.

Although AHAs and BHA have many similar effects on the skin, they have different properties that should be considered when choosing a peeling method. Because BHA is lipophilic, it is able to penetrate the sebaceous material in the hair follicle and exfoliate the pores.[10] AHAs are water soluble and do not have this comedolytic property.[11]

Salicylic acid is in the salicylate family, as is aspirin. Because of its action on the arachidonic acid cascade, it has anti-inflammatory and analgesic properties that make it useful as a peeling agent. Because of the anti-inflammatory and comedolytic properties, salicylic acid is especially useful in

the treatment of acne.[12] Salicylic acid is contraindicated in patients with allergy to aspirin, in pregnant patients, or in patients who are breastfeeding.

There are many indications for superficial chemical peels. Sundamaged skin with wrinkles, actinic keratoses, and seborrheic keratoses can be modified by superficial peels. Topically, salicylic acid has long been used as a keratolytic agent for warts, corns, callus, psoriasis, hyperkeratosis palmaris and plantaris, pityriasis rubra pilaris and acne. It is also found in shampoos for psoriasis, and seborrheic dermatitis of the scalp.[13] A common use is for facial rejuvenation and general improvement of the skin's texture.

When treating the face for wrinkles, hyperpigmentation, or photodamage, similar lesions on the hands, arms, and neck can also be treated to avoid contrast with a younger-appearing face. Swinehart[14] has reported good results with 50% salicylic acid for actinically induced pigmentary changes on the hands and forearms. Melasma, postinflammatory hyperpigmentation and lentigines can be safely and successfully treated with serial repetitive superficial peels in different skin colors. Lim and Tham[15] concluded that 10% glycolic acid and 2% hydroquinone combined with glycolic acid peels at 3-week intervals improves melasma and fine wrinkling in women (Fig. 17.2). There are also reports of its benefit in black patients with different skin disorders.[16] Acne also responds quite well to serial 50–70% glycolic acid and 20–30% salicylic acid, showing even

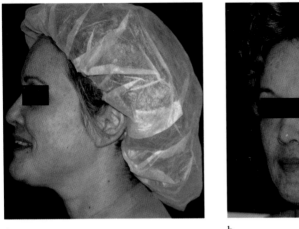
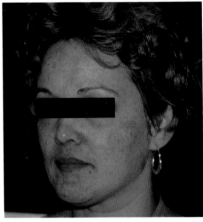

a                                              b

## Figure 17.2

The same patient before (a) and 3 weeks after (b) glycolic acid peel showing improvement in melasma and fine wrinkling.

better results when these are used in combination.[17] AHAs and salicyclic acid can be used as in-office peels every 2–3 weeks or can be used in combination with home-care products containing these acids.

### Trichloroacetic acid

TCA 10–35% is used to improve fine wrinkles, dyschromia and to give the skin a smooth, healthy appearance in facial and nonfacial areas. Careful patient selection is a necessity and darker skin types should not be treated with TCA as they have an increased risk for postinflammatory hyperpigmentation. Low-strength TCA can be repeated every 1 to 3 weeks. However, like other superficial agents, TCA does not affect deeper wrinkles or scars.[18,19] (See also Chapter 15.)

### Jessner's solution

Jessner's solution is a combination of resorcinol 14%, salicylic acid 14% and lactic acid 14% in ethanol 95% to make 100 cc of solution. It can be used with other agents such as glycolic acid, 5-fluorouracil and TCA, enhancing their effects. Resorcinol has long been known to be very effective for acne and melasma but should be used with extreme care in patients with Fitzpatrick skin types of III and greater.

Complications of superficial peelings are minimal. Patients with a history of *Herpes simplex* infection of the face or lips should have prophylaxis with antiviral agents. Postinflammatory hyperpigmentation is the most common complication and usually can be avoided by proper patient selection, broad spectrum sunscreen use, sun avoidance, and use of hydroquinone following the superficial peels. These precautions are especially important in darker skin types.

In summary, superficial peelings are safe and efficacious when used properly. It is important that patients are educated about what peels can and cannot accomplish so that they will have realistic expectations. Patients with more severe photoaging or melasma may need medium peels to achieve the desired result.

## Medium peels

### Trichloroacetic acid

Medium peels are useful for decreasing the depth of scars and wrinkles[20] and for treating melasma in patients with lighter skin types. These peels remove the entire epidermis and the papillary dermis. Fibroblasts are stimulated to grow new collagen and there is an increase in glycosaminoglycan deposition. Medium peels are often performed using TCA at 35–50% strength. Many authors recommend not exceeding 50% in strength. When using TCA, it is important to use weight per volume

(w/v) measurements when calculating strength, otherwise the strength of the peel can be underestimated and scarring may occur.[21] One must purchase TCA in the strength that is desired. For example, dilution of a 50% solution with an equal volume of water does not produce a 25% solution because this type of dilution is volume per volume and the resulting solution would actually be stronger than 25% w/v TCA. When following a protocol from the literature, it is necessary to ensure that the TCA percent is calculated by weight per volume measurements to avoid mistakes.

After application of TCA, denatured protein causes a 'frosting' of the skin. When this frosting has occurred, the peeling is complete. There is a lag of time between the application and the appearance of the frost that varies according to the acid concentration. With the application of 40% TCA the delay may be 5 to 7 s, whereas with more dilute acid, the delay may be as long as 15 to 20 min. This is important to remember in order to avoid overtreatment.

TCA can be used alone or, if a deeper peel is desired, after application of Jessner' solution or glycolic acid. Healing should occur in 5–7 days if TCA is used alone and in 7-10 days when the combination with glycolic acid or Jessner's solution is used.[18,19]

Medium depth peels are contraindicated in patients with darker skin types, and those who have been recently treated with isotretinoin or topical radiation.[22] Because reepithelialization occurs from adnexal structures, it is postulated that after recent treatment with lasers for hair removal healing may be difficult after medium or deep peels.

As with superficial peels, it is important for the patients to use sunscreen and to practise sun avoidance. Patients with darker skin types should use hydroquinone after the peel to decrease the incidence of hyperpigmentation. Patients with a history of *Herpes simplex* infection must receive antiviral medication. Scarring can occur with over-zealous use of TCA or in patients recently treated with isotretinoin.

## Deep peels

Deep peels are rarely performed today because lasers and dermabrasion have shown better results with fewer complications. These methods will be discussed elsewhere.

## Botulinum toxin

Botulinum toxin (BTX) is used to decrease the dynamic wrinkles of the face. The toxin isolated from *Clostridium botulinum*, is a neurotoxin composed of seven serotypes A to G. Type A is the most powerful and the one that has been used for cosmetic indications since 1991 after Carruthers and Carruthers described its use for the correction of glabellar lines.[23] It had been safely used for many years in ophthalmology for patients with strabismus, nystagmus or blepharospasm.[24] BTX blocks neuro-muscular conduction by cleaving the proteins needed for the release of acetylcholine. This causes temporary flaccid paralysis that lasts approximately 3–5 months. Muscle function returns as new neuromuscular junctions are formed. BTX doses are described in units. One unit (U) is the dose that will be lethal to 50% ($LD_{50}$) of a certain kind of mouse. The $LD_{50}$ for a 70 kg human is 2500–3000 U. Approximately 20–75 U doses are used for cosmetic purposes. Doses up to 1000 U have been safely used in cerebral palsy and other neurological disorders.

BTX is most commonly used in the upper half of the face, especially the glabella, crow's feet, and forehead (Fig. 17.3). It has also been used in the lower face, but this must be done with great care because it is possible to interfere with the function of the mouth. BTX has also been injected into the platysma muscle to eliminate neck rhytides, and to improve laxity.[27] BTX is also being used for the treatment of hyperhidrosis of the palms, soles and axillae. Currently, two commercial types of BTX, Botox® and Dysport, are available.

Botox® (Allergan Pharmaceuticals, Irvine, California), although not approved by the US Food and Drug Administration (FDA) for cosmetic use, is the most commonly used form in the United States. Botox® is composed of BTX-A, which functions by cleaving the SNAP-25 protein necessary for the release of acetylcholine into the synaptic cleft. To produce the toxin, cultures of *C. botulinum* are

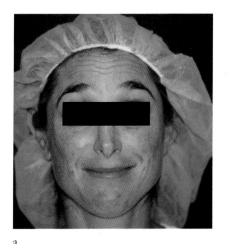
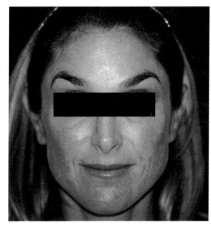

a                                      b

## Figure 17.3

The same patient before (a) and after (b) treatment of the upper face with Botox showing correction of glabellar lines and crow's feet.

fermented and then subjected to autolysis in order to release the toxin complexes. The toxin compound is 900 kDa. Before being placed into the storage vials, the toxin is diluted using human serum albumin, and then freeze-dried and sealed. It is sold in an airtight vial that contains 100 U and must be kept frozen until its use. Prior to injection, it is diluted with preservative-free saline. Although different dilutions may be used, we recommend diluting the vial with 2.5 ml of saline for use in the face and with 5 ml of saline for use in the palms, soles and axillae. The mixture should be used as soon as possible because the toxin loses its potency

rather quickly. Most authors agree the toxin should be used within 7 to 12 h for the best results. (See also Chapter 16.)

Dysport (Ipsen Products, Maidenhead, United Kingdom) is the European source of BTX. It acts on the SNAP-25 protein in a similar manner to Botox®. The Dysport unit is less potent than the Botox® unit.[28] Thus 1 U of Botox® has approximately equivalent potency to 4 U of Dysport. Dysport contains lactose and fixed drug eruptions due to the lactose have been described.[29]

Myobloc (Elan Pharmaceuticals) is a new product that was approved for use in the United States in December

2000. Myobloc is composed of BTX-B, which acts by cleaving the protein synaptobrevin thus preventing acetylcholine release in the synaptic cleft. The drug is available in a ready-to-use solution. It is available in three vial configurations of 2,500 U, 5,000 U and 10,000 U, with a composition of 500 U BTX-B/ml. Myobloc ready-to-use Solution is stable for up to 21 months in refrigerator storage. Myobloc is FDA approved for the treatment of cervical dystonia, but its use in cosmetics has not been approved by the FDA to date. Phase III clinical trials of the use of the drug for the treatment of cervical dystonia have shown its effects to last 12–16 weeks.

Side effects from the use of botulinum toxin are rare when it is used by experienced physicians and most importantly are transitory and reversible. Side effects of botulinum use in the upper face include bruising, ptosis,[30] and very rarely diplopia or ectropion. If ptosis occurs, alpha adrenergic agents such as Iopidine eye drops may improve the symptoms. When injected into the platysma muscle, bruising, drooling, downturning of the corner of the mouth, neck weakness, and dysphagia can occur. When used for hyperhidrosis, BTX must be injected into the superficial dermis because deeper injection may lead to muscle weakness. There is one report in the literature of Botox injections unmasking underlying myasthenia gravis in a patient.[31] An antitoxin is available from the Center for Disease Control in Atlanta, Georgia, USA, but must be administered within 1 h of the BTX to be effective.

# Soft tissue augmentation

The augmentation of soft tissue is a procedure that consists of the injection of an alloplastic material or autologous tissue into the skin. It has been used for wrinkles, scars, atrophic areas, and lip augmentation. There are many different injectable materials available that can be used in patients according to their particular needs. The concept of an ideal filler material has interested physicians for years. Over the past two decades, intense industry research has not yet yielded the perfect filler substance. The perfect material for soft tissue augmentation would be easy to obtain, easy to implant in tissue, inexpensive, easy to store, painless to inject, nontoxic, noncarcinogenic, longlasting, normal appearing, and with no capacity to elicit an allergy or hypersensitivity response. Although many injectable substances are available, none meets all of these properties. We discuss the filler materials currently available worldwide.

## Bovine collagen

Zyderm I (Collagen Corporation, Palo Alto, California) was the first injectable bovine collagen and has been used since 1977, and approved by the FDA in 1981. Zyderm II was approved in 1983 and Zyplast in 1985. In Europe implantable bovine collagen is also available under the name of Resoplast (Rofil Medical International, Breda, The Netherlands).

All of these products are suspensions of bovine dermal collagen. During processing, pepsin digestion removes the more antigenic portions. The products are then suspended in phosphate-buffered physiological saline. Zyderm I and II differ only in the concentration of collagen (35 mg/ml vs 65 mg/ml). Zyplast is crosslinked by the addition of 0.0075% glutaraldehyde (35 mg glutaraldehyde crosslinked per/ml) which makes it more resistant to the action of host collagenases.

Superficial wrinkles are best treated with Zyderm I or II, including horizontal forehead lines, glabellar lines, crow's feet, fine lip lines, and scars. Zyplast is preferred for deeper wrinkles and furrows such as nasolabial folds, marionette grooves, deep scars and to enhance the vermilion border of the lip. Zyderm I can be layered over Zyplast for deeper furrows. Correction is temporary because bovine collagen is displaced from its site in the dermis by host collagenases within 3–6 months following implantation,[32] but up to 30% of patients treated with bovine collagen report some correction lasting up to 18 months.[33]

Bovine collagen treatment has minimal risk of allergy[34] if two skin tests are performed prior to treatment. A positive test consists of redness, swelling or itching, which can occur as early as 6 h after the test but most commonly occurs at 48 h after the test. Despite one negative test, 1.3–6.2% of patients will have treatment-associated hypersensitivity respones,[35,36] therefore a second skin test should be performed to reduce the risk to less than 0.5%. These hypersensitivity reactions resolve within 4 or 24 months in isolated cases.[37,38,39] In the past there was no good treatment and the patient had to wait for the redness and induration to resolve spontaneously. We have recently reported a patient with hypersensitivity to collagen that resolved in 11 days when treated with oral cyclosporine.[40]

Nonallergic adverse reactions include bruising, reactivation of herpetic eruptions, bacterial infections, and superficial local necrosis due to ischemic events caused by a vascular interruption of an arteriole. Cysts at the site of injection have been reported in 0.04% of treated individuals.[41] To avoid these complications, care should be taken to inject only into the dermis,[42] antiviral medications should be used in patients with a history of oral herpes infections, and Zyplast should not be used in the glabellar area. Only Zyderm should be used in this area because it is less likely to develop necrosis due to an ischemic phenomenon caused by a vascular interruption of arterioles.

Some physicians have speculated that exposure to injectable bovine collagen could precipitate autoimmune disease, specifically polymyositis and dermatomyositis. Studies had shown that the antibodies to bovine collagen do not crossreact with human collagen, so the possibility of bovine collagen inducing connective tissue disease in the human host is unlikely.[36,43]

In summary, Zyplast has been used for more than 10 years and is considered as the 'gold standard' injectable material to which all other injectable materials are compared.

Resoplast is a bovine monomolecular collagen solution that comes in 3.5% and 6.5% concentrations. It is very similar to Zyderm and Zyplast and is used with the same technique. It is available in Europe.

Artecoll (Rofil Medical, Breda, The Netherlands) is a solution of bovine collagen combined with polymethacrylate microspheres (PMMA). The collagen is derived from calves up to 6 months old which have been fed only with milk and vegetables and which have been given no hormones or antibiotics. To ensure that the animals were free of bovine spongiform encephalitis (BSE), the collagen is washed with sodium hydroxide to eliminate noncollagen proteins such as viruses. The telopeptide immunogenic ends of the collagen molecule are removed and then the material is filtered to reduce antigenicity. The solution, which contains 3.5% collagen, is mixed with smooth PMMA. PMMA has been used for more than five decades in bone cement and dental prostheses. These microspheres of 30–40 μm in diameter are said to be too large to be phagocytosed or to migrate. In 2–4 months the microspheres become surrounded by a fine fibrous capsule and stay in place as the capsule develops. Lidocaine 0.3% is added to decrease the pain of injection. The material should be stored in the refrigerator.

Artecoll is indicated for wrinkles, large scars and lip augmentation.[44,45] A 27-gauge needle is used to place the material with a tunneling technique in the junction between the dermis and subcutaneous fat. The filler can be modeled by pressure, and the patient should knead the area for 5 days. It is recommended to tape the site for 2 days after the procedure until the fibrous tissue fixes the microspheres in place. Overcorrection is unnecessary if the proper plane of implantation is achieved.

The microsphere implant is an inert and nonbiodegradable material which makes it last longer than fat or collagen. A lasting effect of 1–2 years has been reported by 91% of patients.[34] Out of 60,000 patients, 24 have been reported to have developed granuloma formation, but this is successfully treated with intralesional steroids.[46]

The side-effects of edema, bruising and tenderness fade rapidly in a week. Long-term redness was reported in only 0.5% of patients treated in 1994. Cystic nodules, itching and pain have been reported in a patient 4 months after lip augmentation with Artecoll.[47] Unevenness of the implant has been seen in the 3% of patients and seems to result from higher placement of the Artecoll.[48] Migration of the implant has not been reported.

Artecoll is currently used in South America, Canada and Europe; the

FDA has not approved its use in the US.

## Porcine collagen

FibreI (Mentor Corporation, Santa Barbara, California) was approved by the FDA in 1988 for scars and in 1990 for wrinkles. It is composed of porcine gelatin powder and epsilonaminocaproic acid and is mixed with the patient's plasma and 0.9% sodium chloride. This mixture is injected with the same technique as with bovine collagen implants. In a multicenter clinical trial, 300 patients were treated with Fibrel. In almost 50% of the patients, a 65% improvement was seen without significant loss, no immunological symptoms or any adverse events.[49,50] Patients allergic to bovine collagen may tolerate porcine collagen implants, but must be skin-tested prior to implantation. A positive skin test occurs in 1.9% of tested patients.[51,52] Fibrel is currently not being produced, but the company may bring it back to the market in the future.

Permacol (Tissue Science Laboratories, Hants, UK) is a very recent porcine collagen implant material developed for tissue augmentation. It consists of a porcine dermal collagen that is free from cellular and noncollagenous protein capable of eliciting an immunogenic reaction in the host. Porcine skin is the closest animal tissue to human dermis and provides a more accessible source of donor dermis than human skin. During processing of the implant, an acetone solvent extraction removes epithelial cells, sebaceous glands, hair follicles, sweat ducts and fat deposits, so there is no risk of calcification which has been shown to be linked with the presence of lipids in the dermis. Following, a process of trypsinization that destroys all dermal fibroblasts, it is rinsed in cold sterile saline solution. The lysine residues are then crosslinked in order to improve the longevity of the material. The product is then sterilized by gamma radiation.[53] The elastin fibers are maintained intact within the collagen matrix giving strength and flexibility to the implant. Permacol is available in 5 × 5 cm and 5 × 10 cm sheets and in thicknesses of 0.75 mm and 1.5 mm. It can be cut into any shape.

The advantages of Permacol are that it becomes vascularized by the patient's own blood supply, it allows the treated area to remain soft and flexible, and, according to the company, long-lasting results can be achieved. The permanence of the results is said to be due to crosslinking of the collagen that makes it resistant to collagenase, but there are no studies available supporting this claim. It is not approved by the FDA for use in the US.

## Human-derived collagen

Autologous tissues can be transplanted from one part of the body to another, from the patient or from a donor. Autologous tissue, specifically dermis and fat, has been used with good results for many years.

## Autologous collagen

Autologen (Collagenesis, Beverly, Mass., and Autogenesis Technologies, Boston, Mass.) is composed of collagen fibers derived from skin removed during surgical procedures such as abdominoplasty or mammoplasty. The tissue specimen is frozen and mailed to the company for processing. The material to be injected is mailed back to the physician in a syringe. The collagen concentration ranges from 50 to 120 mg/ml. Two square inches of donor skin will yield approximately 1 ml of Autologen. With this technique, skin testing is not necessary, as there is no risk of a hypersensitivity reaction. This material is ideal for use in a patient under going a surgical procedure who desires soft tissue augmentation.

Isolagen (Isolagen Technologies, Paramaus, New Jersey) is a filling substance consisting of a living system of cultured autologous fibroblasts and extracellular matrix.[54] To obtain the material, a 3 mm skin biopsy is taken from behind the patient's ear. The tissue sample is placed in a container provided by Isolagen and mailed to the company after chilling overnight. The fibroblasts are cultured, and 6 weeks later a 0.1 ml syringe is returned to the physician for skin testing. After a further 2 weeks, a syringe containing 1–1.5 ml of the patient's cells and collagen is sent for implantation. Amounts of 1–1.5 ml of the material are available every 2–3 weeks as needed. The filling material must be injected within 48 h of receipt. Two to five treatments may be needed in a single area in order to achieve the desired correction. Although the risk of hypersensitivity is minimal, a skin test should be performed 2 weeks prior to treatment. This material is said to be longer lasting than Zyderm implants and the company states that patients treated in 1992 have retained their correction for up to 6 years.[55]

Disadvantages of this treatment include high cost, the long processing time (6 weeks) and the painfulness of the injection. Because the implanted fibroblasts are said to grow leading to improvement of the correction with time, patients expecting immediate clinical results may be disappointed.[56] Isolagen is an excellent alternative in subjects who are allergic or uncomfortable using bovine collagen or desire an autologous option. Currently the company has suspended production of Isolagen. (See also Chapter 16.)

## Human cadaver-derived implants

Cymetra (LifeCell Corporation, New Jersey) is an acellular dermal graft material obtained from human cadaver skin. It is freeze-dried which removes all cells from it. The resulting matrix shows undamaged collagens IV and VII, laminin and elastin under the electron microscope. No histocompatibility antigens class I or II are found with immunohistochemical staining. The graft has the ability to integrate the surrounding tissue and is rapidly revascularized by the patient's blood supply. Alloderm, the same product in sheet form, is frequently used as a surface skin graft in burn patients.[57] Cymetra or Alloderm can be used on acne scars, in atrophic areas, and in defects resulting from trauma or surgical resections. They are also useful in areas without adequate bony prominence, in lip reconstruction or augmentation, and in post-rhinoplastic sequelae.[58] They may also be a useful adjuvant in the treatment of facial wasting seen in AIDS patients.

To provide the desired amount of augmentation, Alloderm can be rolled, folded or cut into the necessary shape and length. Cymetra is injected into the areas to be treated. The advantages of both types of implants include no need for skin testing because all antigenic proteins have been removed, and the bovine results may last longer than those with Zyplast. These materials can also be used in patients with bovine collagen allergy. Disadvantages of Alloderm are that preparation of the material (cutting etc) is required prior to implantation, it takes more time to learn than other techniques and some loss of volume of the implant has been reported. The main disadvantage of Cymetra is that the powdered substance must be mixed with lidocaine prior to injection.

Dermalogen (Collagenesis, Beverly, Mass.) is an injectable human tissue matrix implant that is prepared from the dermis of cadaver donor skin from US tissue banks that is tested and virally inactivated. It is a suspension of collagen and elastic fibers as well as proteoglycans. Skin testing is not required. The advantages are that there is no risk of allergy, the graft may last longer because it is of human origin, and it is very easy to use. The disadvantage is that the high viscosity of the material makes the substance painful to inject. Warming the material for 30 min at room temperature prior to implantation, and covering the area to be injected with a topical anesthetic cream will help solve this problem. Dermalogen is an excellent choice in patients allergic to bovine collagen, or in those who feel uncomfortable using animal products. It is also great for use in patients who want the correction performed as soon as possible because they only have to wait 72 h for the skin test results (Fig. 17.4).

## Hyaluronic acid

Hyaluronic acid is a glycosaminoglycan composed of repeating dimeric units of D-glucuronic acid and N-acetyl-glucosamine. It is a component of the normal dermis, and is capable of binding water up to 1000 times its volume. This influences dermal volume and compressibility.[59] Hyaluronic acid has the same molecular and chemical structure in all species. Hyaluronic acid in its natural form would be rapidly degraded, so in order to achieve a long-lasting effect, the polymer needs to be chemically modified. Crosslinking the hyaluronic

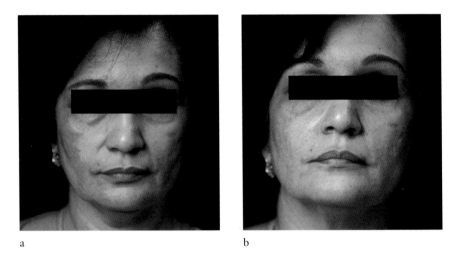

a                                                b

## Figure 17.4

The same patient before (a) and after (b) injection of Dermalogen to the nasolabial folds.

acid makes it more viscous and water-insoluble but maintains the biocompat-ibility. It is injected into the dermis with a threading technique. It is easy to inject, minimally painful, and gives a smooth appearance. Skin testing is unnecessary. Because the product is colorless. Even superficial injections are invisible in contrast to the white bumps sometimes seen with Zyplast or Dermalogen injections. There are cur-rently several types of hyaluronic acid derivatives available on the market. Hylaform and Ial-System are consid-ered second generation hyaluronic acids because they are derived from animals. Restylane is derived from bacterial cultures and is referred to as a third generation hyaluronic acid product. These products are very popular in Europe and Latin America but not yet approved for use in the US.

Hylaform, also known as Hylan Gel or Hylan B (Biomatrix, Ridgefield, New Jersey), is a purified animal hyaluronic acid obtained from rooster combs. It is a very pure gel containing low levels of avian proteins with no reports of toxic or allergic responses.[60] It is available in Europe at a concentration of 6 mg/ml. In order to achieve a complete correc-tion, a series of injections is needed. In a clinical trial, 60% of age-related wrinkles demonstrated some degree of correction after 18 months.[61]

Ial-System (Fidia, Abano Terme, Italy) is made from a highly purified, specific high-molecular weight fraction of hyaluronic acid extracted from rooster combs. It is currently available in sterile prefilled syringes containing 20 mg hyaluronic acid in a volume of 1.1 ml. Ial-System has been shown to be extremely safe and well tolerated. It has been suggested that because of the unique physiological properties of the molecule (it is not crosslinked as the other two types are), it is very easy to handle and to inject. This allows a smooth natural result without the risk of overcorrection.[62]

Restylane (Q-Med, Uppsala, Sweden) is produced in cultures of equine streptococci by fermentation in the presence of sugar. The material is then alcohol-precipitated, filtered, dried and stabilized through epoxidic crosslinks. The material is then heat-sterilized. It is supplied in a disposable syringe containing 0.7 ml of gel that contains 20 mg/ml of hyaluronic acid.

The adverse events associated with all types of hyaluronic acid include transient erythema, bruising, and tenderness at the treatment site. Edema is commonly seen after treatment of the lips. No evidence of systemic side-effects or hypersensitivity have been reported. The advantages of this technique are the ease of use and the ease of storage and transport because it does not have to be refrigerated. (However, it should not be exposed to heat which can lead to the formation of monomers that can lead to inflammation.) In one recent European study, the degree of correction declined from 98% 2 weeks after the treatment to 82% after 3 months, to 69% after 6 months and to 66% after 1 year.[63]

A second study performed in Italy revealed 80% moderate or marked improvement after 8 months as evaluated photographically. Histologically the product persists for a considerable time in the dermis.[64] Hyaluronic acid is an excellent alternative in patients who want implantation performed immediately because skin testing is not required. It is also useful for superficial implantation because it does not show through the skin as the more opaque implants do.

## Fat transplantation

Injection of fat tissue has been used in reconstructive problems since late 19th century. Illouz in the 1980s first began reinjecting fat obtained during liposuction surgery to correct body contour defects. In 1986 Fournier presented a modified technique called micro-lipoextraction and injection which represented a significant advance in cosmetic surgery. Many variations of Fournier's technique are currently used. A study of the behavior of the fat implant in a rabbit model showed that adipose tissue can remain viable even after the effects of mechanical forces on the cells during the harvesting and injection. A study by Skouge et al has shown that the fat graft can reintegrate and become revascularized.[65]

Autologous fat transplantation has been used in the facial areas for correction of wrinkles, for depressed or atrophic areas, for malar, cheek and chin augmentation, and for acne or

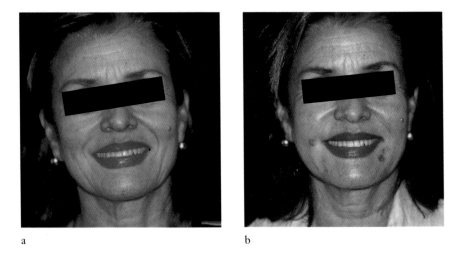

a                                    b

## Figure 17.5

The same patient before (a) and after (b) fat transplantation to the nasolabial folds and
lateral cheek lines.

traumatic scars (Fig. 17.5). It has also
been used in nonfacial areas for rejuvenation of the dorsum of the hands, for
breast enlargement, for defects due to
liposuction, or lipodystrophy, and for
contour defects.[66,67] Fat injections are
most successful when used in facial
areas because in this location, a rich
vascular supply is available to support
the fragile adipose implant.

Various techniques are used for
autologous fat transplantation, but
they are all based on the same idea.
Approximately 15–20 ml of fat is
suctioned with a 13 gauge needle from
the upper outer quadrant of the
patient's hip, medial knee, inner and
outer thigh, abdomen or buttocks. The
harvesting is replaced with a 16 or 18

gauge needle. The same syringe is
used to minimize handling of the graft.
Some physicians use an anaerobic
transfer method to move the fat to a
smaller syringe so that injection is
easier to perform. The syringe is
placed upside down for 5 min in a rack
to allow the separation of the
adipocytes from the serosangineous
fluid. The fat is reinjected into the
desired site at the level of the subcutaneous space and molded in the tissue.
The excess fat tissue is frozen so that it
can be used for touch-up injections
within the next 6 months. Fat transfer
is advantageous because no skin test is
required and there is an unlimited
supply of the injectable material. The
disadvantages of this procedure are

that due to the viscosity of the material, a larger needle is required resulting in temporary visible puncture holes, bruising, swelling and slight tenderness. Although this procedure is considered low-risk, there is one case report of visual loss caused by intravascular injection of fat after fat transfer in the glabellar area.[68]

Survival rates of fresh fat grafts have been reported from 30% to 80% at 1 year.[69,70] Most practitioners estimate survival of the grafts between 40% and 60% 1 year after transplantation as seen in studies by Wetmore.[71]

## Polytetrafluoroethylene or Gore-Tex

Polytetrafluoroethylene (PTFE), under the tradename Gore-Tex (W.L. Gore and Associates, Flagstaff, Arizona), was created in 1969 and has been used since 1972 in vascular surgery. This substance is used as a thread folded as many times as needed to produce the necessary thickness. The guiding needle is advanced into the deep dermis, the two ends of the material are trimmed and the needle removed. The ends are buried deep in the dermis. The main indications for Gore-Tex are deep nasolabial furrows, lip augmentation and deep facial defects.

PTFE manufactured as SoftForm by Collagen Corporation, Palo Alto, California, is now available. SoftForm is PTFE preloaded on a trocar. Under local anesthesia, it can be placed into the deep dermis, the ends trimmed and

buried into the dermis. Gore-Tex and SoftForm are an excellent alternative in patients who desire permanent results. Figure 17.6 shows the results of the use of SoftForm for the correction of facial asymmetry.

Among the problems with these implants are a tendency for extrusion or exposure of the ends, unnatural feel and malalignment of the material which is technique-dependent. A case of nodules with pustules and erosion 6 months after lip augmentation with Gore-Tex has been reported.[47] Infection can occur after placement of this material, so a course of antibiotics is recommended after placement. If infection occurs, the implants must be removed. The implants may also be removed if the patient is not satisfied with the results.[72] (See also Chapter 16.)

## Silicone

Silicone is a family of silicon polymers. It is illegal to use in the US for soft tissue augmentation. Many side-effects have been reported related to impure material or large volumes of this implant,[73,74] such as hypersensitivity reactions, granuloma formation and migration of the material. It is commonly used in some parts of Latin America and in Europe.

Silicone is injected employing the microdroplet technique into the deep dermis and fat.[75] Although the correction seems to be immediate, a delayed hypersensitivity reaction occurs. The inflammation progresses to a local

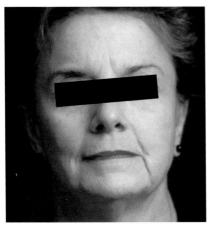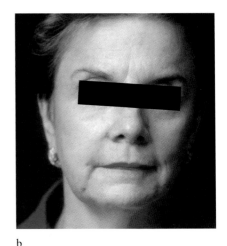

a                                          b

## Figure 17.6

The same patient before (a) and after (b) placement of SoftForm into the left nasolabial fold and marionette line for correction of asymmetry.

fibroblastic reaction which leads to permanent tissue augmentation. Silicone should only be used in small amounts (0.01–0.04 ml) and never in the hip, buttocks or thigh areas because the greatest risk for migration is in these areas. Silicone has been used for nasolabial grooves, glabellar wrinkles, and chin–lip grooves.[76] The authors do not recommend the use of this material because there are many other options that have great results and a better safety profile.

In summary, the field of cosmetic dermatology is rapidly growing with new additions to the armamentarium almost monthly. It is vital that dermatologists performing these cosmetic procedures keep abreast of the latest techniques and insist that the manufacturing companies provide good scientific proof of the safety and efficacy of their products. Many commonly used methodologies are not included in this chapter because good scientific data do not currently exist regarding these procedures. Laser surgery, however, is discussed in a separate chapter.

## References

1  Rubin M, *Manual of chemical peels.* Philadelphia: Lippincott, 1992, pp. 19–20.

2  Lawrence N, Brody HJ, Alt TH, Chemical peeling. In: Coleman (ed), *Cosmetic surgery.* Mosby, 1997, pp. 85–111.

3   Draelos Z, Rediscovering the cutaneous benefits of salicylic acid. *Cosmet Dermatol Suppl* 1997: 4–5.

4   Clark CP III, Alpha hydroxy acids in skin care. *Clin Plast Surg* 1996; 23(1): 49–56.

5   Draelos Z, Hydroxy acids for the treatment of aging skin. *J Geriatr Dermatol* 1997; 5(5): 236–40.

6   Van Scott EJ, Yu RJ, Control of keratinization with alpha hydroxy acids and related compounds. *Arch Dermatol* 1974; 110: 586–90.

7   Van Scott EJ, Yu R, Hyperkeratinization, corneocyte cohesion, and alpha hydroxy acids. *J Am Acad Dermatol* 1984; 11: 867–79.

8   Berardesca E, Distante F, Vignolini GP et al, Alpha hydroxyacids modulate stratum corneum barrier function. *Br J Dermatol* 1997; 137: 934–8.

9   Ditre CM, Griffin TD, Murphy GF et al, Effects of alpha hydroxy acids on photoaged skin: a pilot clinical, histologic and ultrastructural study. *J Am Acad Dermatol* 1996; 344: 187–95.

10   Kligman A, A comparative evaluation of a novel low-strength salicylic acid cream and glycolic acid procedures on human skin. *Cosmet Dermatol* 1997; Suppl Sept: 11–15.

11   Davies M, Marks R, Studies on the effect of salicylic acid on normal skin. *Br J Dermatol* 1976; 95: 187–92.

12   Weirich EG, Longauer JK, Kirkwood AH, Dermatopharmacology of salicylic acid. Topical contra-inflammatory effect of salicylic acid and other drugs in animal experiments. *Dermatologica* 1976; 152: 87–99.

13   Lin AN, Nakatsui T, Salicylic acid revisited. *Int J Dermatol* 1998; 37: 335–42.

14   Swinehart JM, Salicylic acid ointment peeling of the hands and forearms. *J Dermatol Surg Oncol* 1992; 18: 495–8.

15   Lim JTE, Tham SN, Glycolic acid peels in the treatment of melasma among Asian women. *Dermatol Surg* 1997; 23: 177–9.

16   Grimes PE, The safety and efficacy of salicylic acid chemical peels in darker racial-ethnic groups. *Dermatol Surg* 1999; 25: 18–22.

17   Dinardo J, A comparison of salicylic acid, salicylic acid with glycolic acid and benzoyl peroxide in the treatment of acne. *Cosmet Dermatol* 1995; 8: 43–4.

18   Chiarello SE, Resnik BI, Resnik SS, The TCA Masque, A new formulation used alone and in combination with Jessner's solution. *Dermatol Surg* 1996; 22: 687–90.

19   Brody HJ, Skin resurfacing: chemical peels. In: Freedberg IM, Eisen AZ, Wolff K et al (eds), *Fitzpatrick's dermatology in general medicine*, 5th edn. New York: McGraw Hill, 1999, pp. 2937–47.

20   Rubin MG, Trichloroacetic acid and other non-phenol peels. *Clin Plast Surg* 1992; 19(2): 525–35.

21   Bridenstine J, Dolezat J, Standardizing chemical peel solution formulations to avoid mishaps. *J Dermatol Surg Oncol* 1994; 20: 813–16.

22   Dinner MI, Artz JS, The art of the trichloroacetic acid chemical peel. *Clin Plast Surg* 1998; 25(1): 53–62.

23   Carruthers J, Carruthers JA, Botulinum toxin use for glabellar wrinkles. Annual Meeting of the American Society of

Dermatologic Surgery, Orlando, Florida, 1991.

24  Carruthers JDA, Carruthers JA, Treatment of glabellar frown lines with C. botulinum-A toxin. *J Dermatol Surg Oncol* 1992; 18: 17–21.

25  Ocampo J, Indicaciones cosmeticas de la toxina botulinica. *Piel* 1997; 12: 434–41.

26  Carruthers J, Carruthers A, Clinical indications and injection technique for the cosmetic use of botulinum A exotoxin. *Dermatol Surg* 1998; 24: 1189–94.

27  Brandt F, Beliman B, Cosmetic use of botulinum A exotoxin for the aging neck. *Dermatol Surg* 1998; 24: 1232–4.

28  Lowe NJ, Botulinum toxin type A for facial rejuvenation, United States and United Kingdom perspectives. *Dermatol Surg* 1998; 24: 1216–18.

29  Cox N, Duffey P, Royle J, Fixed drug eruption caused by lactose in an injected botulinum toxin preparation. *J Am Acad Dermatol* 1999; 40(2): 263–4.

30  Carynron B, Huddleston SW, Aesthetic indications for botulinum toxin injection. *Plast Reconstr Surg* 1994; 93: 913–18.

31  Borodic G, Myasthenia crisis after botulinum toxin. *Lancet* 1998; 352: 1832.

32  Clark DP, Hanke CW, Swanson N, Dermal implants: safety of products injected for soft tissue augmentation. *J Am Acad Dermatol* 1989; 21: 992–8.

33  Klein AW, Injectable collagen. In: Moschells SL, Hurley HJ (eds), *Dermatology*. Philadelphia: W.B. Saunders Company, 1992, pp. 2455–61.

34  Elson ML. Soft tissue augmentation: update 1997. *J Clin Dermatol* 1998; 25–30.

35  Castrow FF, Krull EA, Injectable collagen implant update. *J Am Acad Dermatol* 1983; 9: 889.

36  Siegle RJ, McCoy JP Jr, Schade W, Swanson NA, Intradermal implantation of bovine collagen: humoral responses associated with clinical reactions. *Arch Dermatol* 1984; 120: 183–7.

37  Klein AW, Rish DC, Injectable collagen: an adjunct to facial plastic surgery. *Facial Plast Surg* 1987; 4: 87.

38  Klein AW, In favor of double testing. *J Dermatol Surg Oncol* 1989; 15: 263.

39  Klein AW, Rish DC, Injectable collagen update. *J Dermatol Surg Oncol* 1984; 10: 519.

40  Baumann L, Kerdel F, The treatment of bovine allergy with cyclosporin. *Dermatol Surg* 1999; 25: 247–9.

41  Hanke CW, Higley HR, Jolivette DM et al, Abscess formation and local necrosis after treatment with Zyderm or Zyplast collagen implant. *J Am Acad Dermatol* 1991; 25: 319–26.

42  Cooperman LS, Mackinnon V, Bechler G, Pharriss BB, Injectable collagen: a six year clinical investigation. *Aesthet Plast Surg* 1985; 9: 145–51.

43  Klein AW, 'Bonfire of the wrinkles'. *J Dermatol Surg Oncol* 1991; 17: 543.

44  Artecoll Product Description. Rofil Medical International BV, Breda, The Netherlands, 1996.

45  Rispin P, PMMA microspheres may make collagen implants permanent. Absence of migration, granuloma formation, and late allergic reactions are also pluses. *Dermatol Times* 1998; Feb; 16–17.

46   Mang WL, Sawatzki K, Complications after implantation of PMMA (polymethyl-methacrylate) for soft tissue augmentation. *Z Hautkr* 1998; 42–4.

47   Hoffmann C, Shuller-Petrovic S, Soyer P, Kerl H, Adverse reactions after cosmetic lip augmentation with permanent biologically inert implant materials. *J Am Acad Dermatol* 1999; 40: 100–2.

48   Lemperle G, PMMA microspheres for long lasting correction of wrinkles. Presented at Int Society Aesthetic Plastic Surgery Congress, New York, September 1995.

49   Millikan L, Long term safety and efficacy with Fibrel in the treatment of cutaneous scars. *J Dermatol Surg Oncol* 1989; 15: 837.

50   Millikan L, Banks K, Purkait B, Chungi V, A 5-year safety and efficacy evaluation with fibrel in the correction of cutaneous scars following one or two treatments. *J Dermatol Surg Oncol* 1991; 17: 223–9.

51   Cohen IS, Fibrel. *Semin Dermatol* 1987; 6: 228–37.

52   Millikan L, Rosen T, Monheit G, Treatment of depressed scars with gelatin matrix implant. A multicentric study. *J Am Acad Dermatol* 1987; 16: 1155–62.

53   Grant RA, Cox RW, Kent CM, The effects of gamma-radiation on the structure and reactivity of native and cross-linked collagen fibers. *J Anat* 1973; 115: 29–43.

54   Alkek DS, Isolagen, a new autologous collagen. *Cosmet Dermatol* 1998; 11: 30–2.

55   Nidecker A, Cultured fibroblasts provide new collagen source. *Skin Allergy News* 1998; March; 43–4.

56   West T, Alster T, Autologous human collagen and dermal fibroblasts for soft tissue augmentation. *Dermatol Surg* 1998; 24: 510–12.

57   Lattari V, Jones LM, Varcelotti JR et al, The use of a permanent dermal allograft in full thickness burns of the hands and foot: a report of three cases. *J Burn Care Rehabil* 1997; 189(2): 147–55.

58   Jones FR, Schwartz M, Silverstein P, Use of non immunogenic acellular dermal allograft for soft tissue augmentation: a preliminary report. *Aesthetic Surg Q* 1996; 196–201.

59   Haake AR, Holbrook K, The structure and development of skin. In: Freedberg IM, Eisen AZ, Wolff K et al (eds), *Fitzpatrick's dermatology in general medicine, 5th edn.* New York: McGraw Hill, 1999, pp. 70–114.

60   Melton JL, Hanke CN, Soft tissue augmentation. In: Roenigk RK, Roenigk HH (eds), *Dermatologic surgery. Principles and practice.* New York: Decker, 1996, pp. 1077–87.

61   Piacquadio D, Cross-linked hyaluronic acid (Hylan gel) as a soft tissue augmentation material: a preliminary assessment. In: Elson ML (ed), *Evaluation and treatment of the aging face,* New York: Springer Verlag, 1995.

62   Cavicchini S, Setaro M, Sparavigna A et al, A clinical trial on the safety and performance of intradermally injected hyaluronic acid (IAL-SYSTEM™) in face contour deficiencies. Presented at the 8th Associazione Italiana Dermatologi Ambulatoriali National Congress, 31 August to 4 September 1999, Domus De Maria, Italy.

63   Olenius M, The first clinical study using biodegradable implant for the treat-

ment of lips, wrinkles and folds. *Aesthetic Plast Surg* 1998; 22: 97–101.

64  Duranti F, Salti G, Bovani B et al, Injectable hyaluronic acid gel for soft tissue augmentation, a clinical and histological study. *Dermatol Surg* 1998; 24: 1317–25.

65  Skouge JW, Canning DA, Jefs RD, Long term survival of perivesical fat harvested and injected by microlipoinjection techniques in a rabbit model. Presented at 16th Annual Meeting of the American Society for Dermatologic Surgery. Fort Lauderdale, Florida, March 1989.

66  American Academy of Dermatology, Guidelines of care for soft tissue augmentation: fat transplantations. *J Am Acad Dermatol* 1996; 34: 690–4.

67  Skouge JW, Ratner D, Autologous fat transplantation. In: Coleman WP III, Hanke CW, Alt T, Asken S (eds), *Cosmetic surgery of the skin, 2nd edn*. St. Louis: Mosby, 1997, pp. 206–16.

68  Teimourian B, Blindness following fat injection, *Plast Reconstr Surg* 1988; 82: 361.

69  Gurney CE, Studies on the fate of free transplants of fat, *Proc Staff Meet Mayo Clin* 1937; 12: 317.

70  Fisher G, Autologous fat implantation for breast augmentation. Workshop on liposuction and autologous fat implant, Isola d'Elba, Sept 1986.

71  Wetmore SJ, Injection of fat for soft tissue augmentation. *Laryngoscope* 1980; 99: 50.

72  Hary C, Baumann LS, Your cosmetic practice. *Skin and Ageing* 1999; 7: 88–94.

73  Merida MT, Vigil QN, Granulomas cutaneos causados por sustancias cosmeticas. *Derm Vencz* 1997; 35: 79–83.

74  Ashley FL, Thompson DP, Henderson T, Augmentation of surface contour by subcutaneous injection of silicone fluid. A current report. *Plast Reconstr Surg* 1973; 51(1): 8–13.

75  Scimanovitz VJ, Orentreich N, Medical-grade fluid silicone: a monographic review. *J Dermatol Surg Oncol* 1977; 3: 597–611.

76  Naoum C, Dasiou-Plakida D, Pantelidaki K et al, Histological and immunohistochemical study of medical-grade fluid silicone. *Dermatol Surg* 1998; 24: 867–70.

# Index